ANNUAL REVIEW OF
PUBLIC HEALTH

ANNUAL REVIEW OF PUBLIC HEALTH

LESTER BRESLOW, *Editor*
University of California at Los Angeles, School of Public Health

JONATHAN E. FIELDING, *Associate Editor*
University of California at Los Angeles, School of Public Health

LESTER B. LAVE, *Associate Editor*
The Brookings Institution

VOLUME 1

1980

ANNUAL REVIEWS INC.   4139 EL CAMINO WAY   PALO ALTO, CALIFORNIA 94306

ANNUAL REVIEWS INC.
Palo Alto, California, USA

REPRINTS   The conspicuous number aligned in the margin with the title of each article in this volume is a key for use in ordering reprints. Available reprints are priced at the uniform rate of $1.00 each postpaid. The minimum acceptable reprint order is 5 reprints and/or $5.00 prepaid. A quantity discount is available.

International Standard Serial Number: 0163-7525
International Standard Book Number: 0-8243-2701-2

Annual Reviews Inc. and the Editors of its publications assume no responsibility for the statements expressed by the contributors to this Review.

PRINTED AND BOUND IN THE UNITED STATES OF AMERICA

PREFACE

Public health workers today are driven to concern themselves with a large array of scientific, technical, organizational, political, and ethical issues that range over many facets of public and private life. The continuing expansion of significant research and professional literature that affects the field of public health and closely related fields has prompted the launching of this latest addition to the growing family of *Annual Reviews*.

We are in the midst of a second American "public health revolution." As a nation we are mobilizing efforts to deal in a more organized way than in the past with a relatively new set of major health challenges, the chronic diseases: cancer, diseases of the cardiovascular system, cirrhosis, chronic respiratory diseases, and injuries caused by accidents and other forms of violence. Also emerging is a general struggle for health enhancement as a whole, by and for persons of all ages. These problems differ from those that were the main province of public health in the past; they have become especially prominent during the second half of the twentieth century.

The first "public health revolution" sought control of communicable diseases in the United States and all industrializing countries. Major advances began in the nineteenth century; communicable diseases have now been largely (but by no means completely) controlled in the United States.

And so the field of public health is changing in several important respects:

1. The diseases considered most significant have changed drastically. Heart disease, cancer, and the other so-called modern diseases have become the focus of professional and public attention.
2. Classical public health arrangements are declining in vigor. The structures erected mainly for communicable disease control have been foundering in recent years, perhaps because their original mission has been largely accomplished.
3. New mechanisms are springing up, often haphazardly. Governments at various levels have created new agencies to deal with the problems that seem most relevant. The Health Care Financing Administration (HCFA) was created to channel funds for public medical care nationally, through Medicare and Medicaid; the Environmental Protection Agency (EPA), to lead the action against ill effects, including health damage, of environmental degradation; the Occupational Safety and Health Administration (OSHA), to make and enforce rules designed to minimize occupational hazards to health; and the National Institutes of Health (NIH), to foster the nation's biomedical research. Although these and other

agencies often operate through state and local organizations, they have grown largely outside the previous federal-state-local structures of public health. They have bypassed the laboratory services, nursing services, epidemiological services, sanitation, health education, and other services that constituted what we previously knew as public health.

Nonetheless, the fundamental nature of public health work is unaltered. At any given time, whether in 1880 or 1980, the field of public health consists of the ways and the extent to which society organizes institutions and means to protect itself against disease and to advance the health of its people. Whenever existing forms of protection are judged inadequate, new forms will emerge. This process has been intense during the last 20 years. When the pressure upon American society for medical care programs for the elderly and the poor became strong enough in the 1960s, Medicare and Medicaid were adopted. A few years later when it was recognized that advancing technology in industry and elsewhere threatened to inflict substantial damage to human health, as well as to cause other losses, the EPA and OSHA were established to safeguard both the general and the working environment. In the 1970s it became clear that the daily behavior of people —their driving, eating, and smoking habits, their use of dangerous drugs, for example—can have harmful effects on their health, and various efforts were undertaken to change this behavior favorably. The scope and impact of the new agencies and measures have made public health concerns far more visible than before.

People in America and other industrialized nations have become increasingly conscious not only of the major diseases that affect them but also of the governmental and other arrangements for mitigating these diseases and their effects. Costs have become an agonizing issue. People have become conscious of the tremendous expenditure for the diagnosis and treatment of disease, which increased from a little over 4% of the US Gross National Product in 1950 to about twice that amount 25 years later. Questions have arisen about the social benefits associated with that cost increase, what the expenditure is doing for health, and how the inflation of costs can be restrained.

Prevention has again thrust itself to the forefront of public health thinking. Although a preventive strategy had proved effective against the communicable diseases earlier, for decades it was not advanced seriously against cardiovascular diseases, cancer, and other current intractable health problems. The prospect of success in preventing these diseases did not seem great until recently.

Several factors changed the situation. One was enhanced knowledge of the factors causing present health problems. Epidemiologic research during the past few decades demonstrated that cigarette smoking causes lung cancer and some other forms of cancer, as well as chronic obstructive lung disease; that inadequate fluoride and excessive sugar result in dental caries; and that male smokers with high blood cholesterol and high blood pressure are 15 to 20 times more likely to develop cardiovascular disease than male nonsmokers with normal blood cholesterol and blood pressure.

Another factor was the successful application of such knowledge. The lung cancer rate of British physicians declined substantially relative to that of other British men, after the physicians began early to quit cigarette smoking; aggressive handling of even moderate degrees of high blood pressure reduced mortality in study groups significantly; fluoridation of public water supplies cut dental caries as much as 50%. These and other preventive interventions have demonstrated the value of such a strategy.

A third and equally important factor is increased public understanding of the controllable hazards to health. By 1975, for example, nine out of ten persons believed that cigarette smoking endangers health and 84% wanted something done about it.

A final buttress to the new emphasis on prevention is the emergence of certain favorable trends both in certain of the major chronic diseases and in the risk factors responsible for them. Coronary heart disease mortality had been increasing steadily from the early part of the century into the 1960s, when it was causing three out of ten deaths. Since the late 1960s it has turned sharply downward, falling about 2.5% per year—an approximately one-fourth drop in a decade. The extent of cigarette smoking, high blood cholesterol, and neglected high blood pressure have also been declining. Although no cause-and-effect relationship between these particular phenomena can yet be asserted, the need for further careful examination of that issue is clear. While we await further knowledge, prudence calls for a public health policy not only against cigarette smoking, but also for finding and dealing appropriately with early high blood pressure and advocating a diet that keeps blood cholesterol low and is otherwise nutritious.

Advances in public health depend upon several approaches. One is to use effectively the core analytic disciplines of the field: biostatistics and epidemiology. These can be applied to delineate the health problems, to isolate the factors likely to be responsible, and to evaluate progress against them. Today, biostatistics and epidemiology can point the way, just as they did in the campaigns against the major diseases of a prior era. Hence it is necessary to give substantial attention to these basic sciences of public health. In 1978, a National Research Council body found that enough scientific personnel had already been trained or were being trained in many facets of biomedical and behavioral research. In three disciplines, however, that body reported a great need: biomathematics/biostatistics, epidemiology, and toxicology. Mounting an effective attack on the nation's current set of diseases will require a sizeable increase in the number of epidemiologists and biostatisticians as well as attention to these disciplines themselves. Several of the chapters in this volume indicate the benefits and problems of applying epidemiology and biostatistics to the present health scene.

Beyond analysis, of course, public health must be concerned with ways to improve the health situation. There are essentially three ways: (*a*) personal health services, (*b*) environmental control measures, and (*c*) influences on behavior. In recent decades personal health services in the form of increasingly expensive medical care have been the predominant approach to health in the United States. We have invested vast sums in building and using both physical and personnel resources to diagnose and treat disease. Only in the past few years has much attention been given to ways of evaluating this tremendous enterprise and its procedures, to considering how economies could be achieved in it, to making it more effective and available to people, and to focus it on preventive measures rather than on conventional diagnosis and treatment.

These and related matters constitute the public health aspects of medical care. Because medical care has become such a prominent feature of American life, so highly regarded but so expensive for individuals, the idea of equity in obtaining it has emerged as a major consideration in public debate. The focus on that idea, important as it is, has tended to submerge the main public health significance of medical care, that is, what it can do for health. Even the term "medical care" tends to obscure implications for public health. Personal and family nursing service, for example, especially that directed toward maintaining health in the community, has long been a mainstay of public health and is adjusting itself to the current situation. It is therefore appropriate that this volume includes attention to some specific aspects of personal health service pertaining to public health.

Many issues that arise from our changing environment are beginning to affect the American people and to arouse their organized action. These include ecological concerns, the preservation of natural "wilderness" areas and the species that are indigenous to them; aesthetic values and their potential loss due to encroachments upon the environment that affect the enjoyment of its natural beauty; and physical discomfort arising from environmental pollution with chemicals, noise, and other factors.

Perhaps no other feature of the changing environment, however, has recently attracted so much attention as the discovery that long-continued exposure to certain man-made chemicals and radiation can cause fatal disease. The events at Love Canal near Niagara Falls, in which improperly handled industrial waste chemicals endangered the health of hundreds of people living nearby, and the Three-Mile Island nuclear reactor accident are only two examples of the kinds of current developments that generate expressions of public concern.

These and other experiences have sensitized people to the serious health hazards created in the environment as a result of human activity, especially industrial activity. Advancing technology obviously brings many improvements to life, but not without dangers. People have begun to understand the adverse impact on health of certain new products for consumption, even certain drugs intended to improve health, and the damage from exposure at work to agents such as asbestos and ionizing radiation—typically discovered only decades after the start of exposure. Public health concern about the environment is shifting rapidly from its previous focus on disease-causing microorganisms in water, milk, and food to chemical and physical pollution of air, water, and soil. Cancer is probably the most dreaded as well as one of the most common conditions attributed in large part to environmental factors. How to assess the carcinogenicity of substances that may enter the environment has therefore become a significant public health concern. Although the technology of environmental protection against cancer and other disease-causing substances will differ from the technology of dealing with microbial causes of disease, the public health strategy will be similar: to identify as precisely as possible the causative factors of disease, to determine their relative significance in the causation of disease, to develop and apply means for their control on a priority basis, and to evaluate the control efforts.

What people typically do each day in their lives, sometimes called lifestyle, is now recognized as another important causative element in the pattern of disease affecting them, including premature mortality. A Canadian study indicates that about one-fifth of the morbidity and about one-fifth of the years-of-life lost between ages one and 70 may be attributed to just two habits: cigarette smoking and excessive use of alcohol. Other common aspects of daily living that have been substantially incriminated in loss of health include too little exercise, too many calories in relation to bodily requirements, and excessive intake of saturated fats, sugar, and salt. One's daily diet, use of alcohol and tobacco, along with usual habits of driving, exercise, and the like constitute lifestyle, which altogether exerts a profound impact on health.

To improve the public's health requires attention to such habits; for example, endeavoring to reduce the use of cigarettes. The most obvious approach is to educate people about the adverse effects and appeal to them to quit smoking. Although useful to some extent, especially for those with high levels of education, this direct appeal must be expanded. It is necessary to take account of the fact that the cigarette habit is deeply ingrained in many people; contributing to that habit are the social pressure from peers and others to start and to continue smoking, and the many forces generated by cigarette companies that encourage cigarette consumption. The latter include public advertising and lobbying in opposition to legislation and other governmental action that would curtail the use of cigarettes through such means as higher taxes and restrictions on the places where one can smoke them. Whether a person uses cigarettes or not thus depends on a special kind of personal choice—a choice influenced largely by how much the social milieu in which one lives encourages or discourages the habit. From the standpoint of public health, to control cigarette smoking one must therefore neutralize those forces in the social situation that favor cigarette smoking. Ignoring those forces, such as the advertising and lobbying by companies that produce and market cigarettes, inclines one to the position sometimes called "blaming the victim." The latter implies that each individual decides by himself and without external influence what habits he adopts. How public health should deal with the issue of cigarette smoking and other habits adverse to health raises political and ethical questions. The form of these questions and answers to them are, in turn, influenced by commercial considerations as well as commitment to improve the public's health. Such problems are difficult but not totally new to public health. In the effort to control communicable diseases, for example, public health had to contend with the narrow interest of dairies and other enterprises that sometimes opposed public health measures because of commercial interest, and even practicing physicians who sometimes refused to report their cases and sought to handle them outside the bounds of what society deemed necessary to protect the health of the public.

As we noted earlier, public health today must explore and keep track of a large array of interdisciplinary problems and issues that relate to many facets of private and public life. As the general interest in health and what should be done to improve it is being refocussed at the present time, and the kinds of problems involved in advancing health are becoming clearer, so is the desirability of a more systematic, organized social effort to improve it.

The *Annual Review of Public Health* will therefore address itself to these issues and the ongoing efforts to achieve progress. Any single volume of the series cannot, of course, encompass the entire field. Each volume can cover only a limited number of specific topics. Over the years, however, the Editors intend to present a rounded view of continuing developments in the field. We shall always welcome comments and suggestions from readers regarding the present and future volumes in the series.

THE EDITORS

Annual Review of Public Health
Volume 1, 1980

CONTENTS

(Note: Future volumes will include a cumulative index of chapter titles arranged in major categories of public health endeavor.)

SOME RELATED ARTICLES IN OTHER *ANNUAL REVIEWS*

Ann Rev. Public Health 1980. 1:1–36

HEALTH AND DISEASE IN THE UNITED STATES[1]

♦12500

L. A. Fingerhut, R. W. Wilson, and J. J. Feldman

National Center for Health Statistics, Hyattsville, Maryland 20782

INTRODUCTION

The characterization of the overall health status of a population or of an individual is not a simple task. Many factors must be considered. Factors relating to mortality, such as life expectancy, mortality rates, both total and cause specific, infant mortality, and maternal mortality, are frequently used to assess the health of the people in an area. These measures are relatively easy to obtain and are available for small geographic areas and often for subgroups of the population. In addition, these measures are frequently available for other countries and, although there are definitional differences, international comparisons can be helpful. Finally, the impact of medical intervention on these measures is generally very direct, i.e. mortality rates should go down and life expectancy should increase—both desirable objectives—with necessary and appropriate medical treatment.

Many other measures of health status have been used to characterize a population. The most common are measures of illness, i.e. the prevalence and incidence of specific diseases and the impact of these diseases as measured by disability (8). In the past much of the information of this type was based on research conducted in hospitals at medical schools. However, because only about 10% of the population in any year is hospitalized and of this group only 10% is in teaching hospitals, much of the health information from examinations was based on only 1% of the population. In 1960 the National Center for Health Statistics (NCHS) initiated a major effort to improve the representativeness of health data by forming the National Health Examination Survey (now called Health and Nutrition Examination

---

[1]Much of the information presented in this chapter has been taken from *Health, United States, 1979* (1) or earlier volumes. This chapter includes selected tables from *Health, United States, 1979*. Reprints are available from NCHS.

1

0163-7525/80/0510-0001$01.00

Survey, or HANES), in which a national probability sample of persons was given an extensive clinical examination with highly standardized procedures in portable clinics that were moved around the country to the various sampling sites. Information has been collected about selected conditions, both known and previously undiagnosed, as well as about a variety of physical, physiological, biochemical, and psychological measures (2a). Data from these surveys have added greatly to the knowledge of our nation's health. Only a limited amount of health data, however, can be collected at any one time, thus necessitating the utilization of other sources of health information.

Health data can also be obtained by simply asking people about their health, either as a part of an examination survey or as a part of separate health surveys. Interview surveys can provide information about what kinds of illnesses people think they have or are willing to report and the presence of various symptoms, as well as the ability of people to perform the routine activities of daily living, the impact of health on their ability to perform these activities, and the use of medical services. These and related questions have been asked for more than 20 years in the National Health Interview Survey conducted by NCHS.

Many of these "nonmortality" health indicators are difficult to interpret, especially when changes are observed over time. For example, does an increase in the prevalence rate of a disease mean that people are less healthy, or does it indicate that doctors are changing a diagnostic procedure? Does an increase in the number of days lost from work as a result of illness mean that employees are getting sicker, or does it mean that employers are providing more liberal sick leave benefits? Does an increase in the number of persons who are unable to work because of a disability indicate a less healthy population, or does it reflect more liberal disability retirement benefits, or possibly a change in the work ethic? Does an increase in the number of people with long-term limitation of activities from chronic diseases indicate a deterioration in health status, or does it reflect improvements in health care that permit a person to survive a heart attack or a stroke, although with some permanent disability? An increase in a health status measure, therefore, does not necessarily mean that the true health status is deteriorating (2b).

Mental and emotional health are now considered to be an aspect of overall health status. This type of measure is usually even more difficult to interpret than the physical illness and disability data. In recent years there has been an increased interest in the development of health status indexes that combine a number of indicators into a single measure of health. Although there are many conceptual problems in the development of health status indexes, there is a frequently expressed desire for a single health index, similar to the Gross National Product or the Consumer Price Index, that will tell us if the health of the country is improving or deteriorating. A number of indexes have been proposed and some have been used to assess the health status of selected populations (3). However, most of the proposed indexes are not composed of indicators that are currently available from national data bases and therefore the collection of new data is required before they can be applied.

One of the best single indicators of general health status is self-assessment of health. The vast majority of the population perceive their own status to be excellent or good when asked the question: Compared with other persons your age, would you say that your health is excellent, good, fair, or poor? Just under half (48%) of the population perceive themselves as in excellent health. Only about 12% report their health to be fair or poor (Table 1). Even though respondents are asked to use other persons their own age as a reference group, respondents perceive their health as declining with age. Whereas only about 8% of young adults see themselves as in fair or poor

Table 1 Health status, utilization, and expenditure measures according to age, United States, 1977[a]

Measure	All ages	Under 17 years	17–44 years	45–64 years	65 years and over
Disability days per person per year	17.8	11.2	14.2	24.4	36.5
Percentage limited in activity	13.5	3.4	8.1	23.1	43.0
Percentage unable to carry on major activity	3.6	0.2	1.2	6.2	17.2
Percentage feeling fair or poor	12.3	4.2	8.5	22.0	29.9
Discharges from short-stay hospitals per 1,000 population[b]	169.2	73.3	159.7	198.4	374.4
Days of care from short-stay hospitals per 1,000 population[b]	1,236.7	308.2	849.2	1,688.3	4,156.3
Surgical operations per 1,000 population[b]	99.7	41.0	104.7	124.6	165.9
Office visits to physicians per person[b]	2.7	2.0	2.5	3.3	4.1
Percentage of office visits at which patient's principal problem judged not serious[b]	51.0	63.0	58.8	41.8	31.9
Per capita personal health care expenditures[c]	$646.00	$253.00	$661.00		$1,745.00

[a] Source: National Center for Health Statistics and Health Care Financing Administration. Data are based on household interviews of a sample of the civilian noninstitutionalized population, on medical records, and on compilations from government sources.
[b] The rates for the under 17 age group are for under 15 age group and rates for 17–44 age group are for 15–44 age group.
[c] The age groups are under 19, 19–64, and 65 years and over.

health, 30% of those 65 or over feel they are in fair or poor health. On the other hand, an equal proportion of the elderly view themselves as being in excellent health. Only minor differences exist between males and females in self-perception of health.

Striking differences are found in self-perceived health status between persons living in families with low income and those with high family incomes, even when the data are adjusted to account for the different age structure of low and high income families. Almost one quarter of persons in low income families (under $5,000) report that they are in fair or poor health, compared with only 5% of those living in high income families (over $25,000) (Table 11). Blacks are twice as likely to perceive themselves in fair or poor health as are whites. Some racial differences remain even within income categories.

In an effort to present a more detailed, although not necessarily comprehensive, picture of the nation's health, this chapter presents data on (a) mortality, including information on life expectancy, infant mortality, and selected causes of death, (b) morbidity, including information on selected chronic diseases, (c) disability, (d) selected data related to prevention of illness, and (e) health care costs and financing.

DEMOGRAPHIC DISTRIBUTION OF THE POPULATION

The size and distribution of the population of the United States have and will continue to have important implications for health status and the use of health resources. Assuming a constant level of health, the more people there are, the more health services will be necessary. However, as the shape of the population changes, so too does the overall health status of the nation. An aging population, for example, will place greater demands on the health care system by virture of its poorer health relative to the younger population.

The population of the United States is aging. A quarter of a century ago, 8% of the country's 152 million people were 65 years of age and over; now close to 11% or 23 million are aged 65 and over. This latter age group is the most rapidly growing population group. Based on various population projections, with each projection assuming different rates of mortality decline, an estimated 11 to 13% of the population, or 32 million people, will be 65 years of age and over in the year 2000. Within that age group, the population over age 75 will grow most rapidly. By 2000, an estimated 14 million people will be at least 75 years of age, 62% more than in 1977 (4).

How will these changes affect health status and health care utilization in the United States? Older people consume more health care than do younger people. They have more chronic illnesses, more disabilities and physical impairments. About 30% of the personal health care dollar, and close to half of the public portion, is spent on people 65 years of age or over. The per capita personal health care expenditure for people aged 65 years and over is almost seven times that of people under 19 years of age (Table 1). Projected changes in the size and age distribution of the population alone will have an impact on health status, on utilization, and consequently on expenditures (5). For example, it is estimated that by the year 2000, 24% of all hospital days will be used by people aged 75 years and over, a third more than in 1977, and 24% of all disability days will be reported by those of at least 65 years of age, an eighth more than in 1977.

In addition to the age distribution of the population, the geographic variation in the residential patterns of the elderly will necessitate selective placement of medical care services. Most elderly people do not change residences. However, those who do move, do so very selectively. For instance, whereas only 5% of all migrants are age 65 and older, about a fifth of Florida's migrants are within this age group. Elderly migrants are likely to seek destinations that have well developed social and medical services and mild climates. In states such as California, Florida, Arizona, and Texas, recreational and health service centers for the elderly are being promoted (6). Further, the rapid growth of "retirement counties"[2] is accounted for primarily by migration. Between 1970 and 1975, growth rates of these counties doubled.

An increasingly older population will also place greater demands on alternative care facilities. For instance, with death rates being much higher for men than for women at older ages, widowed women with chronic or disabling illness may need care they cannot provide for themselves. The need for nursing homes, home health services, adult day care, etc will therefore be heightened.

MORTALITY

The crude death rate in the United States continues its downward trend that has been observed since the early 1930s when national mortality data were first collected.[3] At that time the rate was 10.7 deaths per 1,000 population. After a slight rise in the mid-1950s to mid-1960s, the rate declined every year from 1968 (when the rate was 9.7) to 1977 except for 1971–1972 and 1975–1976. In 1977, there were 8.8 deaths per 1,000 population.

---

[2]Counties characterized by high in-migration of persons 60 years of age and over—360 of them were identified by Calvin Beale in 1970 (7a).

[3]In 1933, the death registration area included all states and the District of Columbia.

Trends in mortality rates differ among age groups. Mortality for infants and age-specific deaths rates for children under 15 years of age decreased at a rate of about 2% per year from 1950 to 1970. By 1977, the pace of the decline increased to about 3% annually overall and to 5% annually for infants under 1 year of age.

Among adolescents and young adults 15 to 19 and 20 to 24 years of age, death rates decreased nearly 2% per year from 1950 to 1960 and then increased at about the same rate during the next 10 years. In the current decade, mortality again decreased, at an overall rate of 1.2 to 1.5% per annum. However, from 1976 to 1977 the death rate for teenagers 15 to 19 years of age increased by 5%. This increase is attributable primarily to increases in death from external causes—particularly suicide, which increased 20%, and motor vehicle accidents, which increased 4%.

Mortality rates for adults in each 5-year age group from 25 to 64 years of age decreased by less than 1% per year from 1950 to 1970, but the pace accelerated to about 2 to 3% per year during the 1970s.

Similarly, changes in mortality for the elderly were very small from 1950 to 1970, but the rate of decline increased to an average of about 2% annually from 1970 to 1977.

Knowledge of changes in specific rates—i.e. rates specific for any number of population characteristics, such as sex, race, and age—is needed to understand the factors affecting mortality. Geographic differences in age- or race-specific mortality rates may reflect inadequate health care services and facilities, or such differences may direct attention to possible environmental problems associated with specific localities.

The change in the death rate, however, is due largely to the changing age structure of the population. For an analysis of trends over time, it is advantageous to look at the age-adjusted death rate, a summary statistic useful for making annual comparisons. This rate shows what the level of mortality would be if no changes occurred in the age composition of the population from year to year. From the beginning of this century, the age-adjusted death rate decreased by 53%, from 17.8 deaths per 1,000 population in 1900 to 8.4 deaths per 1,000 population in 1950, and then by another 27% to 6.1 deaths per 1,000 population in 1977. If the decrease in mortality from 1950 to 1977 were measured only by the crude rate, however, it would be about 9%, a figure that does not reflect the magnitude of the true decline in death rates.

Age-adjusted mortality decreases were much greater for females than for males, both white and black, from 1950 to 1970. During those 20 years, white female mortality decreased at 1.2% per year, whereas white male mortality declined by less than 0.5% per year. Among blacks, the difference was even greater—1.5% per year vs less than 0.5% per year for females and males respectively. These differences are largely a result of decreases in mortality from heart disease and from cancer of the digestive system and peritoneum, and genital organs, all of which have been greater for females than for males. More recently, decreases in mortality rates have accelerated for both males and females. From 1970 to 1977, white mortality rates decreased at an average annual rate of 2.3% per year among females and at 1.9% per year among males. Black female mortality decreased at 2.9% per year and black male mortality decreased at 2.2% per year.

The relative difference between the age-adjusted mortality rates for males and females has been increasing over time. In 1950, the death rate for males was 1.5 times the female rate; by 1977, the ratio increased to 1.8. This increase in the sex ratio in mortality is evident for both whites and blacks. Among whites, the ratio increased from 1.5 in 1950 to 1.8 in 1977; for blacks, it increased from 1.2 to 1.7 during the same 27 years.

Infant Mortality

Infant mortality has shown marked improvements in the last 12 years. From 1965 to 1977, the infant mortality rate decreased by 43% to 14.1 infant deaths per 1,000 live births. For both white and black infants, declines of 5% per year have been observed. During the preceding decade, from 1955 to 1965, the annual rate of decline was much slower, less than 1% per year.

Despite overall decreases, black infant mortality is still considerably higher than white infant mortality. In 1977, the rate for black infants was 23.6 compared with 12.3 for white infants. Furthermore, there is no evidence that the rates are converging.

A number of factors may have influenced the reductions in infant and perinatal mortality: (a) more women receiving prenatal care early in pregnancy, (b) a decreasing proportion of higher order, thus higher risk births, (c) advances in medical science, particularly in neonatology, (d) increasing availability of the most modern care through regional perinatal centers, (e) improvements in contraceptive utilization, allowing women to time and space their pregnancies more effectively, thereby reducing the proportion of high risk births, (f) increasing legal abortion rates, (g) the availability of programs to improve the nutrition of pregnant women and infants, (h) general improvements in socioeconomic conditions.

Geographic variation in infant mortality rates within the United States is substantial. During the periods from 1965 to 1967 and from 1975 to 1977, the New England and Pacific Divisions had the lowest infant mortality rates, and the East South Central Division had the highest infant mortality rate. During the latter period, Maine had the lowest infant mortality rate, 11.2, and the District of Columbia had the highest, 27.2. On the whole, geographic variations were as high from 1975 to 1977 as they were from 1965 to 1967.

During the period from 1975 to 1977, infant mortality among whites ranged from a low of 12.2 in New England to a high of 14.1 in the East and West South Central States. Among blacks the rates ranged from 20.6 in the Pacific Division to 26.5 in the East North Central Division (Table 2).

The infant mortality rate in the United States is higher than the rate in certain other industrialized countries. The 1977 data show Sweden, England and Wales, the Netherlands, and the German Democratic Republic (East Germany), among others, as having lower infant mortality rates than the United States. The average annual decrease in infant mortality from 1972 through the 1975–1977 period for the United States is similar to that observed for other industrialized countries.

Life Expectancy

Life expectancy at birth in the United States reached a record 73.2 years in 1977. During the first half of the century, gains in life expectancy were dramatic, a fact which was attributable to decreases in infectious and parasitic diseases. From 1950 to 1970, 2.7 years were added to the expectation of life. The pace of improvement has accelerated during the present decade, with 2.3 years being added since 1970. Major gains in life expectancy were noted especially for nonwhites whose life expectancy at birth improved by

Table 2 Infant mortality rates, according to race and geographic division: United States, average annual 1965–1967, 1970–1972, and 1975–1977[a]

Geographic division	1965–1967			1970–1972			1975–1977		
	Total[b]	White	Black	Total[b]	White	Black	Total[b]	White	Black
	Infant deaths per 1,000 live births								
United States	23.6	20.6	39.8	19.2	17.1	30.9	15.1	13.3	25.1
New England	21.2	20.4	36.7	16.8	16.2	30.0	12.8	12.2	23.6
Middle Atlantic	22.6	19.7	39.5	18.6	16.3	30.8	15.3	13.2	25.1
East North Central	22.7	20.5	38.7	19.2	17.1	31.7	15.2	13.3	26.5
West North Central	21.3	19.9	40.1	18.1	17.2	30.7	14.0	13.1	25.5
South Atlantic	26.9	21.2	40.6	21.0	17.3	31.0	16.9	13.6	25.2
East South Central	29.1	22.8	44.7	22.3	18.3	33.5	17.3	14.1	26.1
West South Central	25.4	21.6	39.4	20.9	18.8	29.9	16.2	14.1	25.1
Mountain	23.3	21.9	34.2	18.2	17.5	26.3	13.7	13.2	21.1
Pacific	20.9	20.0	32.7	16.8	16.2	26.4	12.8	12.4	20.6

[a] Source: National Center for Health Statistics: Computed by the Division of Analysis from data compiled by the Division of Vital Statistics. Data are based on the national vital registration system.
[b] Includes all other races not shown separately.

4.5 years from 1950 to 1970, compared with 2.6 years for whites. Since 1970, an additional 3.5 years were added for nonwhite people, compared with 2.1 years for whites. Most of the improvement has been among females. There is still a sizable difference—5 years—in life expectancy at birth between whites and nonwhites.

Recent gains in life expectancy for those 65 years of age have been similar for whites and nonwhites. On the average, people reaching 65 years of age in 1977 can expect to live an additional 16.3 years, or 1.1 years more than someone reaching age 65 in 1970.

Expectation of life at birth is influenced heavily by mortality rates for infancy and childhood. It is not surprising, therefore, that life expectancy in the United States does not compare favorably with certain other industrialized countries. However, the recent annual improvements in number of years gained are better in the United States than in most countries, for both males and females.

Leading Causes of Death

Heart disease, cancer, stroke, and accidents have been the leading causes of death since around 1950 (Table 3). In 1900, infectious diseases—particularly pneumonia and tuberculosis—were the leading causes of death, accounting for a fifth of all deaths in the United States. The precipitous decline in the death rates from these causes has been evident throughout the developed world. Social improvements such as sanitation, nutrition, housing, education, and medical care have all contributed to the decline. More recently, however, decreases in death rates from some of the major chronic diseases—mainly the cardiovascular diseases including heart and cerebrovascular diseases—have been evident.

Heart disease continues to be the leading cause of death in the United States and, as such, it is the predominant influence on total mortality. The age-adjusted death rate decreased by 18% in the 20 years from 1950 to 1970, an average of 1% per year; it declined by nearly the same amount in the first 7 years of this decade at an average decline of 2.6% per year. During those 27 years, the age-specific rates declined by more than 40% for each 5-year age group from 25 to 49 years of age, and by more than 30% for each succeeding age group from 50 to 74 years of age. For those in the 5-year age groups from 75 to 85 years of age and over, the decline was more than 20%.

Decreases in age-adjusted heart disease mortality rates have been much greater for females than for males, especially between 1950 and 1970. Among white and black females heart disease mortality dropped 25% and 28%, respectively during this period, compared with decreases of 9% and 10% among white and black males, respectively. During the current

Table 3 Age-adjusted death rates[a] and average annual percentage change, according to leading causes of death in 1950: United States, selected years 1950–1977[b]

			Cause of death			
Year	All causes	Diseases of the heart	Malignant neoplasms	Cerebro-vascular disease	Accidents[c]	Tubercu-losis
			Deaths per 100,000 resident population			
1950	841.5	307.6	125.4	88.8	57.5	21.7
1955	764.6	287.5	125.8	83.0	54.4	8.4
1960	760.9	286.2	125.8	79.7	49.9	5.4
1965	739.0	273.9	127.0	72.7	53.3	3.6
1970	714.3	253.6	129.9	66.3	53.7	2.2
1975	638.3	220.5	130.9	54.5	44.8	1.2
1976	627.5	216.7	132.3	51.4	43.2	1.1
1977	612.3	210.4	133.0	48.2	43.8	1.0
			Average annual percentage change			
1950–77	−1.2	−1.4	0.2	−2.2	−1.0	−10.8
1950–55	−1.9	−1.3	0.1	−1.3	−1.1	−17.3
1955–60	−0.1	−0.1	0.0	−0.8	−1.7	−8.5
1960–65	−0.6	−0.9	0.2	−1.8	1.3	−7.8
1965–70	−0.7	−1.5	0.5	−1.8	0.1	−9.4
1970–77	−2.2	−2.6	0.3	−4.5	−2.9	−10.7
1975–77	−2.1	−2.3	0.8	−6.0	−0.5	−0.9

[a]Note: Age-adjusted rates computed by the direct method to the age distribution of the total U.S. population as enumerated in 1940, using 11 age intervals.
[b]Source: Division of Vital Statistics, National Center for Health Statistics: Selected data. Data are based on the national vital registration system.
[c]Includes motor vehicle and all other.

decade, the rates of decline in heart disease mortality for both races and both sexes have become more nearly equal—18 and 19% for white and black females and 15 and 14% for white and black males. As a result, the relative differences in the death rates for heart disease between males and females have been increasing over time. In 1950, heart disease mortality for white males was 1.7 times that for white females, and by 1977, the ratio widened to 2.1. Similarly, the ratios for the black population increased from 1.2 in 1950 to 1.6 in 1977.

Racial differences in heart disease mortality for males are very large, especially at the younger ages. In each 5-year age group from 25 years of age to 40 years of age, heart disease mortality in 1977 for black males was more than twice as high as that for white males. Between 40 and 64 years of age the relative difference decreased, and for those 65 years of age and over mortality was lower for black males than for white males. Racial differences in heart disease mortality were greater among females than males, especially at the younger ages.

Ischemic heart disease mortality includes about 90% of all heart disease mortality, and as such, the trends are similar. Age-adjusted death rates decreased about 3% per year during the past decade. For each 5-year age group between 25 and 69 years of age, declines of at least 25% during the period from 1968 to 1977 have been noted. Since 1968, the ratio of white male to white female mortality (2.2 : 1) has remained virtually unchanged.

Some of the explanations suggested for the downturn in heart disease mortality are: (a) decreased smoking in general and in smoking of high tar and nicotine cigarettes in particular among adult males, (b) improved management of hypertension, (c) decreased dietary intake of saturated fats, (d) more widespread physical activity, (e) improved medical emergency services, (f) more widespread use and increased efficacy of coronary care units. Unfortunately there is no definitive evidence for determining which of these explanations or which combination thereof can account for the decline (7b).

The second major component of cardiovascular diseases is cerebrovascular disease or stroke, the third leading cause of death in the United States in 1977. Cerebrovascular age-adjusted mortality rates decreased about 25%, to 66 deaths per 100,000 population from 1950 to 1970. By 1977, the rate had decreased an additional 27% to 48 per 100,000 population. Reductions have been observed for males and females, whites and nonwhites, in nearly every age group. In recent years, cerebrovascular death rates have continued to decrease at a greater pace than have heart disease death rates, 4.5% vs 2.6% annually since 1970. This downturn in stroke mortality probably reflects both a decrease in the incidence of stroke and in the fatality rate among stroke victims. Improved management of hypertension has been offered as an explanation of the declining incidence (7c, 7d).

Malignant neoplasms or cancers are the second leading cause of death in the United States. In 1977, the age-adjusted mortality rate was 133 deaths per 100,000 population, 6% higher than in 1950. This overall rise masks significant differences in cancer mortality, not only for individual sites, but also for males and females, white and black people, and the elderly and the young. For example, from 1950 to 1970 the age-adjusted cancer mortality rate increased for males at an average annual rate of 0.8% for whites and 2.3% for blacks; it decreased very slightly for females, 0.5% for whites and 0.3% for blacks. During the 1970s the situation changed somewhat for females, showing annual increases of 0.1% and 0.7% for whites and blacks respectively. The rate of increase decreased slightly for males with increases of 0.5% and 1.6% for whites and blacks, respectively.

Cancer mortality has been increasing for some sites, namely the respiratory system, breast, colon, pancreas, and bladder, and has been decreasing for others, i.e. the stomach, rectum, cervix, and uterus.

Of interest has been the 33% decrease in cancer mortality since 1950 for the population under 45 years of age. In addition, the rate for persons from 45 to 49 years of age has decreased by 5% since 1974. The decreases have come about, in part, through reduced incidence of breast cancer in young women and lung cancer in young men, and through substantial improvements in treatment for childhood leukemias and Hodgkins disease. In the 5-year age groups between 50 and 64 years of age, cancer mortality increased, ranging from 6 to 15%, since 1950. For those aged 65 years and over, the rate has risen 16% since 1950.

Respiratory cancer includes about one quarter of all deaths from malignant neoplasms. The age-adjusted respiratory cancer mortality rate increased by 168% between 1950 and 1977 to 34.3 deaths per 100,000 population while the rates for all other cancers combined actually declined.

The age-adjusted mortality rate for respiratory cancer more than doubled from 1950 to 1970, increasing at average annual rates of 4% for white males and females and 7% and 5% for black males and females, respectively. During the following 7 years, mortality increased an additional 3% per year. The annual rates of increase slowed substantially for males and increased for females.

From 1950 to 1970, the sex ratios (i.e. male mortality to female mortality) in respiratory cancer mortality increased for both whites and blacks; but by 1977, the ratios had decreased, a fact that is accounted for by the faster rate of increase in female mortality. Nevertheless, respiratory cancer mortality for males is significantly higher than for females (56 versus 16 deaths per 100,000 population in 1977 among white people and 78 versus 17 among black people).

The recent slower rates of increase for male mortality are attributed in part to lowered smoking rates and to the growing acceptance of cigarettes with lower tar and nicotine levels. Increases in heavy smoking for females may account for some of the reduction in the sex ratio differences.

Accidents remain the fourth leading cause of death in the United States. They are the leading cause of death for the population from 1 to 34 years of age. The major component within this category is motor vehicle accidents (48% of the total).

As discussed previously, the increase in the motor vehicle accident death rate from 1970 to 1977 contributed to the overall mortality increase among teenagers. Motor vehicle accident death rates are higher for males from 15 to 24 years of age than for any other group.

Recent trends in age-adjusted motor vehicle accident death rates for the total population show a decrease of about 1% per year between 1968 and 1973. The rate dropped 17% from 1973 to 1974 and remained at this low level for 2 additional years. The years with lowered rates correspond to the early stages of the 55 miles per hour speed limit throughout the country. However, the death rate increased by about 4% from 1976 to 1977, which is perhaps an indication of relaxed adherence to, or enforcement of the speed limit. According to recent provisional data, there were 51,130 motor-vehicle-related deaths in the United States in 1978, more than in any year since 1973.

MORBIDITY

Although it is impossible to present a detailed discussion of a wide range of chronic diseases in this paper, a summary comparison of the impact of selected conditions indicates the varying types and levels of impact. Rice et al (8), using data from the National Health Interview Survey, investigated the comparative burden of 15 major chronic conditions (Table 4). Sinusitis and hayfever are prevalent conditions and, although most people with these conditions are bothered by them, the diseases cause very little long-term limitation of activity or short-term bed disability. On the other hand, a large proportion of the persons with heart disease, emphysema, and stroke have long-term limitation of activity and high levels of bed disability.

The data in Table 5 present the relative impact of all disease in the United States. In assessing the total burden of illness, Rice et al compared the major categories of all diseases, both chronic and acute, as grouped by the International Classification of Diseases. The total economic cost of illness was based on the direct costs of medical care as well as on the indirect cost of the losses of input for ill persons who died prematurely. Circulatory conditions ranked either first or second in seven of the eight measures of impact. Respiratory conditions and accidents also consistently ranked relatively high on most measures of impact. Whereas neoplasms were ranked high in terms of potential years of life lost, economic impact, and SSA disability, they were not ranked high on some of the measures of long-term impact because of the fact that a malignancy usually either causes death within a short time after diagnosis, or is considered cured after a period of treatment. Diseases of the blood and blood-forming organs, conditions of childbirth and pregnancy, and diseases of the skin tended to rank consistently low on the different measures of impact, with the exception of physician visits for skin diseases. Most other conditions varied in ranking by the type of impact measure.

Table 4 Impact of selected chronic conditions as measured in health interviews: United States 1970–1976[a]

Condition	Prevalence	Causing limitation of activity	Medical attention in past year	Number of bed days per year	Bothered a great deal or some	Now under treatment or medication recommended by doctor
				(Numbers in 1,000s)		
All heart conditions	10,291	4,281	7,729	129,667	4,847	6,031
Coronary heart	3,307	1,988	2,880	52,912	1,915	2,613
Arthritis	24,573	4,988	12,286	103,206	18,553	9,706
Back problems	8,018	1,964	2,646	32,072	5,573	N/A
Diabetes	4,191	1,245	3,462	24,308	1,425	3,085
Hypertension w/o heart	12,271	1,092	9,890	24,542	3,792	7,301
Asthma	6,031	1,031	3,637	34,980	4,746	3,100
Stroke	1,534	782	1,118	38,503	845	973
Emphysema	1,313	590	785	19,038	847	566
Hernia	3,725	656	2,231	18,252	1,900	1,177
Ulcer	3,955	534	2,369	23,334	2,903	2,587
Bronchitis	6,526	261	4,666	23,494	4,953	1,299
Hayfever	10,826	162	3,800	6,496	8,314	3,692
Sinusitis	20,582	144	6,710	14,407	15,169	4,507
Hemorrhoids	9,744	68	2,777	6,821	5,661	1,871

[a] Source: National Center for Health Statistics, Health Interview Survey. Table modified from (8).

Table 5 Ranking of diagnostic categories according to dimensions of burden, United States 1973–1975[a]

ICD category	Potential years of life lost	Inpatient days	Physician office visits	Work loss days	SSA disability	Limitation of major activity	Bed days	Total economics costs
Infestive and parasitic diseases	10	13	11	7	10	15	7	12
Neoplasms	2	8	13	11	4	10	10	4
Endocrine, nutritional and metabolic diseases	8	11	10	12	8	8	12	11
Diseases of the blood and blood-forming organs	13	15	14	15	—	14	15	16
Mental disorders	12	1	9	10	3	9	11	6
Diseases of the nervous system and sense organs	9	6	3	9	7	5	9	8
Diseases of the circulatory system	1	2	2	4	1	2	2	1
Diseases of the respiratory system	5	9	1	1	6	4	1	5
Diseases of the digestive system	6	7	12	5	9	6	6	3
Diseases of the genitourinary system	11	10	6	7	12	11	8	10
Pregnancy, childbirth, and the puerperium	16	12	—	14	—	—	13	13
Diseases of the skin and subcutaneous tissue	15	14	8	13	—	13	14	14
Diseases of the musculoskeletal system and connective tissue	14	5	7	6	2	3	5	9
Congenital anomalies	7	16	—	16	11	12	16	15
Accidents, poisonings and violence	3	4	4	2	5	7	4	2
Other	4	3	5	3	13	1	3	7

[a] Source: (8).

Hypertension

High blood pressure is relatively common in the United States today. It was estimated from the 1971–1974 HANES that 23.2 million adults aged 18 to 74 had elevated blood pressure (i.e. blood pressure readings of at least 160 mmHg systolic or 95 mmHg diastolic[4] (Table 6). Hypertension is more prevalent among blacks and more frequently found among older people than young people. At the younger ages, the rates of hypertension are higher among men, whereas at older ages they are higher for women, with the crossover occurring at earlier ages for blacks (9). These estimates do not include persons who have their hypertension under control through the use of medication or diet, nor do they include persons with borderline hypertension or institutionalized persons with hypertension. The National Heart, Lung, and Blood Institute, using data from NCHS and other sources, estimated that approximately 35 million Americans have definite hypertension and another 25 million have borderline hypertension (9b).

Studies have demonstrated that people with high blood pressure have a greater risk of acquiring or dying from cardiovascular disease (10), but if the initially very high blood pressure is lowered, the risks of stroke and congestive heart failure are reduced (11, 12). People may be unaware that they have high blood pressure because there are no distinctive physical or psychological symptoms. In fact, data from HANES indicated that only 45% of the examinees with elevated blood pressure had been previously diagnosed. Although there has been no significant change in the proportion of the population with elevated blood pressure, there has been some increase in the proportion that had previously been diagnosed as hypertensive (13).

The different estimates of the number of people with hypertension offer a good illustration of many of the problems involved in estimating how many people in the country have specific diseases. Even when available national data are based on clinical examinations, there is often a lack of agreement on how to define a condition. One of the definitional problems with measuring hypertension is whether the presence of an elevated blood pressure reading is in itself an indication of the condition called hypertension. Does the person who has his blood pressure "under control," by whatever means, still have the condition hypertension? Furthermore, if estimates of hypertension are based solely on interviews, as in the National Health Interview Survey (14a), information can only be reported for those cases that people know they have (this can be further confounded by self-diagnoses vs physician diagnoses) and are willing to report to interviewers.

---

[4]The phrase "elevated blood pressure" is referred to as "definite hypertension" in publications on blood pressure from HANES.

Table 6 Adults aged 18 to 74 with elevated blood pressure,[a] according to sex, race and age: United States, 1971–1974[b]

	Total	Male		Female	
		White	Black	White	Black
			(Number per 100 persons)		
Total 18–74 years	18.1	18.5	27.8	17.1	28.6
18–24 years	3.1	4.9	4.6	1.4	2.9
25–34 years	6.6	8.2	17.7	3.7	10.2
35–44 years	15.5	17.3	38.2	10.1	28.3
45–54 years	24.2	25.8	36.2	18.9	50.9
55–64 years	33.2	31.1	49.9	31.7	54.5
65–74 years	40.7	35.3	50.1	42.3	58.8

[a] Elevated blood pressure is referred to as "definite hypertension" in published reports on blood pressure from HANES.
[b] Source: (9a). Data are based on physical examinations of a sample of the civilian noninstitutionalized population.

As more people become aware of the presence of a condition, as is happening with hypertension, estimates of the disease based on interviews will increase, even though the number of actual cases may not have changed. Diagnostic procedures can improve and physicians can become more aware of the importance of diagnosing and treating certain conditions, especially as more effective treatment methods become known. Each of these factors makes the estimation of the prevalence of a disease difficult and in many cases makes comparisons over time or between different data sources quite questionable. Finally, there is the additional problem of measuring the incidence of a disease, i.e. the number of new cases in a given period (usually a year). Such measures require information on the onset of a condition—information which is often difficult, if not impossible, to obtain, either with clinical data or interview data.

Heart Disease

Although heart disease continues to be the leading cause of death in the United States today, there are no national data on its incidence. The most recent estimate, based on physical examinations, of the prevalence of heart disease dates back nearly two decades to 1960–1962. At that time the National Health Examination Survey estimated that 14.6 million adults had definite heart disease and another 13 million had suspect heart disease. More recent estimates from HANES (1971–1974) are forthcoming, thus permitting some indication of the changes in the prevalence of heart disease.

The 1972 Health Interview Survey questioned the adult civilian noninstitutionalized population on whether they ever had heart disease or heart trouble. The prevalence of heart disease based on these interview data was 10.2 million persons in 1972. No trend should be interpreted from the examination and interview data. However, when the 1971–1974 examination data become available from HANES, estimates of the trend in heart disease can be made as well as an assessment of the relative difference between interview and examination data.

Acknowledging the uncertainty in the interview data, it is still instructive to look at the differentials in heart disease prevalence. The prevalence of heart conditions increased with age from about 2% for people under 45 years of age, to 9% for people aged 45 to 64, and to nearly 20% for those 65 years of age and over. Among those 65 years of age and over, prevalence was reportedly similar for males and females, and for white and nonwhite people (Table 7).

Numerous epidemiologic studies have been made of heart disease (e.g. Framingham, Massachusetts) (14b). Most studies have agreed upon a number of risk factors associated with heart disease, of which the major ones

Table 7 Prevalence of heart disease conditions, according to sex, color, and age: United States, 1972[a]

Color and age	Both sexes	Male	Female
	(Prevalence per 100 population)		
Total			
All ages	5.0	4.8	5.3
Under 17 years	1.1	1.2	0.9
17–44 years	2.5	2.0	2.9
45–64 years	8.9	9.7	8.1
65 years and over	19.9	19.9	19.8
White			
All ages	5.2	5.0	5.4
Under 17 years	1.1	1.2	0.9
17–44 years	2.4	2.0	2.9
45–64 years	8.8	10.0	7.9
65 years and over	20.0	20.1	19.9
Nonwhite			
All ages	4.1	3.6	4.6
Under 17 years	0.9	1.1	0.7
17–44 years	2.8	1.9	3.5
45–64 years	9.2	8.3	9.9
65 years and over	18.5	18.2	18.8

[a]Source: National Center for Health Statistics: Division of Health Interview Statistics, selected data. Data are based on household interviews of a sample of the civilian non-institutionalized population.

are age, male sex, hypertension, cigarette smoking, plasma LDL (low density lipoprotein), and blood glucose. Other hypothesized risk factors include obesity, sedentary lifestyle, water hardness, family history of heart disease before age 65, personality type, and stress (15a, 15b).

Indirect knowledge about the prevalence and incidence of heart disease comes from the Health Interview Survey and the Hospital Discharge Survey. From the former, it is estimated that in 1977, 2% of the civilian noninstitutionalized population, or 4.7 million people, were limited in their usual activity due to heart disease, including nearly 11% of the population 65 years of age and over. From another perspective, of all people who report a limitation of activity, 17% attribute their limitation to heart disease, followed closely by arthritis and rheumatism. Heart disease and arthritis and rheumatism have been the leading causes of activity limitation since the data were first collected in 1957.

According to the Hospital Discharge Survey, 3.2 million persons whose diagnosis was chronic ischemic heart disease were discharged from short-stay hospitals in 1977. An additional 740,000 had an acute myocardial infarction, a crude measure of its incidence. It is somewhat surprising that, given the rapidly decreasing death rate from heart disease, the discharge rate is increasing. (For example, among persons 45 to 64 years of age the increase in the discharge rate between 1972 and 1977 was about 29%, whereas the mortality rate dropped about 15% during the same period.) One explanation is that people are better educated about the symptoms of heart disease and are entering the hospital with milder symptoms. After separating the discharge rate into people discharged alive and those discharged dead, it is the rate for surviving patients that is increasing.

The lack of precise data on the incidence of heart disease makes it difficult to determine the relative contributions of changes in the incidence of heart disease and of changes in improved cardiovascular treatment to the downward trend in heart disease mortality.

Cancer

Cancer, the second leading cause of death, is one of the few chronic conditions for which adequate incidence data are available. The Surveillance, Epidemiology, and End Results Reporting (SEER) Program, conducted by the National Cancer Institute, covers about 10% of the US population and estimates that the average annual cancer incidence rate from 1973 to 1976 was 324.4 cases per 100,000 population. The rates varied from a low of 277.8 in Utah to a high of 358.0 in the San Francisco area. The cancer mortality rate for the SEER geographic areas was 167.7 per 100,000 population, ranging from a low of 122.6 in Utah to a high of 200.4 in New

Orleans. Mortality for the SEER areas combined is remarkably similar to the total US mortality for all cancer sites and for each of the selected sites.

There was considerable variation by site of cancer in the relationship between incidence and mortality (16). For cancers of the breast and prostate, for example, the incidence rate was approximately three times the mortality rate, whereas for lung cancer, incidence was only 25% higher than mortality. This differential can be explained by differences in survival rates for these various forms of cancer. Among those persons diagnosed with cancer of the lung in 1973, the percentage surviving three years was only 12% compared with 78% for those with cancer of the breast and 68% for those with cancer of the prostate.

During the 1970s, the incidence of cancer has been increasing more rapidly than mortality. Cancer incidence for white males and females increased at average annual rates of 1.0 and 1.8% respectively compared with mortality increases of 0.5 and 0.1%. Increases in incidence reflect, in part, improvements in treatment and earlier diagnosis. Even when smoking-related lung cancers are removed from all cancers, incidence is still increasing more rapidly than mortality.

Whereas the incidence of lung cancer in males appears to be leveling off and even decreasing for males under age 65, the incidence is still increasing for women.

Other sites with decreasing incidence among males include rectum (black males), leukemia, stomach, and pancreas. Among females the incidence of leukemia, cancer of the stomach (white females), cervix, and ovary is decreasing (Table 8).

Infant Health: Birth Weight

An important measure of infant health is birth weight. A low-birth-weight infant, one weighing less than 2,500 grams at birth, experiences higher morbidity and mortality (18, 19) (Table 9). Although only 7% of all infants are low-birth-weight, data from the 1960 birth cohort study show that about 75% of all neonatal deaths are of low-birth-weight infants (17).

Birth weight depends on many factors directly related to the mother—height, weight, age, marital status, parity, race, nativity, educational attainment, smoking habits, nutrition, and morbidity during pregnancy. Socioeconomic status appears to be a critical determinant of birth weight. Differences in level of education are at least as important as many demographic or health differences (NCHS report in preparation).

Black infants are in much greater risk of being low-birth-weight. In 1977, 13% of black infants compared with 6% of white infants weighed less than 2,500 grams at birth. Black low-birth-weight infants appear to do better in terms of mortality than white infants (Table 9).

Table 8 Trends in cancer incidence and mortality from 1969 to 1976 and 3 year patient survival rates from 1960 to 1973[a]

Site	Average annual percentage change in incidence from 1969–1976	Average annual percentage change in mortality from 1969–1976	Average annual percentage change in 3 yr survival from 1960–1973
Breast			
White females	1.4	0.3	0.2
Black females	1.7	0.7	0.8
Lung			
White males	1.0	2.6	1.5
White females	8.3	7.6	1.1
Black males	4.2	4.1	1.0
Black females	9.8	5.9	5.8
Colon			
White males	1.0	1.3	0.3
White females	0.4	0.0	0.5
Black males	3.0	2.7	0.6
Black females	1.4	1.3	1.2
Prostate			
White males	1.8	1.2	0.9
Black males	1.2	1.9	2.0
Corpus			
White females	7.5	2.3	0.6
Black females	3.3	2.8	1.0
Bladder			
White males	2.4	0.6	0.9
White females	2.7	−1.4	0.6
Black males	0.2	−0.4	1.2
Black females	6.4	−0.4	0.7
Rectum			
White males	0.9	−3.0	0.9
White females	1.0	−3.1	1.1
Black males	−3.3	−1.0	0.5
Black females	1.9	−3.6	3.5
Leukemia			
White males	−0.8	−0.4	2.8
White females	−1.3	−1.7	2.0
Black males	−1.5	0.8	0.4
Black females	−0.4	0.5	2.6
Stomach			
White males	−2.9	−2.9	0.6
White females	−3.9	−3.6	0.5
Black males	−0.6	−2.6	3.2
Black females	2.1	−1.3	−1.2

[a] Source: (16).

Table 9 Infant and neonatal mortality rates and fetal death rates, according to race and birth weight: United States, selected years 1959–1965[a]

Race and birth weight	Infant mortality rate, 1964–1965[b]	Neonatal mortality rate, 1959–1965[c]	Fetal death ratio, 1959–1965[d]
White, total	21.0	13.6	21.8
2,500 grams or less	184.0	111.4	113.0
2,501 grams or more	8.7	4.4	4.7
Black, total	40.7	19.7	22.7
2,500 grams or less	188.7	90.9	71.0
2,501 grams or more	16.4	5.8	5.9

[a] Sources: (18, 19).
[b] Infant deaths per 1,000 legitimate live births.
[c] Infant deaths under 28 days per 1,000 live births.
[d] Fetal deaths of 20 weeks or more gestation per 1,000 live births.

From 1950 to the mid-1960s the incidence of low birth weight gradually increased from 7.5% to 8.3%, followed by a decline to 7.1% by 1977 (Figure 1). Just about all of the increase was among nonwhite births. During this time period, two interrelated phenomena were taking place. First, there was a sharp decrease in the proportion of nonwhite births delivered by midwives and other nonphysician personnel from 26% to 4%. Second, there was an increase in the proportion of nonwhite births born in hospitals from 58% to 93%. Given these phenomena, various hypotheses have been suggested for the increase in low-birth-weight ratio for nonwhites (20). Part of the increase is attributed to poorer reporting practices during the earlier period. Midwives might have overstated birth weight in nonhospital births, thereby resulting in artifically high birth weight distributions or midwives might have failed to register low-birth-weight infants, thus yielding higher average weights among those who were registered. Part of the increase can be considered real, i.e. there was an actual shift toward lower weight infants. Increased prenatal care among nonwhite women might have resulted in lower weight infants because of efforts made by physicians to restrict the weight of the mother, and thereby of the fetus, in order to avoid complications associated with the delivery of large infants.

The increase in low-birth-weight ratios cannot be attributed to changes in the age or birth order distributions of childbearing. Teenage girls and older women are more likely than other age groups to have a low-birth-weight baby. Similarly, there is an increased risk of low birth weight for first births and fourth or higher order births. Since 1950 there have been compensatory changes in the proportion of births in these high risk groups (NCHS report in preparation). From 1969 to 1977 the proportion of low-

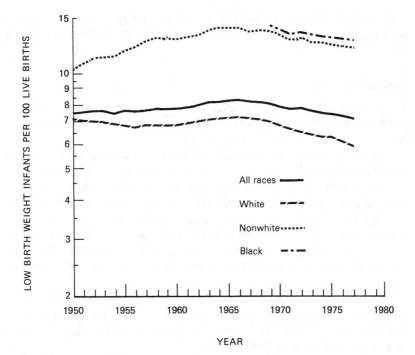

Figure 1 Low-birth-weight ratios: United States, 1950–1977. (Source: National Center for Health Statistics, Division of Vital Statistics, Selected data.)

birth-weight white infants decreased 16% compared with a 9% decrease among black infants[5] (Figure 1).

Geographic variation in low-birth-weight ratios exists across the United States. For the period from 1975 to 1977, the ratios varied from a low of 5.2% in North Dakota to highs of 9.1% in Mississippi and 12.6% in the District of Columbia. In both periods, 1965–1967 and 1975–1977, the ratios were lowest in the West North Central and Pacific Divisions and highest in the South Atlantic Division. The relative difference between the highest and lowest ranking divisions remained the same during the 10 years.

Large variations in low-birth-weight ratios persist even when race-specific data are considered. For example, the ratios for white infants ranged from 5.4% in the Pacific States to 6.9% in the Mountain States. Among blacks, the Pacific States had the lowest ratio (11.5%) and the Middle Atlantic and East North Central States the highest (13.4%).

[5]Prior to 1969 birth weight data were available for blacks and other nonwhite races combined, but not for blacks only.

From 1965–1967 to 1975–1977, the largest relative decreases in low-birth-weight ratios have been in the Mountain and Pacific Divisions (Table 10).

Dental Health

The presence of dental disease reflects both the condition of the teeth and gums and the extent to which needs are met. Dental treatment begun early in life can prevent future dental disease.

According to examinations (1971–1974), 64% of those examined needed some kind of dental care (21). About one fifth needed to have their teeth cleaned and two fifths needed work on decayed teeth. There were pronounced age and family income differences in the need for dental care. For each age group, people with lower incomes had greater dental care needs than those who were more affluent. For example, 78% of children from 12 to 17 years of age in families with incomes of less than $5,000 needed dental care compared with 54% in families with incomes of $15,000 or more.

Among the dentulous population 65 to 74 years of age, about 76% needed dental care.[6] Among these people, the need for care likewise varied by family income—80% of those with family incomes of less than $5,000 vs 66% with incomes of at least $15,000.

Periodontal disease and dental caries are two of the leading causes of tooth loss. Dental caries are a chronic destructive disease of the teeth which, if left untreated, results in loss of affected teeth. Periodontal disease designates a variety of conditions of the supporting structures of the teeth.

The prevalence of periodontal disease is associated with advancing age, sex (it is more prevalent in males), and race (in blacks). These sex and race differences occur throughout all age groups. Of the 54% of the population 65 to 74 years of age who had their natural teeth, 28% were found to need periodontal treatment. In the early 1970s, about 16% of young children 1 to 5 years of age and more than 50% of children 6 to 17 years of age needed dental work on decayed teeth, according to findings of examinations (36).

There are marked differences by socioeconomic status in the use of dental services (1). In 1977, people in families with incomes of $25,000 or more made twice as many visits to the dentist as people with annual incomes of less than $10,000. Furthermore, of those people seeing the dentist, more than two thirds of the highest income group made a visit within the last year compared with less than two fifths of the lower income group.

[6]Three fifths of those 65 to 74 years of age were missing at least half of their permanent teeth, with three fourths of them having lost all of their permanent teeth.

Table 10 Infants weighing 2,500 grams or less at birth, according to color or race and geographic division: United States 1965–1967, 1970–1972, and 1975–1977[a]

Geographic division	1965–1967			1970–1972			1975–1977		
	Total	White	Non-white[b]	Total[c]	White	Black	Total[c]	White	Black
	(Infants weighing 2,500 grams or less at birth per 100 total live births)								
United States	8.3	7.2	13.7	7.8	6.6	13.6	7.2	6.1	13.3
New England	7.9	7.6	14.2	7.2	6.8	14.1	6.6	6.2	12.3
Middle Atlantic	8.6	7.4	15.5	8.2	6.9	14.4	7.7	6.4	13.4
East North Central	7.8	6.9	14.5	7.5	6.4	13.9	7.0	5.9	13.4
West North Central	6.9	6.4	13.1	6.6	6.1	13.3	6.1	5.6	13.2
South Atlantic	9.4	7.5	13.7	8.7	6.9	13.5	8.2	6.3	12.9
East South Central	9.0	7.4	13.0	8.5	6.9	12.8	8.0	6.4	12.3
West South Central	8.7	7.3	13.8	8.2	6.8	13.6	9.5	6.5	13.2
Mountain	8.8	8.5	11.1	7.9	7.7	14.3	7.1	6.9	13.3
Pacific	7.4	6.7	11.3	6.6	6.0	12.3	6.1	5.4	11.5

[a] Source: National Center for Health Statistics: Computed by the Division of Analysis from data compiled by the Division of Vital Statistics. Data are based on the national vital registration system.
[b] Data by birth weight for the black population not available for these years. In the Middle Atlantic, East North Central, South Atlantic, East South Central, and West South Central Divisions, more than 95% of the births in the "nonwhite" color category were black. However, in the Mountain and Pacific States most of the births in the "nonwhite" color category were not black. Overall, 91% of the births in the "nonwhite" color category were black for the 3-year period.
[c] Includes all other races not shown separately.

DISABILITY

The impact of illness can be short-term or temporary, such as the disability caused by a bout with the flu or the common cold, or by an acute episode of chronic disease such as chronic bronchitis or ulcers; or the impact can be long-term and more permanent, such as a person's inability to work as the result of a stroke or the need to reduce the type or amount of work as the result of a heart attack. One of the major indicators of general health status is the proportion of a population with a long-term limitation of activity as a result of chronic illness. Limitation of activity is defined as the inability to carry on the major activity for one's age-sex group, such as working, keeping house, or going to school; restriction in the kind or amount of major activity; or restriction in relation to other activities, such as recreational, church, or civic interests. In 1977 an estimated 28.5 million Americans (excluding the institutionalized population), or 13.5%, had some degree of activity limitation. About three quarters of these were limited in their major activity, i.e. either unable to perform that activity or limited in the kind or amount of that activity. The proportion of the population 45 to 64 years of age with such limitations has been gradually increasing over the past two decades (22a, 22b, 22c). The reason for this increase is not clear, but at least part of the increase can be attributed to more liberal disability retirement plans.

Increased levels of disability can also be expected as mortality rates decline, i.e. people are surviving serious illnesses, but with some degree of disability. As expected, the proportion of persons with a limitation of activity increases markedly with age. Only 3% of children are limited, whereas 43% of the elderly are limited in activity.

There are also major differences in activity limitation by family income, with 22% of the persons in low income families being limited compared with only 9% in high income families. These estimates by family income are age-adjusted, so the observed income differences are not a result of there being more elderly persons in the low income group. It cannot be determined from these data the extent to which low income persons are more likely to be limited because they are poor, or the extent to which they are poor as a result of their health conditions. Among children, where the income depressing effect of illness should be minimal, and among the elderly, where aging probably has more effect on health than does family income, the differences between income groups is the smallest, indicating that the income depressing effect of illness may indeed be a major factor among young and middle-aged adults.

The major causes of limitation of activity are heart conditions and arthritis and rheumatism. About 15% of the limitation of activity is caused by these two groups of conditions. Among the elderly these conditions each cause one quarter of the limitation of activity. Other major causes are hypertension, diabetes, mental and nervous conditions, asthma, impairments of the back or spine, impairments of the lower extremities and hips, and visual limitation.

Limitation of activity is an indicator of the long-term impact of chronic illness; it does not reflect the impact of illnesses of short duration. Another measure, days of disability, refers to any temporary or short-term reduction of a person's daily activities as a result of acute or chronic illness. Illness or injury caused an estimated 3.8 billion restricted activity days in 1977, or an average of 17.8 days per person. A day of restricted activity is one during which a person reduces his or her normal activity for all or most of the day because of illness or injury. Included in this estimate of restricted activity days are 1.5 billion bed days or 6.9 days per person (Table 11). The average number of bed days per person ranges from a little over 5 days for children and young adults to almost 15 days for the elderly.

As with other impact-of-illness indicators, persons in low income families have many more restricted activity days and bed days than do those in higher income families. Income differences in disability days are generally

Table 11 Self-assessment of health, limitation of activity, and disability days, according to selected characteristics: United States, 1977[a]

Selected characteristics	Self-assessment of health as fair or poor (Percentage with)	Limitation of activity	Restricted activity days per person per year	
			Total	Bed days
Total	12.3	13.5	17.8	6.9
Age				
Under 17 years	4.2	3.4	11.2	5.2
17–44 years	8.5	8.1	14.2	5.4
45–64 years	22.0	23.1	24.4	8.2
65 years and over	29.9	43.0	36.5	14.5
Sex[b]				
Male	11.4	14.1	15.9	5.9
Female	12.5	12.0	18.8	7.6
Race[b]				
White	10.9	12.8	17.1	6.6
Black	20.8	15.9	21.6	8.9
Family income[b]				
Less than $5,000	24.2	22.2	29.6	11.9
$5,000–$9,999	16.1	15.8	20.3	7.9
$10,000–$14,999	10.9	12.0	15.8	6.1
$15,000–$24,000	7.5	10.0	14.0	5.3
$25,000 or more	5.2	8.8	12.6	4.9

[a] Source: (1). Data are based on household interviews of a sample of the civilian noninstitutional population.
[b] Age-adjusted by the direct method to the 1970 civilian noninstitutional population using four age categories.

less marked for children and the elderly. About half of all bed disability days are the result of acute illnesses and one quarter of the bed days are due to acute respiratory conditions—primarily influenza, the common cold, and other upper respiratory conditions. Influenza, or at least what people report to be influenza, alone causes more bed days than do heart conditions and arthritis combined.

PREVENTION

The upward spiral of health care cost has created a renewed interest in the role of disease prevention and health promotion as a means of improving health status and reducing the burden of illness. The Department of Health, Education, and Welfare has established the Office of Disease Prevention and Health Promotion. The Surgeon General has recently released a special report on prevention (23). *Health, United States, 1978* contained a chapter on prevention (24). The limitations of the practice of medicine are being recognized, as are the roles of the environment and life styles in the determination of health status (25). The control of infectious diseases during the later part of the nineteenth century and the early twentieth century occurred largely as a result of changes in the environment and life styles, e.g. changes in food supplies and nutrition, improved hygiene, and safer food and water. The first effective drug treatment for tuberculosis, streptomycin, was not introduced until 1947.

The major causes of mortality today—heart disease, cancer, stroke, and accidents—can be prevented, at least in part, by changes in the environment and life style behavior (smoking, eating, exercise, etc) (24). The evidence for the specific role of individual health behavior in the determination of health status is varied, ranging from conclusive as in the case of heavy cigarette smoking, to tenuous as in the case of snacking between meals. Although direct evidence of the extent of the relationship between specific behaviors and health status requires considerably more research, it will not be difficult to measure changes in the health behaviors themselves. A longitudinal study in one county in California has shown that persons having good health practices have a longer life expectancy than do those with poor health practices. The seven health practices studied included cigarette smoking, weight in relationship to height, drinking, hours of sleep, regularity of eating breakfast, eating between meals, and physical activity (26, 27). Information on these seven health practices has been collected on a recent Health Interview Survey and a national study is currently being conducted by NCHS to investigate these and other health promotion practices.

The relationship between eating habits and health status has become an area of attention for those interested in health promotion, even though the precise nature of this relationship is still unknown. There are no national estimates of how many Americans eat a "prudent" diet, although considerable information is available from the Health and Nutrition Examination Survey on the quantity of specific types of food intake (28). [Also see the nutrition chapter in (1).]

Individual concern for the effect of dietary habits is shown by the fact that almost one third of adult males and half of adult females perceive themselves to be overweight. When examination data were assessed to determine obesity (based on triceps skin-fold measurements) it was found that 13% of the adult males and 23% of adult females were obese. Over 40% of the middle-aged black females were found to be obese.

Health promoters have urged people to engage in more physical activity. In 1975 it was found that half of the American adults did not engage in any regular exercise (29a). One of the estimates from HANES (1971–1975) indicated that 53% of persons 18 to 74 years of age reported that they were "very active" in their usual daily activities or that their recreational activities involved "much exercise." The proportion of those exercising has undoubtedly increased since that time.

The use of common drug-like substances (such as sleeping pills) and alcoholic beverages is coming under increasing scrutiny in order to determine their impact on health. One person in twenty uses sleeping pills at least once a week. Most Americans drink alcoholic beverages. One quarter of males 35 to 54 years of age drink every day and more than 10% of the male drinkers 18 to 64 years of age have more than five drinks a day.

Preventive health behavior also includes the judicious use of medical services. About 15% of the population report that they do not have a regular source of medical care. Over 30% of the adult population have not had a blood pressure test within the past year (29b). A third of the persons 40 years of age and over have never had an electrocardiogram (EKG), and two fifths have never had a glaucoma test. One in five women 17 years of age or older has never had a pap smear test (29c). One out of four women who subsequently have live births does not see a doctor during the first three months of pregnancy. Less than half of the population see a dentist in any given year and one in five persons 5 years of age or older has not seen a dentist for at least five years (1).

Dental caries are a very common condition for which a safe, efficacious and cost effective preventive measure is available, i.e. fluoridated drinking water. However, only about 60% of the US population served by public water supplies have adequate levels of fluoridation (30).

Immunization against childhood diseases is one of the safest and most cost effective measures available, yet 30 to 40% of the nation's children 1 to 4 years of age are incompletely immunized against measles, rubella, diphtheria, tetanus, pertussis, and poliomyelitis, and less than half are immunized against mumps.

Cigarette Smoking

Cigarette smoking is one of the major public health problems in this country (31). Mortality from certain diseases, such as coronary heart disease, appears to be affected primarily by an individual's current cigarette smoking practices, whereas mortality from other diseases, such as lung cancer and emphysema, is markedly affected by past cigarette smoking history.

Cigarette use did not begin to spread steadily and rapidly among males in the United States until the early years of this century. Prior to that time, chewing tobacco, snuff, and cigars were the characteristic forms of tobacco consumption. The historical timing is reflected in cohort differences in the penetration of cigarette smoking. Smoking became most common among men born between 1900 and 1940, with three quarters of these individuals becoming cigarette smokers.

Smoking did not gain popularity among women until the early decades of this century. By the 1920s the trend had caught on, with over half of the women born between 1921 and 1945 becoming cigarette smokers. Cigarette smoking has always been less common among females, although in recent years the gap in smoking between the sexes has narrowed, especially among older cohorts. Most of the changes can be attributed to more men than women having quit smoking in recent years.

Although it may be premature to predict the eventual penetration level of cigarette smoking among people born in the 1950s, the fact that in 1978 only about half of the males and two fifths of the females 20 to 24 years of age had ever smoked is encouraging.

Data on trends in teenage smoking confirm the trend that the probability of taking up cigarette smoking is decreasing. Given the rapidity with which the probability of starting to smoke cigarettes increased over several succeeding generations, beginning with males born approximately a century ago, the recent intergenerational declines may presage a substantial change in social norms or fashion with regard to cigarette smoking.

After reaching a peak at about age 30, the proportion of current smokers in any cohort has tended to decline with increasing age. For instance, of the males born during the 1913–1933 period who had ever been cigarette smokers, fully half were no longer smoking cigarettes by 1978. There has thus been an appreciable change in the life cycle pattern of smoking among men; a much larger proportion of smokers are stopping and those who stop are doing so at younger ages. Among women, the pattern is similar—although the proportion of those who have stopped is consistently lower.

Even though the proportion of current smokers has decreased, the amount smoked per person appears to have increased. Some of this increase is explained by the fact that the lighter smokers may have been the ones who quit. It may also be explained by increased smoking levels among persons who smoke low tar and nicotine cigarettes.

The heaviest smokers are those in the 1921–1945 cohorts of males, about 45% of whom smoked between one and two packs a day in 1978. Among females, there has been a much smaller increase in the proportion of heavy smokers: about a fourth of the 1921–1945 cohorts smoked more than a pack of cigarettes per day.

Industrial and Environmental Exposure

Occupational exposure to hazardous substances and exposure to pollutants in the air are two environmentally related factors that can have a detrimental impact on health status. The attention accorded to these problems has increased greatly since the passage of the Occupational Safety and Health Act of 1970. Based on data from the National Occupational Hazard Survey (1972–1974), it was estimated that 1 in 4, or approximately 20 million American workers may have, at the time of the survey, been exposed to hazardous substances regulated by the Occupational Safety and Health Administration (OSHA). In total, as many as 50 million people, nearly one quarter of the population, may have been exposed to one or more such regulated hazardous substances at some time during their working life-times.

Most occupational exposures are to multiple rather than single chemical agents. Workers are also exposed to chemical and physical hazards in the general, non-workplace environment and as a result of smoking and consumption of alcohol and drugs (31). There are probably at least three different categories of occupational diseases: (a) those that are caused solely by occupational factors, (b) those in which occupation is one of the causal factors, (c) those in which occupation affects the course of a preexistent disease. There are many examples of ill health effects of industrial exposure that can be cited:

Exposure to asbestos is perhaps the most serious known occupational health problem in the United States. An estimated 8 to 10 million people have been or are currently exposed to asbestos in the workplace. Asbestosis and mesothelioma are two diseases associated with this exposure (A. Robbins, unpublished).

At least 35,000 textile workers in the United States are permanently disabled as a result of occupational exposure to cotton dust. More than 300,000 people are likely to have been exposed to the agents in the workplace which are presumed to cause byssinosis.

Workplace exposure to toluene diisocyanate (TDI), used in the manufacture of polyurethane, is a cause of both respiratory and dermatologic conditions. An estimated 100,000 people are exposed to TDI vapor, a potent respiratory irritant and sensitizer; severe symptoms can develop from exposure to very low concentrations (A. Robbins, unpublished).

A recent US Department of Health, Education, and Welfare paper (K. Bridbord, P. Decoufle, J. F. Fraumeni, unpublished) suggests that 20 to 38% of all cancers may be related, in part, to occupational factors. Although occupational exposure is a factor in virtually every field of clinical medicine, it is seldom taken into account in diagnosing disease. Thus, the full extent of occupational diseases suffered by American workers today is not known. However, many workers continue to be exposed to well-known hazards, such as lead, mercury, and silica, and suffer from diseases that have been known for centuries to be of occupational origin. At the same time, little is known about the health effects of chemicals that have been developed in recent years and continue to be introduced into commerce at the rate of several hundred per year.

Air quality estimates from the Environmental Protection Agency (EPA) show that the levels of particulate matter and sulfur oxides have improved during this decade, primarily as a result of improvements in industrial processes. EPA estimates that 29% fewer people in 1977 than in 1972 were exposed to annual mean particulate matter levels in excess of the standards. Most of the decrease occurred prior to 1975 (32). On the other hand, nitrogen oxide emissions have increased as a result of increased fuel use by electric utilities and increased highway motor vehicle travel.

NATIONAL HEALTH EXPENDITURES

National health expenditures are compiled and published on a yearly basis by the Health Care Financing Administration (HCFA) (33). Included are the sum of expenditures for personal health care, prepayment and administration, government public health activities, and research and medical facilities construction. Excluded are expenditures for education and training of physicians and other health workers and nonmedical activities generally related to industrial and environmental health hazards, such as pollution control and occupational safety.

In 1978, health expenditures in the United States totaled $192.4 billion, an average of $863.01 per person (Table 12). During the 1970s, national health expenditures have more than doubled with an average annual increase of 12.6%. Price controls, imposed during the Economic Stabilization Program (August 1971 to April 1974), were briefly successful in holding down health care costs. In 1978 the trend of rapidly rising health expenditures continued with an annual increase of 13.2% (33).

The Nation's total health care bill continues to represent an increasing proportion of the Gross National Product (GNP). During the past three decades, national health care expenditures increased from 4.5% of the GNP in 1950 to 9.1% of the GNP in 1978. Moreover, per capita personal health care expenditures for 1978 were 10.7 times the level for 1950, an increase from $70.37 to $752.98 per person. Much of this increase is due to inflation. In constant dollars, the 1978 expenditures were only 2.6 times the level for 1950.

The level of health care spending is determined by the quantities of various purchased services and the price of each service. Quantities change as a result of changes in the size and characteristics of the population and changes in the utilization patterns of various population groups. Rapid

Table 12 National health expenditures: United States, selected years 1929 to 1978[a]

Year	All health expenditures in billions	National health expenditures — Percentage of gross national product	National health expenditures — Amount per capita	Source of funds — Private — Amount in billions	Source of funds — Private — Amount per capita	Source of funds — Private — Percentage of total	Source of funds — Public — Amount in billions	Source of funds — Public — Amount per capita	Source of funds — Public — Percentage of total
1929	$ 3.6	3.5	$ 29.49	$ 3.2	$ 25.49	86.4	$ 0.5	$ 4.00	13.6
1935	2.9	4.0	22.65	2.4	18.30	80.8	0.6	4.34	19.2
1940	4.0	4.0	29.62	3.2	23.61	79.7	0.8	6.03	20.3
1950	12.7	4.5	81.86	9.2	59.62	72.8	3.4	22.24	27.2
1955	17.7	4.4	105.38	13.2	78.33	74.3	4.6	27.05	25.7
1960	26.9	5.3	146.30	20.3	110.20	75.3	6.6	36.10	24.7
1965	43.0	6.2	217.42	32.3	163.29	75.1	10.7	54.13	24.9
1966	47.3	6.3	236.51	34.0	169.81	71.8	13.3	66.71	28.2
1967	52.7	6.6	260.35	33.9	167.61	64.4	18.8	92.24	35.6
1968	58.9	6.8	288.17	37.1	181.40	63.0	21.8	106.76	37.0
1969	66.2	7.1	320.70	41.6	201.83	62.9	24.5	118.87	37.1
1970	74.7	7.6	358.63	47.5	227.71	63.5	27.3	130.93	36.5
1971	82.8	7.8	393.09	51.4	244.12	62.1	31.4	148.97	37.9
1972	92.7	7.9	436.47	57.7	271.78	62.3	35.0	164.69	37.7
1973	102.3	7.8	478.38	63.6	297.17	62.1	38.8	181.22	37.9
1974	115.6	8.2	535.99	69.0	319.99	59.7	46.6	216.00	40.3
1975	131.5	8.6	604.57	75.8	348.61	57.7	55.7	255.96	42.3
1976	148.9	8.8	678.79	86.6	394.73	58.2	67.3	284.06	41.8
1977	170.0	9.0	768.77	100.7	455.29	59.7	69.3	313.50	40.8
1978[b]	192.4	9.1	863.01	114.3	512.62	59.4	78.1	350.40	40.6

[a] Source: (33). Data are compiled by the Health Care Financing Administration.
[b] Preliminary estimates.

increases in health care prices, however, have been the primary force behind the huge growth in health expenditures.

Funds for health care expenditures are derived from both private and public sources. Private expenditures are those paid primarily by private health insurance carriers, consumers, and by industry and philanthropic organizations. Public expenditures are those made by federal, state, and local governments and include Medicare and Medicaid (which pay for health care services provided to the aged, disabled, and poor) and programs that provide services directly to specified beneficiaries.

When the Medicare and Medicaid programs went into effect in 1966, public spending began to grow rapidly. In 1978 public per capita expenditures were $350.40, or 6.5 times the pre-Medicare-Medicaid level of $54.13 in 1965 (Table 12). Total public expenditures have increased 1.6 times as fast as private expenditures. Moreover, whereas public funds accounted for one fourth of all health expenditures in 1965, they accounted for 40.6% in 1978.

Data from the National Medical Care Expenditure Survey conducted by National Center for Health Statistics (NCHS) and the National Center for Health Services Research (NCHSR) are currently being analyzed. This new survey will provide detailed information on health expenditures, including out-of-pocket cost, by a wide range of sociodemographic variables.

NEW SOURCES OF HEALTH INFORMATION

This chapter presents a summary of some of the current data and issues in the measurement of health status. In the process, a number of data sources have been mentioned. *Health, United States,* from which much of the material in this chapter was drawn, was legislated by Congress in 1974. In doing so, Congress recognized the need to draw together what is known about the health of the American people. The legislation specifically required that the report cover four areas: the health status of the American people, the use of health services, health care resources, and health care financing (1, 34, 35, 36).

The NCHS is playing a leading role in the development of data sources needed for monitoring research into environmental health. Additional information useful for describing the nation's health status will be available from new surveys currently in process or in the planning stages by the NCHS. These include (*a*) the National Natality and Fetal Mortality Surveys, (*b*) the National Medical Care Utilization Expenditure Survey, (*c*) a follow-back to a sample of respondents from the Health and Nutrition Examination Survey I, (*d*) the National Survey of Personal Health Practices and Health Consequences.

Literature Cited

1. DHEW 1980. *Health, United States, 1979.* DHEW (PHS) 80–1232. Washington: GPO. In press
2a. Miller, H. 1973, 1977. Plan and operation of the health and nutrition examination survey, United States, 1971–1973. In *Vital and Health Statistics.* Ser. 1:10a,b. Natl. Cent. Health Stat. DHEW (HSM)73–1310, 77–1310. Washington: GPO
2b. Gruenberg, E. M. 1977. The failures of success. *Milbank Mem. Fund Q.* 55:(1) 1–24
3. Amundson, J. D., ed. 1976. Health status indexes—work in progress. *Health Serv. Res.* 11:330–528
4. U.S. Bur. Census 1977. Projections of the population of the United States: 1977 to 2050. *Curr. Popul. Rep.* Ser. P–25:704
5. Rice, D. P. 1978. Projection and analysis of health status trends. Presented at Ann. Meet. Am. Public Health Assoc., 106th, Los Angeles
6. Biggar, J. C. 1979. The sunning of America: Migration to the sunbelt. *Popul. Bul.* 34:8
7a. Beale, C. L. 1976. A further look at nonmetropolitan population growth since 1970. *Am. J. Ag. Econ.* 58:953–58
7b. Havlik, R. J., Feinleib, M., eds 1979. Proc. Conf. Decline in Coronary Heart Disease Mortality. (NIH)79–1610
7c. Garraway, W. M., Whisnant, J. P., Furlan, A. J., Phillips, L. H. II, Kurland, L. T., O'Fallon, W. M. 1979. The declining incidence of stroke. *New Engl. J. Med.* 30:449–52
7d. Levy, R. I. 1979. Stroke decline: Implications and prospects. *New Engl. J. Med.* 30:490–91
8. Rice, D. P., Feldman, J. J., White, K. L. 1976. The current burden of illness in the United States. Presented at Inst. Med., Natl. Acad. Sci., Washington, DC
9a. Roberts, J., Maurer, K., 1977. Blood pressure levels of persons 6–74 years—United States, 1971–1974. In *Vital and Health Statistics.* Ser. 11:203. Natl. Cent. Health Stat. DHEW (HRA)78–1648. Washington: GPO. 103 pp.
9b. Levy, R. I. 1978. National high blood pressure conference: Speech by R. I. Levy at the national conference on high blood pressure control, April 2–4 1978, Los Angeles, California. *Urban Health: J. Health Care in the Cities,* pp. 10ff
10. Kannel, W. B., Gordon, T., eds. 1974. *The Farmingham Study, An Epidemiological Investigation of Cardiovascular Disease,* Sect. 30. DHEW (NIH): 74–599. Washington: GPO
11. Veterans Adm. Coop. Study Group on Antihypertensive Agents 1970. Effects of treatment on morbidity in hypertension. II. Results in patients with diastolic blood pressure averaging 90 through 114 mm. Hg. *J. Am. Med. Assoc.* 213:1143–52
12. Veterans Adm. Coop. Study Group on Antihypertensive Agents 1967. Effects of treatment on morbidity in hypertension results in patients with diastolic blood pressure averaging 115 through 129 mm. Hg. *J. Am. Med. Assoc.* 202:1028–34
13. Wilson, R. W., Danchik, K. M., Monk, M. 1977. Hypertension. In *Health, United States, 1976–1977.* DHEW (HRA):77–1232, pp. 27–41. Washington: GPO
14a. Moss, A. J., Scott, G. 1978. Characteristics of persons with hypertension: United States, 1974. In *Vital and Health Statistics.* Ser. 10:121. Natl. Cent. Health Stat. DHEW (PHS):79–1549. Washington: GPO. 176 pp.
14b. Kannel, W. B., Gordon, T. 1973. Assessment of coronary vulnerability. In *The Framingham Study in Early Phases of Coronary Heart Disease, the Possibility of Prediction,* ed. J. Waldenstrom, T. Larsson, N. Ljungstedt, pp. 123–143. Stockholm: Nordiska Bokhandelns
15a. Levy, R. T. 1978. Progress in prevention of cardiovascular disease. *Prev. Med.* 7:464–75
15b. Kuller, L. I. 1976. Epidemiology of cardiovascular diseases: Current perspectives. *Am. J. Epidemiol.* 104:425–56
16. Schneiderman, M. A. 1979. Trends in cancer incidence and mortality in the United States. Natl. Cancer Inst. Presented before Subcomm. Health Sci. Res., Senate Comm. Hum. Resour.
17. Armstong, R. J. 1972. A study of infant mortality from linked records. In *Vital and Health Statistics.* Ser. 20:12. Natl. Cent. Health Stat. DHEW (HSM)72–1055. Washington: GPO. 90 pp.
18. MacMahon, B., Kovar, M. G., Feldman, J. J. 1972. Infant mortality rates: Socioeconomic factors United States. In *Vital and Health Statistics.* Ser. 22:14. Natl. Cent. Health Stat. DHEW (HSM)72–1045. Washington: GPO. 68 pp.
19. (NINDS) Natl. Inst. of Neurol. Dis. Stroke 1972. Collaborative Perinatal Study. *The Women and Their Pregnan-*

cies. DHEW (NIH)73–379. Washington: GPO. 540 pp.

20. Chase, H. C. 1972. Trends in "prematurity," United States: 1950–67. In *Vital and Health Statistics.* Ser. 3:15. Natl. Cent. Health Stat. DHEW (HSM)72–1030. Washington: GPO. 51 pp.

21. Kelly, J. E., Harvey, C. R. 1979. Basic data on dental examination findings of persons 1–74 years, United States, 1971–1974. In *Vital and Health Statistics.* Ser. 11:214. Natl. Cent. Health Stat. DHEW (PHS) 79–1662. Washington: GPO. 33 pp.

22a. Wilder, C. S. 1977. Limitation of activity due to chronic conditions, United States, 1974. In *Vital and Health Statistics.* Ser. 10:111. Natl. Cent. Health. Stat. DHEW (HRA)77–1537. Washington: GPO. 65 pp.

22b. Wilder, C. S., 1971. Chronic conditions and limitations of activity and mobility, United States, July 1965–June 1967. In *Vital and Health Statistics,* Ser. 10:61. Natl. Cent. Health Stat. DHEW 1000–10–61. Washington: GPO

22c. Gleeson, G. A. 1959. Limitation of activity and mobility due to chronic conditions, United States, July 1957–June 1958. In *Health Statistics from the U.S. National Health Survey,* Ser. B-11. Public Health Serv. DHEW 584–B11. Washington: GPO

23. DHEW 1979. *Healthy People—The Surgeon General's Report on Health Promotion and Disease Prevention.* DHEW (PHS) 79–50071A. Washington: GPO. 484 pp.

24. Elinson, J., Wilson, R. W. 1978. Prevention. In *Health, United States, 1978.* DHEW (PHS)78–1232, pp. 21–45. Washington: GPO

25. McKeown, J. 1978. Determinants of health. *Hum. Nat.* 1:60–67

26. Belloc, N. B. 1973. Relationship of health practices and mortality. *Prev. Med.* 2:67–81

27. Belloc, N. B. 1976. Health practices and mortality—nine-year follow-up. Res.

Grant No. HS00368. Natl. Cent. Health Serv. Res.

28. Dresser, C. M. V., Carroll, M. D., Abraham, S. 1978. Selected findings: Food consumption profiles of white and black persons 1–74 years of age in the United States, 1971–74. In *Advance Data from Vital and Health Statistics,* No. 21. Natl. Cent. Health Stat. DHEW (PHS)78–1250. Washington: GPO. 11 pp.

29a. Choi, J. W. 1978. Exercise and participation in sports among persons 20 years of age and over: United States, 1975. In *Advance Data from Vital and Health Statistics.* No. 19. Natl. Cent. Health Stat. DHEW (PHS)78–1250. Washington: GPO. 11 pp.

29b. Moss, A. J., Scott, G. 1978. Characteristics of persons with hypertension, United States, 1974. In *Vital and Health Statistics,* Ser. 10:121. Natl. Cent. Health Stat. DHEW (PHS) 79–1549. Washington: GPO

29c. Moss, A. J., Wilder, M. H. 1977. Use of selected medical procedures associated with preventive care, United States, 1973. In *Vital and Health Statistics,* Ser. 10:110. Natl. Cent. Health Stat. DHEW (HRA)77–1538. Washington: GPO

30. Cent. Dis. Control 1977. *Fluoridation Census. 1975.* Washington: GPO. 407 pp.

31. DHEW 1979. *Smoking and Health, a Report of the Surgeon General.* DHEW (PHS)79–50066. Washington: GPO

32. U.S. Environ. Prot. Agency. Air quality, planning, and standards of division, 1978. *Natl. Air Qual. Emission Trends Rep.* EPA–450/2–78–052

33. Gibson, R. M. 1979. National health expenditures, 1978 *Health Care Fin. Rev.* 1(1):1–36

34. DHEW 1976. *Health, United States, 1975.* DHEW (HRA)76–1232. Washington: GPO 612 pp.

35. DHEW 1977. *Health, United States, 1976–1977.* DHEW (HRA)77–1232. Washington: GPO. 441 pp.

36. DHEW 1978. *Health, United States, 1978.* DHEW (PHS)78–1232. Washington: GPO. 488 pp.

Ann. Rev. Public Health 1980. 1:37–68
Copyright © 1980 by Annual Reviews Inc. All rights reserved

QUALITY ASSESSMENT AND QUALITY ASSURANCE IN MEDICAL CARE

♦12501

P. J. Sanazaro

University of California, San Francisco, School of Medicine, San Francisco, California 94143

INTRODUCTION

Throughout this century, quality assurance has been the explicit purpose of the medical profession in reforming medical education, establishing certification of specialists, initiating peer review, and promoting continuing medical education. During this period, hospital standards have been upgraded, first by the Hospital Standardization Program and, since 1952, by its successor organization, the Joint Commission on Accreditation of Hospitals (JCAH). Despite these manifestations of self-regulation, the effectiveness of these measures in upgrading the quality of care has been sharply questioned (1–4). Within the past 15 years, political, social, and legal forces have combined to abruptly supplant traditional professional autonomy with regulation, mandating explicit accounting for the quality of care. The result has been rapid, nation-wide implementation of medical auditing in hospitals, using methods developed independently of fundamental principles and concepts established by earlier students of quality assessment and quality assurance. The major issues surrounding this turn of events have been addressed at length in statements of policy (5, 6), in symposia and conferences (7–9), and in a major private sector study (10).

This review is limited to a small portion of the literature on quality assessment and assurance of personal medical care, i.e. services given by or at the direction of a physician to individual patients and the results of that care. Some important, highly relevant subjects are omitted. Practical constraints also dictate the exclusion of literature pertaining to the performance

37

of other health professionals and of the medical system generally and its effects on health status, cost-benefit and cost-effectiveness, and ethics of medical care. These subjects are increasingly intertwined in public policy but require separate consideration.

Extensive reviews of the literature on quality assessment and quality assurance have been published, notably those of Donabedian (11a, 11b) Brook (12, 13), and Greene (14). Williamson (15) has abstracted and usefully classified 3500 articles relevant to this subject. Collections of papers have been published on peer review (16) and quality assurance in ambulatory care (17).

No attempt is made to define "quality" in this review, beyond the commonly accepted understanding that quality of medical care connotes correct evaluation and efficacious treatment of each patient's medical condition with minimum possible risk, combined with educational and caring functions that together enable the patient to attain the optimum achievable clinical, functional, and psychosocial results.

The review begins with a consideration of quality assessment and an account of how social and political forces have brought about widespread implementation of medical auditing. Basic concepts and principles are then reviewed, with emphasis on criteria and standards and use of outcomes as measures of quality. A section is devoted to physician performance specifically because of its central importance to this subject. The final section considers current programs of quality assurance, available evidence on their effectiveness, and an interpretation of the state of the art. The review concludes with an overview and recommendations for needed research and development.

QUALITY ASSESSMENT

Much recent research in quality assessment has been strongly influenced by the practice of performing medical audits based on explicit criteria. The circumstances responsible for the general use of this method of evaluation and for the kinds of criteria used by audit committees are briefly summarized.

Medical Auditing

The two basic features of medical auditing are (a) selecting an important element of performance and (b) comparing the observed level of performance with predetermined criteria or standards. This concept of auditing dates from work performed early in this century that demonstrated the feasibility of assessing the quality of surgical care by examining end-results and taking into account other factors that could influence the outcomes (18,

19). Ponton (20) introduced the current approach in which record librarians abstract specific items of information from medical charts and refer designated records to physicians for peer review. By 1952, the many hospital-related factors other than physician performance that may influence care and its results were well-known: administration, equipment, essential services to support physicians, competent personnel, supervision of patient care, and personnel policies affecting morale (21).

Lembcke (22) described the definitive state of the art of audit as applied to surgical care, but did not publish a comparable report on the application of his principles to the assessment of medical (as opposed to surgical) treatment. This vacuum was filled by the Commission on Professional and Hospital Activities (CPHA) (23) and by the work of Payne (24–28).

COMMISSION ON PROFESSIONAL HOSPITAL ACTIVITIES Established in 1953, the Commission conducts a Professional Activity Study (PAS), which provides forms on which subscribing hospitals' record librarian staffs abstract medical records of all discharged patients. CPHA then processes these and furnishes summaries to each hospital, together with comparison data on other hospitals in the same geographical region. PAS reports put into practice the use of empirical norms (29, 30). The Commission promoted medical auditing, beginning in the late 1950s, on the premise that a substantial difference between a subscribing hospital's performance level and the empirical median or range was an indication of need for that hospital to audit its performance. The Commission recently has added a "Quality Assurance Monitor" (QAM). In this, panels of specialists in the various fields of medicine define normative standards for the expected frequency of diagnostic and therapeutic procedures and outcomes. Any hospital that finds its level of performance falling outside that normative range is expected to examine the original medical records to determine whether performance is actually substandard. No systematic studies have been published on the actual use of CPHA data by hospitals, but its programs have spurred the adoption of auditing.

A recent study has analysed the reliability of the abstracts produced for CPHA and a number of other private hospital discharge abstracting systems by reabstracting records and comparing the items with those on the original abstracts (31). Discrepancies were found in 35% of common principal diagnoses and in 27% of common principal procedures. The quality of the data was thought adequate for reporting on utilization but unsuitable for use in health services research or evaluation of care.

EVOLUTION OF OPTIMAL CARE CRITERIA It was the work of Payne (24–27) that determined the approach to auditing used by most hospitals at the beginning of the 1970s. In 1961, Payne adapted previously developed utilization criteria to the purpose of auditing medical, gynecologic, and surgical care by incorporating criteria for the adequacy of physicians' recording in medical charts (24). This was expanded by Payne, working with panels of practicing specialists, into sets of criteria for optimal performance in 51 different conditions covering 135 ICDA diagnoses. The intent of auditing with these criteria was to promote change in diagnostic and therapeutic behavior of the medical staff (27). The auditing was educational and self-evaluative, not punitive, and not directed to individual physicians (24). This approach engendered physician acceptance and implementation.

The Hawaii Medical Association next commissioned a study by Payne of the quality of personal medical care in all Hawaii hospitals and in a sample of private offices (26). The concept of *optimal care criteria* was further extended by panels of local physicians to include pre- and post-hospitalization care and outcomes. In 3316 cases covering 21 diagnostic hospital categories, the overall rate of physician adherence to the criteria was 71%. For a smaller sample of cases receiving office care, the adherence rate was 41%.

Consequently, by 1972, it was already known that adherence by physicians to their own optimal care criteria was low, especially in office practice, but this finding had not been critically examined. Two sequences of events in the meantime combined to bring about widespread adoption of medical auditing based on this class of consensually set criteria.

DISSEMINATION OF AUDITING BY OPTIMAL CARE CRITERIA   The first impetus toward widespread adoption of medical auditing based on optimal care criteria was the federal government's regulations based on the Medicare legislation of 1965, which required each hospital to appoint a committee responsible for the retrospective review of records of all patients whose hospital stay exceeded a specified number of days. Periodic reports on utilization by Medicare patients were required, and many hospitals then subscribed to the services of CPHA to fulfill this requirement. In addition, committees throughout the country ordered over 6000 copies of the Hospital Utilization Review Manual prepared at the University of Michigan (25, 27). These guidelines were useful to newly formed utilization review committees that were required to determine whether patients' admission and stay and the procedures in the hospital were medically justified. These determinations were important because, without them, the hospital would not be reimbursed for that hospital stay. In that sense, the utilization review criteria were "pay or no pay" guidelines directed to third-party payers. The manual also contained recommended items in the medical history and physical examination, the recording of which was believed to be indicative of the quality of care. By this means most hospital committees in the United

States were first introduced to the idea of conducting medical audits based on optimal care criteria.

By 1970, Congress had concluded that the Medicare requirements for utilization review were ineffective in controlling unnecessary hospital use and in 1972 enacted PL 92–603 (6). This law established the Professional Standards Review Organizations (PSRO) program, in which local PSROs composed entirely of practicing physicians were set up in each of approximately 200 geographical areas that blanketed the United States. Their mandated function was to assure that the care given Medicare and Medicaid patients (a) was medically necessary, (b) conformed to acceptable professional standards, and (c) was provided in the most efficient manner possible. The PSROs were required to carry out a more stringent form of utilization review and to conduct medical care evaluation studies (MCEs) (6, 32). These were defined as medical audits to determine whether or not the care of Medicare and Medicaid patients conformed to acceptable standards. A national committee, established to develop guidelines for the use of PSROs in concurrent utilization review and medical care evaluation, initially endorsed empirical or optimal care criteria, but then proposed the use of essential criteria (33), i.e. valid criteria as originally defined by Lembcke (22) and adapted by Sanazaro (10). However, by this time the majority of hospitals were using optimal care criteria. The general model for MCEs promoted by the PSRO program was a modification of Payne's early work: determine study objective, establish criteria and standards, design study, collect data, develop reports, analyze results, identify deficiencies, develop a corrective plan, and restudy (6). Two field studies have shown that the implementation of this model by hospital medical staffs falls considerably short of the objectives, especially the identification and correction of important deficiencies in medical care (34, 35).

The second major circumstance that fortuitously accelerated the application of medical auditing as the main form of quality assessment was a series of court decisions that held that the hospital had separate corporate liability for malpractice on the part of a staff member (36). These court decisions established the principle that the hospital governing board is legally liable if a patient suffers adverse outcomes by virtue of the board allowing an incompetent physician to care for patients in that hospital. The net effect of these rulings was to prompt hospitals to strengthen their procedures for reviewing the quality of care. It also motivated the Joint Commission on Accreditation of Hospitals in 1970 to place more emphasis on the direct assessment of quality of care. Hospitals responded by doing audits based on optimal care criteria.

Dissatisfied with this state of auditing, the JCAH staff adopted Williamson's (37) concept of first assessing diagnostic outcomes (accuracy of diagnosis) to determine whether there is a need to examine the diagnostic process, and then examining the outcomes of care to determine whether there is a need to evaluate the adequacy of patient management. This principle was incorporated into the Performance Evaluation Procedure (PEP) (36, 38a). When in 1975 the Joint Commission required hospitals to perform a specified number of audits each year, it was this form of audit or its equivalent that many hospitals attempted to adopt. The effect of the JCAH requirement, along with the PSRO requirement, was to expedite national implementation of medical auditing. By 1976, 93% of all hospitals were conducting audits (38b). Pertinent here is the fact that neither of the most prevalent forms—those based on optimal care criteria or outcomes— had been systematically evaluated for reliability, sensitivity, or validity.

Basic Concepts and Principles of Quality Assessment

This summary of the practice of medical auditing throughout the country can be compared with the basic principles of quality assessment that were laid down in a series of papers published between 1950 and 1968. Sheps (39) made explicit the view that assessing the quality of hospital care involves application of general principles of measurement and evaluation, especially reliability and validity. Quality can only be inferred from the interpretation of a number of different reliable and valid measurements that amount to a "profile." Appraisal of quality may be directed to three aspects: assumed prerequisites for quality care (facilities, organization, staff, standards); elements of performance; and effects of care or outcomes, taking into account the many factors besides treatment that influence health status. The validity of empirical or normative standards for any of these three aspects must be independently established. Standards should be periodically revised in accord with the advances of medical knowledge.

Lembcke (22) described the use of valid criteria to evaluate individual cases and the use of independently set standards to evaluate overall medical staff performance. The purpose of auditing is to assure that benefits of modern medical knowledge are being successfully applied to patients. It is advisable to "single out and concentrate on a few features that are essential to achievement of the desired end-result of hospital care." Availability of scientific knowledge on which to base criteria determines the scope of the medical audit. Confirmation of clinical diagnosis, justification of surgery, proper use of antibiotics, and judging whether death may have been preventable are elements of care susceptible to scientific auditing.

The papers of Sheps (39) and Lembcke (22) described evaluation of hospital-based medical care in operational terms. Scientific validity of criteria was emphasized; standards of good practice were defined as the level of performance observed in a reference group of hospitals, usually teaching hospitals. The approach was empirical, descriptive, and practical.

Ten years later, Donabedian (40) published his classic paper, which reformulated Sheps' three categories of elements within which to evaluate quality, calling them simply "structure," "process," and "outcome." He carefully pointed out the complexity of interrelationships among these categorizations, which were not mutually exclusive, and the need to validate their relationship to quality. In 1968, he further elaborated his views (41).

In 1967, Shapiro (42) described the difficulties of assessing quality by examining outcomes of care because of the multiple factors other than treatment that influence outcomes favorably or unfavorably. He stated that as the known efficacy of treatment increased, criteria for such treatment could be used as indirect means of assessing the adequacy of outcome.

In 1967, Williamson (43) illustrated the use of auditing to identify specific educational needs that should be addressed by targeted continuing education. In 1968, he proposed a set of principles for setting priorities in quality assessment: specific diagnoses of high frequency that have important adverse impact on patients and high social costs if untreated and are amenable to preventive, curative, or rehabilitative treatment (44). He reported a series of heuristic studies in which practitioners and clinical experts estimated the clinical and functional outcomes that should be attained by patients with specified conditions who received proper treatment. Interview and follow-up examination of patients with those conditions were then conducted to determine the patients' actual status after discharge from the hospital. The finding of substantial discrepancies between most estimates and actual patient status led to his later formulation of the health-accounting system (45).

The above papers and perspectives define the major concepts and principles of evaluation that should be applied in formal efforts to assess the quality of medical care. As noted above, the most prevalent forms of medical auditing do not adequately embody these principles (34, 35).

CRITERIA OR STANDARDS IN MEDICAL AUDITING   In addition to Payne et al (26), six major efforts have been mounted to evaluate ambulatory or office care on the basis of consensually set criteria that incorporate the "optimal care" concept (46–51). Observed rates of adherence to optimal care criteria ranged approximately from 30 to 60%. Higher values in two studies were perhaps attributable to having solicited supplementary data beyond that appearing in participating practitioners' records (46, 48).

These results have been interpreted to mean that the technical quality of care is at a generally low level. However, optimal care criteria are not valid indicators of the actual quality of care received by patients (52). The criteria represent physician opinions concerning the information on symptoms and signs that ideally ought to be recorded in patients' charts. Donabedian has held that this is an important dimension of the quality of care (11a). Rosenfeld (53) and Lyons & Payne (54) reported some association between the amount of recording in the chart by physicians and the technical quality of care. The most definitive evidence bearing on this question is that presented by Sanazaro & Worth (55). Their study, based on hospital records of 6946 cases with confirmed diagnoses, found that 30% of cases met all documentation criteria for predisposing or etiologic factors, stage or severity of condition, important associated conditions, and prior treatment; however, 73% of these same cases met all criteria of scientifically validated treatment. There was no significant correlation between the amount of documentation of important clinical information and the provision of correct treatment, or between documentation and outcomes attributable to treatment received. The postulated relationship between chart content and results of diagnosis and treatment has been challenged by others (56). A relationship has been reported between the amount of recorded information on educational aspects of care and degree of patient knowledge and compliance (57).

The second criticism of optimal care criteria stems from such criteria sets having incorporated utilization criteria that define all procedures that might be necessary in diagnosing or treating patients with a particular diagnosis. These criteria are useful to third party payers in deciding whether or not to pay for a procedure because their only consideration is that the procedure be consistent with the diagnosis. But when such items are used in medical auditing, there is no way of knowing which of the listed procedures is essential for the diagnosis or treatment of any particular patient. This is the fundamental requirement for any criteria used in assessing the quality of medical care.

Brook demonstrated the futility of relying on optimal care criteria as a means of assessing quality (12). He reported that implicit judgments of adequacy of care and of outcome were discrepant: 63% of the cases were rated as having received adequate care on the basis of actual clinical outcomes, but the medical management was rated adequate in only 27% of these same patients. When detailed explicit criteria of optimal care were used as the basis for assessing care, only 1 to 2% of 296 records met all criteria: the more extensive the list of items that "ought to be recorded" in order to provide documentation of good quality care, the lower the ratings of quality that resulted from abstracting records in accord with those criteria.

In recognition of the central importance of valid criteria in assessing quality, guidelines were issued to experimental medical care review organizations in 1971 to assist them in evolving such criteria (58). The guidelines stated that criteria should 1. assure accuracy of diagnosis, 2. incorporate procedures that conform to results of scientific studies, 3. define means of determining whether or not efficacious therapy was given correctly, 4.

incorporate only those end results that are entirely attributable to medical treatment received, 5. be continually revised in keeping with results of clinical research, and 6. be extended as resources permit to include psychosocial aspects of care and its results. Enactment of PSRO legislation overtook this effort, and in the rush to implement MCE requirements, these guidelines were not generally followed.

A second cluster of recent studies has addressed the relationship between "process" and "outcome" (12, 50, 59–61). Generally weak or absent correlations were found between assorted processes and clinical outcomes. McAuliffe (62) has critiqued the assumptions, design, and methods of analysis used in some of these studies. He pointed out that some confused the requirements of analytic (experimental) research with those of descriptive research or evaluations. Properly designed evaluations can demonstrate associations that have been previously established as causal in clinical trials, provided that samples are large enough. In their large scale study, Sanazaro & Worth (55) found strong statistical associations between validated procedures and clinical outcomes in patients with acute bacterial pneumonia and between validated contraindicated treatment and death in patients with acute myocardial infarction. The Kaiser-Permanente study (63) found some associations between specific medical treatment and specific medical outcomes. The discussion in the latter report emphasizes the importance of validity, sample size, and intervening variables in attempting to find associations between treatment and clinical outcomes. An earlier study illustrated the feasibility of detecting a significant association in an outpatient setting between administering oral iron for iron deficiency anemia and the resulting increase in hemoglobin (64).

USE OF OUTCOME MEASURES IN QUALITY ASSESSMENT   Outcomes attributable to care received are generally considered the ultimate indicators of the quality of medical care. The principle of assessing quality through study of adverse outcomes has been followed for over 60 years by surgical departments in hospitals (19, 20, 22). Committees have judged the appropriateness of operations through study of tissue removed and have reviewed deaths and complications in order to identify possible shortcomings in skill or judgment that might have been responsible. In the study of surgical services in the United States (65), committees of participating hospitals differed greatly in their judgments concerning whether surgeon-, hospital-, patient-, or community-related factors were responsible for preventable deaths and complications.

Systematic research in outcome assessment has been hampered by a lack of agreement on basic premises and a lack of precision in definition. Sanazaro & Williamson derived inductively an empirical classification of beneficial and detrimental patient effects from reports of 19,900 end results attributed to specified physician actions (66). Major categories were (a) clinical outcomes (mortality, longevity, change in disease status and symptoms, risk of adverse effects); (b) outcomes attributable to education, counseling, and caring (knowledge and understanding of patient's own condition and self-management; outlook and attitude toward patient's own condition; satisfaction with physician and with medical care generally; compliance); (c) outcomes defining patient's function as an individual, family member, or member of the community; and (d) the effects of incurring costs and hospitalization.

Brook et al (13) offer a detailed conceptual overview of the subject and propose four categories of generic outcome criteria: (a) physical (e.g. activities of daily living), (b) physiological (e.g. morbidity, mortality), (c) psychosocial (e.g. role performance), and (d) general (e.g. stress/tension). The report proposed alternate methods of controlling for the effects of intervening variables outside the influence of the medical care system that could affect outcomes favorably or unfavorably. The disease-specific outcomes defined by panels of experts for eight common conditions were published separately (67). Starfield has proposed the use of seven classes of outcomes: resilience, achievement, disease, satisfaction, comfort, activity, and longevity (68).

Sanazaro & Worth analysed immediate outcomes of hospital treatment that were recorded concurrently for 5600 Medicare and Medicaid patients prior to discharge and retrospectively for another 1300 Medicare and Medicaid patients with common medical and surgical conditions (55). The categories of outcomes were (a) clinical status at discharge, (b) functional status at discharge, (c) preventable complications, and (d) death. Because of the advanced average age of patients and the unavailability of information on relevant prognostic factors, death and functional status were not found to be useful indicators of the technical quality of care. The most valid indicators were preventable complications and failure to attain expected clinical status. Incidence of these indicators after appendectomy and cholecystectomy varied from less than 10% to more than 40% among the 68 hospitals in the study.

The most detailed study of adverse surgical outcomes is that of the Stanford Center for Health Care Research (69). Controlling for identifiable factors that can influence outcomes (patient and disease characteristics, type of operation), the group confirmed in 17 hospitals the earlier findings of the National Halothane Study (70) that up to 350% differences exist in adjusted rates of postoperative mortality and morbidity.

Williamson (71) has reported his experience in applying a broad range of outcome measures in his health accounting projects. Trained health accountants obtain information from medical records, interview or examine patients, or obtain specimens to provide the desired follow-up information on patients' clinical and functional status. Williamson has used a "health status scale" that ranks patients at one of six levels of function between "asymptomatic" and "dead." The results of the outcome evaluation are then compared with the estimates of expected outcome status made by the medical staff of the particular hospital or clinic conducting the study. Any discrepancy between expectations and findings is termed an "achievable benefit not achieved," which calls for further study of the factors responsible for failure to attain the full expected benefit. (See section on quality assurance.)

The general literature on assessment of ambulatory care has been recently reviewed (72a, 72b). Mushlin et al (73) applied a "problem status index" in assessing the adequacy of outcomes of ambulatory care. By follow-up interview of patients, the level of symptoms, activity and anxiety related to the condition for which the patient received treatment were defined and used to supplement chart review.

Ware et al (74) reviewed comprehensively the recent literature on measurement of patient satisfaction. Based on his own work and that of others, he identified eight dimensions of satisfaction: art of care (the caring function), technical quality of care, accessibility and convenience, finances, physical environment, availability, continuity, and efficacy and outcomes of care. He noted that satisfaction with the art of care and with the technical quality of care are highly interrelated, that satisfaction is a predictor of patient compliance, and that the full effects of satisfaction on health and illness behavior are not yet known. One major study reported a striking disparity between patient satisfaction and quality of hospital care judged by chart review (75).

Several reports have documented the importance of patient education or counseling—and the resultant knowledge, understanding, and attitudes—in achieving the full therapeutic benefit of medical treatment (76–78). The impressive results achieved in significantly better control of hypertension through this means (77, 78) are not matched by experience in adult patients with diabetes. Williams' (79) early observation that patient knowledge and compliance did not correlate with degree of control has been replicated (60b, 80). The control of diabetes, as is true of the management of many medical conditions for which efficacious treatment exists, is manifestly more difficult to achieve than the control of blood pressure, because the regimen that diabetic patients must follow is more complex and demanding. This underscores the need to interrelate evaluation of medical outcomes with assessment of the technical adequacy of causally related medical treatment and all intervening patient behavior variables.

Gonnella and associates (81, 82) have proposed that clinical staging, as has been applied to patients with cancer, be applied more generally as one means of measuring outcomes. They have developed provisional classifications of three stages of severity for common diagnoses, and these are now being tested empirically. This principle has been followed implicitly for many years by surgical committees reviewing death and complications, but without benefit of a standard classification of disease severity. The principle was also incorporated in the Performance Evaluation Procedure of the JCAH (38a), in which complications were identified and adequacy of adherence to "critical management criteria" (i.e. valid treatment criteria) was then determined. If valid treatment criteria have been met, then the complication or progression of disease to a greater degree of severity is considered nonpreventable, or at least not attributable to deficiencies in medical management. Testing "clinical staging" in the hospital setting will provide needed studies of reliability and validity of current techniques for examining preventability of common complications and deaths. On the other hand, use of this approach in evaluating the technical adequacy of ambulatory medical care encounters formidable difficulties. Among these is the necessity of distinguishing among all nonmedical-care-related factors that can account for patients progressing to advanced stages of disease. The method may better lend itself in this setting to community-based analyses of medical care and should perhaps be regarded as an extension of the tracer approach developed by Kessner (83).

PROTOCOLS, ALGORITHMS, AND CLINICAL DECISION MAKING
The use of clinical algorithms or protocols (85–88) and clinical decision making (89–90) in evaluating the appropriateness of diagnosis and treatment is a development primarily of the 1970s, though predicted and pilot tested earlier by Peterson (84). Algorithms display the logic of sequential decision making based on the findings produced by antecedent steps in the diagnostic process. Depending upon which of the potential clinical manifestations of the problem or disease are present in the individual patient, further diagnostic steps or therapeutic interventions are specified. The substantive content of these decision trees is based on the results of clinical observations and is subject to the same considerations as other forms of criteria: The validity of the defined sequences should be scientifically substantiated.

Algorithms have been used primarily in the training or supervision of physician extenders or nurse practitioners. The general expectation that physicians would resist imposition of such algorithms has been confirmed (91). However, after physicians agreed in an emergency room service to use structured recording forms that corresponded to the contents of algorithms, the amount of missing data was reduced from 20% to 1%.

The principle of algorithms, when combined with prospective determination of the frequency of associations in diagnosis, can be transformed into mathematically defined clinical decision making instruments (88–90, 92, 93). The degree of uncertainty with respect to sensitivity and specificity of diagnostic tests can be translated into mathematical terms, and the conditional probabilities of the consequences of alternate courses of action are stated. The application of these probabilities prospectively to decisions involving individual patients merits further study.

These principles have been adapted to the retrospective assessment of quality in a technique called "criteria mapping" (94). The algorithmic logic followed by physicians in evaluating presenting clinical manifestations is embodied in the criteria used to review diagnosis and treatment. One value of this approach is that only data that pertain to the individual patient's actual clinical status need to be abstracted. This approach also eliminates the main difficulty posed by optimal care criteria in evaluating care: Only a few criteria may actually apply in a given case, thus yielding a low adherence score that hears no necessary relationship to actual technical quality of care. Algorithm-based evaluation is also superior in being applicable to nonspecific problems such as back pain or chest pain.

It is to be expected that further experience with clinical decision making in its various forms will materially advance the reliability and validity of methods of evaluating the quality of technical care.

PHYSICIAN PERFORMANCE

Based on her review of the literature, Barro (95) concluded that physician performance has two main components: technical skills (psychomotor and cognitive) and interpersonal skills. Sanazaro & Williamson (66) used a modification of the critical incident method to develop an empirical classification of physician performance and its effects on patients. The five elements of performance reported most frequently by internists as having a demonstrable effect on patients were, in order: arriving at a diagnosis, use of drugs and biologicals, patient education, manner in dealing with patients, and use and interpretation of laboratory tests. Of 6300 end results of care attributed by internists to physician actions, 50% related to clinical effects (longevity, risks, and changes in the disease process or physical symptoms); 28% concerned psychological symptoms, attitudes toward medical care, attitudes toward and understanding of patients' own condition, and compliance; and 12% pertained to patient functioning (96).

The American Academy of Pediatrics (97) and the American Board of Internal Medicine (98) have used results from other critical incident studies to derive formulations of clinical competence as the basis for revising their testing and measuring procedures. The underlying dimension of competence was identified as "problem solving." The relationship of such measures to physician performance is not yet known.

Price and associates (99) compiled a list of 116 qualities of physicians: 87 positive or desirable and 29 negative or undesirable. Obtained initially from physicians' opinions regarding "the basic factors of success," the list was then reviewed and modified by medical educators, college and medical students, administrators, clergymen, a variety of other professional people, and patients. The relative importance assigned to most factors by various representatives of the public differed from those assigned by physicians. "Thorough up-to-date knowledge of his own field of medicine" was ranked first by the general public and ranked 18.5 by physicians. The general public rated "able to be his own teacher" 19.5 on the list and physicians rated this second in importance.

Methods of Assessment

No large scale observational studies of physicians caring for patients have been conducted in the United States since the original report by Peterson et al (100). Instead, most assessment of physician performance has relied upon peer review of records or on criteria-based record auditing. Morehead (75, 101, 102a, 102b) has reported extensive experience with the use of expert physician reviewers who examine the entire medical record in order to judge the quality of care provided by physicians. Morehead considers this method more valid because physician reviewers take into account all disease- and patient-related factors that bear on management decisions and on the results of care. In her view, these can never be fully encompassed by any set of explicit criteria that ostensibly provide a more objective determination of quality. A directly opposite view has been taken by others because they observed low reliabilities of implicit judgments by peer reviewers (28, 103). This latter position is supported by results obtained by using the Kappa coefficient, which represents the rate of agreement corrected for the rate that could be expected by chance alone (63, 104). Whether reviewing entire records or abstracts of records, physicians agree with one another on judged quality of care at or near the level expected by chance alone. This finding dictates that physician judgments should not be used to make fine discriminations among levels of performance by physicians. However, peer review may still be the best practical method of identifying serious deficiencies in care (105a).

Most studies of physician performance based on office record data have disclosed low rates of adherence to explicit normative criteria, as discussed in the section on quality assessment. Hulka et al (50) attempted to determine whether there is a distinction between "good record keeping" (which is all that a high adherence score may reflect) and actual satisfactory performance. Of the observed variability in recording performance, 50% was attributed to lack of information in the records. There was no relationship between the adherence scores and particular characteristics of physicians or their practice. It was hypothesized that the unexplained systematic variation in the adherence scores might be due to "differences in the quality of care."

To answer the question of whether doctors actually collect more information and do more with patients than they habitually write down, two studies compared the content of records with the results of tape recorded physician-patient visits (57) or observational checklists (51). Items pertaining to history, physical examination, laboratory or other procedures, drugs prescribed, and referrals were adequately recorded (with up to 90% concordance between observation and recording). However, advice to patients and instructions regarding side effects of drugs were poorly recorded (10% or less). Important information on diagnosis, major drugs, and abnormal test results was recorded in 94 to 96% of instances in one study (105b).

Performance of physicians in providing technical care will continue to be assessed largely on the basis of adherence to explicit criteria. The content of normative or consensual criteria used in medical auditing differs considerably, depending upon the expertise of the particular group setting the criteria. This is reflected in the report by Wagner et al (106) in which pediatricians specializing in infectious disease, as compared with family physicians and general pediatricians, were most restrictive in defining indications for use of antibiotics. Consensus by clinically active experts appears to be a workable method of defining the most scientifically valid criteria that are applicable nationally (55, 107, 108). Adherence rates to such criteria have much more significance than adherence rates to norms or normative criteria generally. Similar reasoning has been applied in proposing modifications of profile data obtained on hospitals (109a).

PATIENT SURVEYS   The known variability in content of physicians' records has long made it evident that the full range of physician performance and its effects on patients cannot be assessed on the basis of record content alone. This is particularly true of the nonmedical elements of care and its results. Based on the observation that internists reported a high proportion of nonclinical outcomes in a critical incident study (109b), a before-and-after study was conducted of 102 patients receiving office care in a New York group practice (P. J. Sanazaro and J. W. Williamson 1967, unpublished data). Patients appearing for an unscheduled "urgent" appointment were interviewed in person before seeing one of eight internists and again by telephone one week after termination of that episode of care. In contrast to the office records, the interviews identified significant changes in symptoms, functional status (work or usual activities, sexual function, role as parent), knowledge of and attitudes toward the condition and its treatment, satisfaction with the physician and medical care, and concerns over costs. Using a similar technique, Mushlin et al (73) incorporated the principles developed by Williamson (37) to demonstrate the value of post-treatment symptoms, disability, and anxiety in pinpointing deficiencies of care that were not detected on routine chart audit. The evidence is mounting that patient interviews combined with chart review based on valid criteria provide a more complete assessment of physician performance. This is particularly so in office care, because the importance of inducing appropriate patient behavior to achieve the full benefit of care is well documented (45, 60b, 74, 76–78), and information on this critical element is usually not available in office records.

Level of Performance

The technical quality of care provided by medical staffs of hospitals varies substantially. In an unpublished report of the American College of Surgeons in 1918, only 89 of over 692 hospitals met the barest standard of care (110). Hospital standards were then progressively raised. In more recent studies, hospital staffs are still shown to vary with respect to rates of unjustified hysterectomy (111, 112, 113), unjustified appendectomy (29, 114), postoperative death rates (69, 70), postoperative morbidity (55, 69), and provision of scientifically validated medical treatment (55).

Studies by Morehead and colleagues provide extensive data on quality of care provided by physicians in hospitals, as judged by clinical experts. Care for 43% of 684 cases was rated as fair or poor (75, 101); 36% of 792 cases in a separate study were judged to have received unsatisfactory care (113). Variations in incidence of operations unexplained by differences in case mix are considered by some to reflect adversely on the technical quality of care (115). Physician performance in ambulatory care has not been systematically evaluated since Peterson et al (100) documented extensive deficiencies in basic skills. Evaluations based on chart audits suggested considerable variability in performance, but the criteria differed from study to study and did not support uniform conclusions (26, 46–51). Williamson (71) has reported high rates of missed diagnoses and substandard control of hypertension. Kessner (116a) found that 45% of 248 patients receiving treatment for high blood pressure had no clear indication for such treatment. A critical review has been published of literature on physician performance and its correlates "which may serve as indicators of quality of medical care" (116b).

Of particular interest are reviews that document surprising degrees of unreliability of data obtained by physicians in examining patients and interpreting results of X-rays and other common diagnostic procedures (104, 117).

VARIABILITY OF PHYSICIAN PERFORMANCE   A growing body of data indicates that the performance of individual physicians varies under different circumstances. Stapleton (118) reported a higher level of performance by staff physicians caring for patients in a teaching service than when the same physicians cared for comparable patients in a nonteaching service of the same hospital. De Dombal et al (93) observed that surgeons, required as part of a study to provide critical data upon which they based their diagnosis and decision to operate, substantially reduced the incidence of ruptured appendices and of nonindicated operations during the study. After the study ended, performance of the same surgeons promptly reverted toward previous less satisfactory levels.

Introduction of protocols for the guidance of physician's assistants was also shown to improve the performance of physicians (119). McDonald (120) reported on the effectiveness of computer-printed reminders to residents in outpatient clinics that certain observations, tests, or changes in treatment were indicated for their patients. Residents receiving the alert abided by the suggestions in 51% of all instances; a control group of residents caring for comparable patients made indicated changes in only 21%. A similar principle is embodied in the use of an algorithm-based encounter form (91) and a computer-generated summary (121a, 121b); these significantly increased both the recording of pertinent data and the carrying out of indicated procedures.

Another form of surveillance is that reported in Canada after the College of Physicians and Surgeons of Saskatchewan concluded that the incidence of hysterectomy was disproportionate to the number of women aged 15 years or above in the population (112). Representatives of the college visited seven hospitals and held consultative discussions with the staff. Subsequently the rates of such operations declined in six of the seven hospitals.

Lembcke's (22) report presented definitive evidence that surgeons could dramatically improve their surgical judgment on being advised that their rates of unjustified operations were unacceptable to the medical staff, administration, and board of the hospital.

A physician's fund of medical knowledge may not directly correlate with his habitual performance. Members of a medical staff who used antibiotics inappropriately in 70% of their cases showed on a written test that they knew how to use antibiotics appropriately in most of those same cases (122). Gonnella et al (123) more definitively documented the lack of association between low actual performance in diagnosing urinary tract infection and high scores on tests of knowledge on diagnosis of urinary tract infection. McDonald (120) noted that physicians did not sustain their higher level of performance when they no longer received reminders, just as surgeons' accuracy of diagnoses and judgments decreased promptly after termination of a study (93).

The consistency of physician performance in different diseases or procedures has not been adequately analyzed. Observational studies suggested that individual physicians carried out the basic skills of patient evaluation and treatment at the same general level regardless of the patients' presenting problems (100). However, this finding may have been influenced by the halo effect, a problem that pervades attempts to evaluate clinical performance by observation. The performance of physicians within individual hospitals in treating patients with bacterial infections appeared to be homogeneous but did not correlate with the level of management of patients with acute myocardial infarction (55). Studies of performance based on adherence to normative criteria have concluded that there is a significant but low inter-diagnosis correlation (124). Expert peer review studies suggest a high degree of consistency in quality of care provided by physicians to the majority of their cases (102a), but the reliability of these observations is not known. No conclusions can be drawn from these few studies because the data cannot be directly compared.

MEASUREMENT OF CLINICAL JUDGMENT   Physicians' clinical judgment is widely regarded as the central determinant of the quality of care. Yet surprisingly few studies of this attribute have been reported. Information from a simple self-administered patient questionnaire, scored according to explicit decision rules, identified more potential diagnoses than did specialists or general practitioners eliciting the history themselves from the same patients (125). The one area in which physicians excelled was in recognizing psychophysiologic disorders. In another study, empirically determined probabilities were used in a computer program for the diagnosis of patients with severe abdominal pain admitted to a surgical service. The computer-based program consistently outperformed the senior surgeons in arriving at the diagnosis that was verified at operation (91.8% vs 79.6%) (92). When the program was revised to use the surgeons' estimates of frequencies of manifestations in the various diagnoses, the accuracy of computer-based diagnosis decreased significantly. It has been suggested that physicians may not be using a specific "diagnostic process" that can be mathematically modelled (126). The same may be true of physicians' clinical judgment.

QUALITY ASSURANCE

"Quality assurance" connotes a systematic effort to maintain satisfactory performance or improve medical care and its results. Continuing medical education (CME) is the most pervasive professionally initiated activity intended to maintain or improve the quality of care provided by physicians throughout their practice years (127, 128). The American Medical Association now offers a Physician's Recognition Award to those physicians who complete 150 credit hours of CME within a three year period. About 10 states require CME as a condition of reregistration of license to practice. Major specialty societies offer self-education and self-assessment programs as companion efforts to the recertification examinations of their counterpart specialty boards.

That some form of CME is required by physicians who wish to remain abreast of new knowledge and techniques is self-evident. The fact that physicians pass recertification examinations after variable years in practice is de facto evidence that CME can be effective. But few formal evaluations of CME have been published.

A recent review found that most of the published evaluations were weak in design, limiting possible conclusions (129a). In 113 studies that were judged to meet several criteria of validity, neither attendance nor satisfaction with the CME course correlated with learning. Acquisition of knowledge was strongly, positively associated with younger age and greater length of training of participants. The overall conclusion was that "a significant and consistent documentation of the existence of benefits (from CME) is absent." Another review found distinct improvement in physician competence, physician performance, and patient health status reported in "about half of the evaluation studies published since 1960," but shortcomings in the data made it "impossible to conclude that the improvements were caused by the CME" (129b).

Systematic information is lacking about the relationship of knowledge to performance. Despite abundant anecdotal evidence that there exists a substantial disparity between knowledge and performance, only fragmentary data to this effect have been published (120, 122, 123). Other data can be taken to infer that considerable improvement can be achieved in performance without recourse to CME (22, 93, 119, 121a). CME appears to be one of many necessary but not sufficient conditions for achieving genuine quality assurance.

The most extensive, formally organized activities directed to explicit quality assurance are conducted in individual hospitals in response to requirements of JCAH (38a) and PSRO (6). In general, these activities conform to the "bi-cycle model" developed by Brown (122), based on the earlier work of Williamson (43). In this model, deficiencies identified by auditing are corrected by some form of direct action or, more commonly, by continuing medical education. The problem is reexamined at a later date to make certain that it has been resolved. Documentation of this model's effectiveness in bringing about improvement in medical care is uneven (26,

43, 122, 127, 130, 131). A study of seventeen hospitals that employ this model found widespread inadequacies in the design of medical care evaluation studies, selection of criteria, and implementation of the program (35). Important findings were generally not followed up in an organized or appropriate manner. The conclusions of the investigators were, first, that those responsible for carrying out these programs did not have sufficient technical knowledge, and second, that the activities were carried out primarily to fulfill external requirements rather than as part of a professional commitment to upgrade the quality of hospital care.

Another report of hospital-based quality assurance programs found that substandard staff performance was the least frequent basis for corrective actions (34). The lack of adequate information about the effectiveness of such programs was cited, and the view was expressed ". . . that many of the changes (that were observed) should be the routine responsibility of a competent hospital or health professional and should not depend on the imposition of a special quality review program."

Williamson (71) details 50 outcome deficiencies in his studies, 30 of which were attributable to correctable determinants involving the patient, physicians, or institutions. Plans for correcting these were actually implemented in only 18 instances and on reevaluating 15 of these, 8 were shown to have produced improvement. There was no explanation of this desultory corrective response to "serious health care deficiencies."

An extension of this method in eight institutions has carefully evaluated the reliability of data generated by the health accounting approach, the validity of conclusions regarding efficacy of corrective actions, and cost-effectiveness (J. W. Williamson, unpublished information).

A set of suggested prerequisites for effectively correcting deficiencies found by medical audits within a large prepaid group plan including minimizing the retrospective aspect of audits, focusing on poorer-than-expected outcomes or failure to adhere to scientifically validated treatment elements, assuring physicians that valid data have been obtained, and prompt and direct feedback of performance (63). Ratification of criteria by participating physicians had no effect on willingness to change behavior in response to demonstrated nonadherence to those criteria.

The PSRO program contains within its requirements the potential for area-wide or regional quality assurance in hospital care. All hospitals that are to be reimbursed by Medicare or Medicaid programs must eventually comply with the requirements of the local PSRO that a specified number of medical care evaluation studies (MCEs) be carried out. The guidelines define MCEs broadly, encompassing both administrative and clinical areas, and indicate that continuing education is the expected approach for bringing about needed improvements (6). A brief report from one PSRO concluded that broadside feedback of information on deficiencies of recording were ineffective in improving the performance of practitioners, but that more immediate and direct notification of inappropriate use of whole blood in transfusions produced definite response in the desired direction (131). An early assessment of eight PSROs, identified as leaders in the movement, found little documentation of their effectiveness to bringing about improvements in care (34). The investigators questioned the appropriateness of the organization for quality assurance, technical comprehension of the tasks, designs of the methods of assessing quality, and adequacy of follow-through. Brook & Williams (132) reviewed studies of PSRO precursor organizations, most commonly Foundations for Medical Care, and noted little evidence of impact on quality. Detailed evaluation of one such organization found that such impact occurred only in the reductions in the number of unnecessary injections given in office care, and this may have resulted more from threatened denial of payment than from CME.

Private Initiative in PSRO conducted five case studies and concluded that the potential of PSROs for upgrading the quality of care in hospitals was limited (10). Although PSROs can require area-wide studies in which important differences in quality of care among hospitals might be identified, it remains the responsibility of the individual hospital's governing board and medical staff to decide whether and how to react to the findings. Using 24 experimental and 26 control hospitals, this same study evaluated the feasibility of conducting concurrent quality assurance within the PSRO-hospital framework, i.e. monitoring the care of patients while they were in the hospital in accord with valid criteria that defined a basic standard of care (133). The slightly better adherence to validated treatment criteria in the experimental group was attributed to the posting of the criteria on the records. Tension between hospital medical staffs and the PSRO organization, combined with the sensitive nature of the surveillance process, militated against effective intervention on the part of physician monitors (who were usually members of the hospital staff) when important deviations from the criteria were observed. Definite improvements in hospital staff performance were observed in six hospitals in which the staff or a key member gave strong and continuing support to the study.

The Department of Health, Education, and Welfare made a preliminary study of the impact of MCEs on the quality of care (134). More than 3500 MCEs were reported quarterly, but the report made no distinction between MCEs conducted by hospitals purely in response to the PSRO requirements and those conducted for purposes of accreditation by JCAH but also submitted to the PSRO. Using a "variation rate method," the study found slight increases in adherence to locally set criteria of good care between the time of initial audit and any subsequent reaudit. A separate study questions the impact of MCEs on quality of care (38b).

Determinants of Quality Assurance

It is generally believed that the organization, staffing, and facilities of a hospital or clinic have a substantial effect on quality of care, and accreditation by JCAH rests heavily on this premise. Early studies reported no discernible relationship between these elements and quality of care as determined by chart review (135, 136). Roemer & Friedman (137), using sociologic analysis, case studies, and international comparisons, concluded that the aggregate results "point to a positive association between higher levels of medical staff structuring and hospital performance." Empirical data on 42 hospitals in Massachusetts tend to support this conclusion (138). Investigators at Stanford have tested the relationship of hospital structure to performance most rigorously (139a). Using data from 17 acute care hospitals on postoperative morbidity (on the seventh day) and mortality up to 40 days after operation, corrected for patient and disease factors, they found a strong association between lower rates and stringency of requirements that govern the appointment of surgeons to the staff and the awarding of surgical privileges.

When the sociologic data were compared in a subsequent study with partially corrected in-hospital death rates for medical and surgical patients, these associations were no longer present (139b). In-hospital death rates have been criticized as an invalid basis for comparing performance among hospitals (140).

With respect to practitioners in office care, Freidson & Rhea (141) concluded that the assumed collegial control of performance was generally nonexistent among physicians. Technical quality of care has been reported to be higher in one group practice setting than in an independent practice setting, even when care for both groups of patients is fully prepaid (49). Donabedian has reviewed earlier literature on quality assurance and has provided a definitive formulation of key issues and principles (11a).

These principles have not been followed in the rush of the 1970s to implement various forms of quality assurance. Medical audit committees were assigned responsibility for corrective action, as in Payne's purely educational approach (24). The published models for both JCAH and PSRO begin with the steps needed to assess care and end with steps that call for corrective administrative and professional action (6, 36). The function of quality assurance is presented as an extension of the audit committee's responsibility. Abundant antecdotal and formal evidence exists that this formulation and its attempted implementation have generally failed to achieve the expected results (34, 35, 38b, 52, 63, 130, 131). One reason is that auditing, as it is generally conducted, has not identified important problems in medical care or used valid criteria, relying instead on statistical or optimal care criteria. Second, taking action to protect patients from substandard physician performance is an executive function, carried out at the level of department chairmen or the medical executive committee. Proper institutional and medical staff organization and commitment are prerequisites to effective executive action in assuring quality of care through matching of clinical privileges to objectively documented, satisfactory performance of each staff member.

In recognition of these various circumstances, JCAH has now revised its earlier requirements for a set number of outcome-oriented audits and the usual audit model, substituting a new standard on quality assurance in hospitals (142). The standard emphasizes a written plan, organization and integration of all activities that monitor quality, and documentation of effectiveness in improving patient care or clinical performance. The intended result is to return primary responsibility for quality assurance to the executive and policy levels of the staff and hospital. Medical auditing is then relegated to its proper place as one of many alternate mechanisms for evaluating important aspects of care in accord with valid criteria and standards.

A variety of modalities have been shown to be effective in promptly improving important aspects of care. One technique was simply obscuring abnormal laboratory results, thereby calling attention to their presence (43). A common denominator in many instances was a professionally acceptable form of surveillance or monitoring. The surveillance may be indirect, reflecting the expectations of a responsible or authoritative body (22, 112). More direct methods involve the use of protocols (119), use of special data forms (91, 93), computer-generated reminders (120, 121a, 121b), or direct concurrent monitoring (55, 131). These interventions serve as stimuli to the physician at the moment of providing care or making a decision regarding an individual patient. The result appears to be a more accurate or complete perception of the patient's clinical status and requirements for care, and a more effective application by the physician of his clinical knowledge. This amounts to de facto quality assurance.

SUMMARY AND RECOMMENDATIONS

This review, in summarizing the social, professional, and political circumstances that recently brought about widespread implementation of untested forms of medical auditing for purposes of quality assessment and quality assurance, points out that basic concepts and principles of quality assessment were not adequately embodied in the techniques that were adopted. The preoccupation of some investigators with untested concepts of quality rather than sound evaluation design and validity of criteria was noted in studies of relationships between care processes and outcomes. Studies of physician performance have not produced standardized methods of reliably evaluating actual performance in the care of patients. Variability in the technical quality of care is well documented. The data so far available question the effectiveness of current quality assurance mechanisms, specifically, continuing medical education and hospital-based auditing linked to continuing education. The prevalent model of medical auditing, designed to implement educational concepts rather than to protect patients from substandard care, should be discarded. Commitment and better organization of medical and hospital staff to implement needed changes in care, well-known prerequisites for effective programs of quality assurance, are receiving renewed attention.

The past decade has been an unsettling one for all participants in quality assurance. Government agencies have discovered the enormity of challenge in attempting to regulate the quality of medical care. National organizations developed and promoted methods of examining the quality of hospital care without subjecting them to formal testing and evaluation. Physicians and hospitals accepted these methods in the belief that they must work or they would not have been promoted by such prestigious organizations. Physicians generally failed to appreciate that auditing is merely one technique of evaluating medical care, and came to believe that having a medical audit committee would satisfy externally imposed requirements for quality assurance. The effect has been to replicate a much criticized practice in medical literature: publication of ideas or premature conclusions based on small, uncontrolled, or biased studies, leading to widespread application of methods that are subsequently discredited or found to be ineffective. Donabedian (143), Kessner (116a), and Komaroff (144) agree that expectations of quality assurance have exceeded present capability and urge more experimental and empirical studies. Other research agendas have been proposed (5, 11b, 13, 14, 34, 74).

The capacity for discriminating between clearly adequate and clearly inadequate medical care has existed throughout this century. The desired capability is that of reliably assessing performance of individual physicians, groups and clinics, and hospital medical staffs so that an acceptable sample of technical care and the caring functions can be compared with valid standards over time. The dynamic nature of contemporary medical care is evident in the emergence of increasingly large systems of hospitals and hospital-based care as well as systems of nonhospital-based care. Methods of quality assessment and assurance will have to be adaptable to these changing circumstances.

The achievement of these capabilities will require both research and development, as was planned in the implementation of the experimental medical care review program (58). The combination of research and development can better respond to the pressing, immediate problem of designing better approaches to quality assessment and assurance. Some of the more important agenda items include:

1. The development of efficient, professionally acceptable methods of reliably monitoring the application of efficacious medical treatment and the attainment of outcomes that have been shown to be the direct results of that treatment (13, 55, 58)
2. Further evaluation of the general applicability of the staging concept in objectively assessing technical adequacy of care in hospitals (81)
3. More extensive application of the principles and techniques of clinical decision making to the prospective evaluation of medical care given individual patients
4. Use of combined approaches to quality assessment in keeping with the principle of concurrent validation (62)
5. Systematic determination of the sampling requirements for monitoring the technical and psychosocial aspects of care of patients in hospitals
6. Development of methods of assessing the performance of medical staff members to assure with stated high probability that their performance conforms to valid standards of care for medical and surgical patients
7. Further testing the use of adjusted rates of postoperative morbidity and mortality, including that occurring after discharge, in objectively comparing the performance of surgeons in given geographic areas (69)
8. Exploration of the causes of interhospital differences in post-operative morbidity and mortality (69)
9. Evaluation of emerging models of hospital-based quality assurance, including organizational components, design of technical procedures, and relation to quality assurance responsibilities (The new JCAH standard will promote innovation and flexibility, providing an important opportunity to study a "natural" experiment.)
10. Better information on physician performance across the various diseases and conditions most prevalent in his practice
11. Refinement of methods of evaluating physician performance, in both technical and interpersonal skills, on the basis of observable patient outcomes attributable to physicians' care

12. Continued exploration of professionally acceptable methods of promoting more complete recording of basic clinical and psychosocial data in medical records
13. Better understanding of the relationship between physicians' level of knowledge and their performance
14. Further exploration of professionally acceptable methods of surveillance that elicit a higher level of performance at the physician's given level of knowledge
15. Systematic study of key factors in hospital-based and area-wide quality assurance mechanisms (5, 34).

The ultimate objective is to design methods that can maintain currency with scientific and technologic advances and be applied to the major components of medical care in all settings. The technical requirements for these methods have yet to be specified. In this period of realistic reappraisal, it is evident that both descriptive and analytic research, in parallel with research and development (145), must be more deliberately responsive to professional and societal mandates for effective systems of quality assessment and quality assurance. The medical and hospital professions, policy makers and investigators alike, must acknowledge the magnitude of the task, the time it will take to accomplish, and the amount of scientific effort it will require.

Literature Cited

1. McCleery, R. S., Keelty, L. T., Lam, M., Phillips, R. E., Quirin, T. M. 1971. *One Life—One Physician: An Inquiry into the Medical Profession's Performance in Self-Regulation.* Washington DC: Public Affairs Press. 167 pp.
2. Worthington, W., Silver, L. H. 1970. Regulation of quality of care in hospitals: The need for change. *Law Contempor. Probl.* 35:305–33
3. Derbyshire, R. C. 1969. *Medical Licensure and Discipline in the United States.* Baltimore: Johns Hopkins Press. 183 pp.
4. Ellwood, P. M., O'Donoghue, P., McClure, W., Holley, R., Carlson, R. J., Hoagberg, E. 1973. *Assuring the Quality of Health Care.* Minneapolis: Interstudy. 134 pp.
5. Institute of Medicine. 1974. *Advancing the Quality of Health Care: Key Issues and Fundamental Principles.* Washington DC: NAS. 56 pp.
6. Goran, M. J., Roberts, J. S., Kellogg, M., Fielding, J., Jessee, W. 1975. The PSRO hospital review system. *Med. Care* 13 (4):Suppl., pp. 1–33

7. Committee on Medicine in Society. 1976. Professional responsibility for the quality of health care. *Bull. NY Acad. Med.* 52:5–184
8. Egdahl, R. H., Gertman, P. M., eds. 1976. *Quality Assurance in Health Care.* Germantown, Md: Aspen Systems. 355 pp.
9. Symposium: Federal Regulation of the Health Care Delivery System. 1975. *Univ. Toledo Law Rev.* 6:577–836
10. Sanazaro, P. J., ed. 1978. *Private Initiative in Professional Standards Review Organizations (PSRO).* Ann Arbor: Health Adm. Press. 388 pp.
11a. Donabedian, A. 1969. Medical Care Appraisal: Quality and Utilization. In *A Guide to Medical Care Administration,* Vol. 2. New York: Am. Public Health Assoc., 221 pp.
11b. Donabedian, A. 1978. *Needed research in the assessment and monitoring of the quality of medical care.* Hyattsville, Md: Nat. Cent. Health Serv. Res. DHEW Publ. No. (PHS) 78–3219. 35 pp.

12. Brook, R. H. 1973. *Quality of Care Assessment: A Comparison of Five Methods of Peer Review.* Natl. Cent. Health Serv. Res. Dev. US Dep. of Health, Education, and Welfare. 343 pp.

13. Brook, R. H., Davies-Avery, A., Greenfield, S., Harris, L. J., Tova, L., Solomon, N. E., Ware, J. E. Jr. 1977. Assessing the quality of medical care using outcome measures: An overview of the method. *Med. Care* 15 (9):Suppl., pp. 1–165

14. Greene, R. ed. 1976. *Assuring Quality in Medical Care: The State of the Art.* Cambridge, Ma: Ballinger. 293 pp.

15. Williamson, J. W. 1977. *Improving Medical Practice and Health Care.* Cambridge, Ma: Ballinger. 1035 pp.

16. Ertel, P. Y., Aldridge, M. G., eds. 1977. *Medical Peer Review: Theory and Practice.* St. Louis: Mosby. 421 pp.

17. Giebink, G. A., White, N. H. 1977. *Ambulatory Medical Care Quality Assurance 1977.* La Jolla, CA: La Jolla Health Science Publ. 181 pp.

18. Codman, E. A. 1918. *A Study in Hospital Efficiency as Demonstrated by the Case Report of the First Five Years of a Private Hospital.* Boston: Thomas Todd. 179 pp.

19. Ward, G. G. 1947. Audits measure our results. *Mod. Hosp.* 69(1):86ff.

20. Ponton, T. R. 1928. Gauging the efficiency of the hospital and its staff. *Mod. Hosp.* 31(2):64–68

21. MacEachern, M. T. 1952. Examining the present status of the medical audit. *Hospitals* 26(12):49ff

22. Lembcke, P. A. 1956. Medical auditing by scientific methods: Illustrated by major female pelvic surgery. *J. Am. Med. Assoc.* 162:646–55

23. Bremer, M. A., Slee, V. N. 1977. Information systems in peer review. See Ref. 16, pp. 287–95

24. Payne, B. C. 1967. Continued evolution of a system of medical care appraisal. *J. Am. Med. Assoc.* 201:536–40

25. Payne, B. C., ed. 1968. *Hospital Utilization Review Manual.* Ann Arbor: Univ. Michigan Med. School. 112 pp.

26. Payne, B. C., Lyons, T. F., Dwarshius, L., Kolton, M., Morris, W. 1976. *The Quality of Medical Care: Evaluation and Improvement.* Chicago: Hospital Research and Educational Trust. 146 pp.

27. Payne, B. C. 1973. From performance measures to utilization review to quality assurance. In Regional Medical Programs Service, *Quality Assurance of Medical Care,* 241–60. DHEW Publ.

No. (HSM) 73–7021. Washington DC: GPO. 483 pp.

28. Payne, B. C. 1977. Research in quality assessment and utilization review in hospital and ambulatory settings. See Ref. 16, pp. 335–55

29. Eisele, C. W., Slee, V. N., Hoffman, R. G. 1956. Can the practice of internal medicine be evaluated? *Ann. Intern. Med.* 44:144–61

30. Myers, R. S. 1959. The misuse of antibacterials in inguinal herniorrhaphy. *Surg. Gynecol. Obstet.* 108:721–25

31. Institute of Medicine. 1977. *Reliability of Hospital Discharge Abstracts.* Washington DC: NAS. 113 pp.

32. Goldberg, G. A., Needleman, J., Weinstein, S. L. 1972. Medical care evaluation studies: A utilization review requirement. *J. Am. Med. Assoc.* 220: 383–87

33. Welch, C. E. 1975. PSRO: Guidelines for criteria of care. *J. Am. Med. Assoc.* 232:47–50

34. Institute of Medicine. 1976. *Assessing Quality in Health Care: An Evaluation.* Washington DC: NAS. 144 pp.

35. Escovitz, G. H., Burkett, G. L., Kuhn, J. C., Zeleznik, C., Gonnella, J. S. 1978. The effects of mandatory quality assurance: A review of hospital medical audit processes. *Med. Care* 16:941–49

36. Jacobs, C. M., Christoffel, T. H., Dixon, N. 1976. *Measuring the Quality of Patient Care: The Rationale for Outcome Audit.* Cambridge, Ma: Ballinger. 183 pp.

37. Williamson, J. W. 1971. Evaluating quality of patient care: A strategy relating outcome and process assessment. *J. Am. Med. Assoc.* 218:564–69

38a. Joint Commission on Accreditation of Hospitals. 1974. *The PEP Primer: Performance Evaluation Procedure for Auditing and Improving Patient Care.* Chicago: Joint Comm. Accreditation Hosp. 298 pp.

38b. Gertman, P. M., Monheit, A. C., Anderson, J. J., Eagle, J. B., Levenson, D. K. 1979. Utilization review in the United States: Results from a 1976–1977 national survey of hospitals. *Med. Care* 17 (8):Suppl. pp. 1–148

39. Sheps, M. C. 1955. Approaches to the quality of hospital care. *Public Health Rep.* 70:877–86

40. Donabedian, A. 1966. Evaluating the quality of medical care. *Milbank Mem. Fund Q.* 44 (3): Part 2, pp. 166–203

41. Donabedian, A. 1968. Promoting quality through evaluating the process of patient care. *Med. Care* 6:181–202

64   SANAZARO

42. Shapiro, S. 1967. End result measurements of quality of medical care. *Milbank Mem. Fund Q.* 45(2): Part 1, pp. 7–30
43. Williamson, J. W., Alexander, M., Miller, G. E. 1967. Continuing education and patient care research: Physician response to screening test results. *J. Am. Med. Assoc.* 201:938–42
44. Williamson, J. W., Alexander, M., Miller, G. E. 1968. Priorities in patient care research and continuing medical education. *J. Am. Med. Assoc.* 204: 303–8
45. Williamson, J. W., Aronovitch, S., Simonson, L., Ramirez, C., Kelly, D. 1975. Health accounting: An outcomebased system of quality assurance: Illustrative application to hypertension. *Bull. NY Acad. Med.* 51:727–38
46. Hare, R. L., Barnoon, S. 1973. *Medical Care Appraisal and Quality Assurance in the Office Practice of Internal Medicine.* San Francisco: Am. Soc. Intern. Med. 432 pp.
47. Thompson, H. C., Osborne, C. E. 1976. Office records in the evaluation of quality of care. *Med. Care* 14:294–314
48. Hulka, B. S., Kupper, L. L., Cassel, J. C. 1976. Physician management in primary care. *Am. J. Public Health* 66: 1173–78
49. LoGerfo, J. P., Efird, R. A., Diehr, P. K., Richardson, W. C. 1976. Quality of Care. In *The Seattle Prepaid Health Care Project: Comparison of Health Services Delivery,* ch. IV. Springfield, Va: Natl. Tech. Info. Service PB 267 492. 260 pp.
50. Hulka, B. S., Romm, F. J., Parkerson, G. R. Jr., Russell, I. T., Clapp, N. E., Johnson, F. S. 1979. Peer review in ambulatory care: Use of explicit criteria and implicit judgments. *Med. Care* 17 (3):Suppl. pp. 1–73
51. Riedel, R. L., Riedel, D. C. 1979. *Practice and Performance: An Assessment of Ambulatory Care.* Ann Arbor: Health Adm. Press. 306 pp.
52. Sanazaro, P. J. 1976. Medical audit, continuing medical education and quality assurance. *West. J. Med.* 125:241–52
53. Rosenfeld, L. S. 1957. Quality of medical care in hospitals. *Am. J. Public Health* 47:856–65
54. Lyons, T. F., Payne, B. C. 1974. The relationship of physicians' medical recording performance to their medical care performance. *Med. Care* 12: 463–69
55. Sanazaro, P. J., Worth, R. M. 1978.

Concurrent quality assurance. See Ref. 10, pp. 87–131
56. Fessel, W. J., Van Brunt, E. E. 1972. Assessing quality of care from the medical record. *N. Engl. J. Med.* 286:134–38
57. Zuckerman, A. E., Starfield, B., Hochreiter, C., Kovasznay, B. 1975. Validating the content of pediatric outpatient medical records by means of taperecording doctor-patient encounters. *Pediatrics* 56:407–11
58. Sanazaro, P. J., Goldstein, R. L., Roberts, J. S., Maglott, D. B., McAllister, J. W. 1972. Research and development in quality assurance: The experimental medical care review organization program. *N. Engl. J. Med.* 287:1125–31
59. Lindsay, M. I., Hermans, P. E., Nobrega, F. T., Ilstrup, D. M. 1976. Quality-of-care assessment: I. Outpatient management of acute bacterial cystitis as the model. *Mayo Clin. Proc.* 51:307–12
60a. Romm, F. J., Hulka, B. S., Mayo, F. 1976. Correlates of outcomes in patients with congestive heart failure. *Med. Care* 14:765–76
60b. Romm, F. J., Hulka, B. S. 1979. Care process and patient outcome in diabetes mellitus. *Med. Care* 17:748–57
61. Nobrega, F. T., Morrow, G. W. Jr., Smoldt, R. K. 1977. Quality assessment in hypertension: Analysis of process and outcome methods. *N. Engl. J. Med.* 296:145–48
62. McAuliffe, W. E. 1978. Studies of process-outcome correlations in medical care evaluations: A critique. *Med. Care* 16:907–30
63. Baker, T. H., Klitsner, I. N., Sadoff, C. N., Cummings, M. A., Sapin, S. O., Weil, H. M., Kovner, J. W. 1978. *Quality of Medical Care: Research in Methods of Assessment and Assurance.* Kaiser-Permanente Medical Care Program, Southern Calif. Reg. 162 pp.
64. Starfield, B., Scheff, D. 1972. Effectiveness of pediatric care: The relationship between processes and outcome. *Pediatrics* 49:547–52
65. Subcommittee on Quality of Surgery. 1976. The critical incident study of surgical deaths and complications. In *Surgery in the United States: A Summary Report of the Study on Surgical Services for the United States,* 3:2132–2282. Am. Coll. Surg. and Am. Surg. Assoc. 729 pp.
66. Sanazaro, P. J., Williamson, J. W. 1970. Physician performance and its effects on patients: A classification based on reports by internists, surgeons, pediatri-

cians, and obstetricians. *Med. Care* 8:299–308

67. Davies-Avery, A., Lelah, T., Solomon, N. E., Harris, L. J., Brook, R. H., Greenfield, S., Ware, J. E. Jr., Avery, C. H. 1976. *Quality of Medical Care Assessment Using Outcome Measures: Eight Disease-Specific Applications.* Santa Monica, Ca: Rand Corporation. 758 pp.

68. Starfield, B. 1974. Measurement of outcome: A proposed scheme. *Milbank Mem. Fund Q.* 52(3):39–50

69. Stanford Center for Health Care Research. 1976. Comparison of hospitals with regard to outcomes of surgery. *Health Serv. Res.* 11:112–27

70. Moses, L. E., Mosteller, F. 1968. Institutional differences in postoperative death rates: Commentary on some of the findings of the National Halothane Study. *J. Am. Med. Assoc.* 203:492–94

71. Williamson, J. W. 1978. *Assessing and Improving Health Care Outcomes: The Health Accounting Approach to Quality Assurance.* Cambridge, Ma: Ballinger. 327 pp.

72a. Christoffel, T., Loewenthal, M. 1977. Evaluating the quality of ambulatory health care: A review of emerging methods. *Med. Care* 15:877–97

72b. Shortridge, M. H. 1974. Quality of medical care in an outpatient setting. *Med. Care* 12:283–300

73. Mushlin, A. I., Appel, F. A., Barr, D. M. 1978. Quality assurance in primary care: A strategy based on outcome assessment. *J. Community Health* 3:292–305

74. Ware, J. E. Jr., Davies-Avery, A., Stewart, A. L. 1978. The measurement and meaning of patient satisfaction. *Health and Med. Care Serv. Rev.* 1 (1):1–15

75. Ehrlich, J., Morehead, M. A., Trussell, R. E. 1962. *The Quantity, Quality and Costs of Medical and Hospital Care Secured by a Sample of Teamster Families in the New York Area.* New York: Columbia Univ. School of Public Health and Adm. Med. 83 pp.

76. Colcher, I. S., Bass, J. W. 1972. Penicillin treatment of strepococcal pharyngitis: A comparison of schedules and the role of specific counseling. *J. Am. Med. Assoc.* 222:657–59

77. Inui, T. S., Yourtee, E. L., Williamson, J. W. 1976. Improved outcomes in hypertension after physician tutorials: A controlled trial. *Ann. Intern. Med.* 84:646–51

78. Levine, D. M., Green, L. W., Deeds, S. G., Chwalow, J., Russell, R. P., Finlay, J. 1979. Health education for hypertensive patients. *J. Am. Med. Assoc.* 241:1700–3

79. Williams, T. F., Martin, D. A., Hogan, M. D., Watkins, J. D., Ellis, E. V. 1967. The clinical picture of diabetic control, studied in four settings. *Am. J. Public Health* 57:441–51

80. Hulka, B. S., Kupper, L. L., Cassel, J. C., Mayo, F. 1975. Doctor-patient communication and outcomes among diabetic patients. *J. Community Health* 1:15–27

81. Gonnella, J. S., Goran, M. J. 1975. Quality of patient care—a measurement of change: The staging concept. *Med. Care* 13:467–73

82. Gonnella, J. S., Cattani, J. A., Louis, D. Z., McCord, J. J., Spirka, C. S. 1977. Use of outcome measures in ambulatory care evaluation. See Ref. 17, pp. 91–125

83. Kessner, D. M., Kalk, C. E., Singer, J. 1973. Assessing health quality: The case for tracers. *N. Engl. J. Med.* 288:189–94

84. Peterson, O. L. 1963. Medical care: Its social and organizational aspects: Evaluation of the quality of medical care. *N. Engl. J. Med.* 269:1238–45

85. Sox, H. C., Sox, C. H., Tompkins, R. K. 1973. The training of physician's assistants: The use of a clinical algorithm system for patient care, audit of performance and education. *N. Engl. J. Med.* 288:818–24

86. Komaroff, A. L., Flatley, M., Knopp, R. H., Reiffen, B., Sherman, H. 1974. Protocols for physician assistants: Management of diabetes and hypertension. *N. Engl. J. Med.* 290:307–12

87. Greenfield, S., Anderson, H., Winickoff, R. N., Morgan, A., Komaroff, A. L. 1975. Nurse-protocol management of lowback pain: Outcomes, patient satisfaction and efficiency of primary care. *West. J. Med.* 123:350–59

88. Komaroff, A. L., Pass, T. M., McCue, J. D., Cohen, A. B., Hendricks, T. M., Friedland, G. 1978. Management strategies for urinary and vaginal infections. *Arch. Intern. Med.* 138:1069–73

89. McNeil, B. J., Keeler, E., Adelstein, S. J. 1975. Primer on certain elements of medical decision making. *N. Engl. J. Med.* 293:211–15

90. Pauker, S. G., Kassirer, J. P. 1975. Therapeutic decision making: A cost-benefit analysis. *N. Engl. J. Med.* 293:229–34

91. Frazier, S. H., Brand, D. A. 1979. Quality assessment and the art of medicine:

The anatomy of laceration care. *Med. Care* 17:480–90

92. Leaper, D. J., Horrocks, J. C., Staniland, J. R., de Dombal, F. T. 1972. Computer-assisted diagnosis of abdominal pain using "estimates" provided by clinicians. *Br. Med. J.* 4:350–54

93. de Dombal, F. T., Leaper, D. J., Horrocks, J. C., Staniland, J. R., McCann, A. P. 1974. Human and computer-aided diagnosis of abdominal pain: Further report with emphasis on performance of clinicians. *Br. Med. J.* 1:376–80

94. Greenfield, S., Lewis, C. E., Kaplan, S. H., Davidson, M. B. 1975. Peer review by criteria mapping: Criteria for diabetes mellitus: The use of decision-making in chart audit. *Ann. Intern. Med.* 83:761–70

95. Barro, A. R. 1973. Survey and evaluation of approaches to physician performance measurement. *J. Med. Educ.* 48(11):Suppl., pp. 1051–93

96. Sanazaro, P. J., Williamson, J. W. 1968. End results of patient care: A provisional classification based on reports by internists. *Med. Care* 6:123–30

97. American Academy of Pediatrics, Inc. 1974. *Foundations for Evaluating the Competency of Pediatricians.* Chicago: Am. Acad. Pediatr. 91 pp.

98. Committee on Evaluation in General Internal Medicine 1979. Clinical competence in internal medicine. *Ann. Intern. Med.* 90:402–11

99. Price, P. B., Taylor, C. W., Nelson, D. E., Lewis, E. G., Loughmiller, G. C., Mathiesen, R., Murray, S. L., Maxwell, J. G. 1971. Measurement and Predictors of Physician Performance: Two Decades of Intermittently Sustained Research. Salt Lake City: LLR Press. 166 pp.

100. Peterson, O. L., Andrews, L. P., Spain, R. S., Greenberg, B. G. 1956. An analytical study of North Carolina general practice: 1953–1954. *J. Med. Educ.* 31(12):Part 2, pp. 1–165

101. Morehead, M. A., Donaldson, R. S., Sanderson, S., Burt, F. E. 1964. *A Study of the Quality of Hospital Care Secured by a Sample of Teamster Family Members in New York City.* New York: Columbia Univ. School of Public Health and Adm. Med. 98 pp.

102a. Morehead, M. A. 1967. The medical audit as an operational tool. *Am. J. Public Health* 57:1643–56

102b. Morehead, M. A., Donaldson, R. 1974. Quality of clinical management of disease in comprehensive neighborhood health centers. *Med. Care.* 12:301–15

103. Richardson, F. M. 1972. Peer review of medical care. *Med. Care* 10:29–39

104. Koran, L. M. 1975. The reliability of clinical methods, data and judgments. *N. Engl. J. Med.* 293:642–46, 695–701

105a. Peters, E. N. 1972. Practical versus impractical peer review. *Med. Care* 10:516–21

105b. Starfield, B., Steinwachs, D., Morris, I., Bause, G., Siebert, S., Westin, C. 1979. Concordance between medical records and observations on coordination of care. *Med. Care* 17:758–66

106. Wagner, E. H., Greenberg, R. A., Imrey, P. B., Williams, C. A., Wolf, S. H., Ibrahim, M. A. 1976. Influence of training and experience on selecting criteria to evaluate medical care. *N. Engl. J. Med.* 294:871–76

107. Report of the Joint National Committee on Detection, Evaluation, and Treatment of High Blood Pressure: A cooperative study. 1977. *J. Am. Med. Assoc.* 237:255–61

108. Veterans Administration Ad Hoc Interdisciplinary Advisory Committee on Antimicrobial Drug Usage 1977. Guidelines for peer review. *J. Am. Med. Assoc.* 237:1001–2

109a. McAuliffe, W. E. 1978. On the statistical validity of standards used in profile monitoring. *Am. J. Public Health* 68:645–51

109b. Sanazaro, P. J., Williamson, J. W. 1968. End results of patient care: A provisional classification based on reports by internists. *Med Care* 6:123–30

110. Schlicke, C. P. 1973. American surgery's noblest experiment. *Arch. Surg. Chicago* 106:379–85

111. Doyle, J. C. 1953. Unnecessary hysterectomies: Study of 6,248 operations in thirty-five hospitals during 1948. *J. Am. Med. Assoc.* 151:360–65

112. Dyck, F. J., Murphy, F. A., Murphy, J. K., Road, D. A., Boyd, M. S., Osborne, E., deVlieger, D., Korschinski, B., Ripley, C., Bromley, A. T., Innes, P. B. 1977. Effect of surveillance on the number of hysterectomies in the Province of Saskatchewan. *N. Engl. J. Med.* 296:1326–28

113. Fine, J., Morehead, M. A. 1971. Study of peer review of inhospital patient care. *NY State J. Med.* 71:1963–73

114. Sparling, J. F. 1962. Measuring medical care quality: A comparative study. *Hospitals* 36:62ff.

115. Lewis, C. E. 1969. Variations in the incidence of surgery. *N. Engl. J. Med.* 281:880–84

116a. Kessner, D. M. 1978. Quality assessment and assurance: Early signs of cognitive dissonance. *N. Engl. J. Med.* 298:381–86

116b. Palmer, R. H., Reilly, M. C. 1979. Individual and institutional variables which may serve as indicators of quality of medical care. *Med. Care* 17:693–717

117. Garland, L. H. 1960. The problem of observer error. *Bull. NY Acad. Med.* 36:570–84

118. Stapleton, J. F., Zwerneman, J. A. 1965. The influence of an intern-resident staff on the quality of private patient care. *J. Am. Med. Assoc.* 194:877–82

119. Grimm, R. H. Jr., Shimoni, K., Harlan, W. R. Jr. 1975. Evaluation of patient-care protocol use by various providers. *N. Engl. J. Med.* 292:507–11

120. McDonald, C. J. 1976. Protocol-based computer reminders, the quality of care, and the non-perfectability of man. *N. Engl. J. Med.* 295:1351–55

121a. Johns, C. J., Simborg, D. W., Blum, B. I., Starfield, B. H. 1977. A minirecord: An aid to continuity of care. *Johns Hopkins Med. J.* 140:277–84

121b. Barnett, G. O. 1976. *Computer-stored ambulatory record (COSTAR).* NCHSR Res. Dig. Ser., Washington DC: DHEW Publ. No. (HRA) 76–3145. 40 pp.

122. Brown, C. R. Jr., Uhl, H. S. M. 1970. Mandatory continuing education: Sense or nonsense? *J. Am. Med. Assoc.* 213:1660–68

123. Gonnella, J. S., Goran, M. J., Williamson, J. W., Cotsonas, N. J. Jr. 1970. Evaluation of patient care: An approach. *J. Am. Med. Assoc.* 214:2040–43

124. Lyons, T. F., Payne, B. C. 1974. Interdiagnosis relationships of physician performance measures. *Med. Care* 12:369–74

125. Brodman, K., van Woerkom, A. J. 1966. Computer-aided diagnostic screening for 100 common diseases. *J. Am. Med. Assoc.* 197:901–5

126. Leaper, D. J., Gill, P. W., Staniland, J. R., Horrocks, J. C., de Dombal, F. T. 1973. Clinical diagnostic process: An analysis. *Br. Med. J.* 3:569–74

127. Symposium on Continuing Medical Education 1975. *Bull. NY Acad. Med.* 51:701–88

128. Egdahl, R. H., Gertman, P. M., eds. 1977. *Quality Health Care: The Role of Continuing Medical Education.* Germantown, Md: Aspen Systems. 245 pp.

129a. Bertram, D. A., Brooks-Bertram, P. A. 1977. The evaluation of continuing medical education: A literature review. *Health Educ. Monograph* 5:330–62

129b. Lloyd, J. S., Abrahamson, S. 1979. Effectiveness of continuing medical education: A review of the evidence. *Eval. Health Prof.* 2:251–80

130. Cayten, C. G., Tanner, L. A., Riedel, D. C., Williams, K. H. Jr. 1974. Surgical audit using predetermined weighted criteria. *Conn. Med.* 38:117–22

131. Nelson, A. R. 1976. Orphan data and the unclosed loop: A dilemma in PSRO and medical audit. *N. Engl. J. Med.* 295:617–19

132. Brook, R. H., Williams, K. N. 1976. Evaluation of the New Mexico Peer Review System 1971–73. *Med. Care* 14(12): Suppl., pp. 1–122

133. Sanazaro, P. J., Worth, R. M. 1978. Concurrent quality assurance in hospital care. *N. Engl. J. Med.* 298:1171–77

134. Office of Policy, Planning and Research, Health Care Financing Administration 1979. Section 5. Quality assurance activities: Medical care evaluation studies. In *Professional Standards Review Organization 1978 Program Evaluation,* pp. 182–229. Washington DC: H.E.W. Publ. No. HCFA-0300. 309 pp.

135. Makover, H. B. 1951. The quality of medical care: Methodological survey of the medical groups associated with the Health Insurance Plan of New York. *Am. J. Public Health* 41:824–32

136. Colwell, A. R. Sr., Fenn, G. K. 1959. Standards of practice of internal medicine: Methods of judging its quality in hospitals. *Ann. Intern. Med.* 51:821–32

137. Roemer, M. I., Friedman, J. W. 1971. *Doctors in Hospitals: Medical Staff Organization and Hospital Performance,* pp. 281–82. Baltimore & London: Johns Hopkins Press. 322 pp.

138. Shortell, S. M., Becker, S. W., Neuhauser, D. 1976. The effects of management practices on hospital efficiency and quality of care. In *Organizational Research in Hospitals,* ed. M. Brown, S. M. Shortell, pp. 90–107. Chicago: Blue Cross Assoc. 112 pp.

139a. Scott, W. R., Flood, A. B. 1978. Professional power and professional effectiveness: The power of the surgical staff and the quality of surgical care in hospitals. *J. Health Soc. Behav.* 19:240–54

139b. Scott, W. R., Flood, A. B., Ewy, W. 1979. Organizational determinants of services, quality, and cost of care in hospitals. *Milbank Mem. Fund Q.* 57:234–64

140. Goss, M. E. W., Reed, J. I. 1974. Evaluating the quality of hospital care

through severity-adjusted death rates: Some pitfalls. *Med. Care* 12:202–13

141. Freidson, E., Rhea, B. 1963. Processes of control in a company of equals. *Soc. Problems* 11:119–31

142. Joint Commission on Accreditation of Hospitals 1979. New JCAH quality assurance standard for hospitals. *Perspectives on Accreditation* 3:1–9

143. Donabedian, A. 1977. Evaluating the quality of medical care. See Ref. 16, pp. 50–73

144. Komaroff, A. L. 1978. The PSRO, quality-assurance blues. *N. Engl. J. Med.* 298:1194–96

145. Sanazaro, P. J. 1973. Federal health services R & D under the auspices of the National Center for Health Services Research and Development. In *Health Services Research and R & D in Perspective,* ed. E. F. Flook, P. J. Sanazaro, pp. 150–183. Ann Arbor: Health Admin. Press. 311 pp.

Ann. Rev. Public Health 1980. 1:69–82

TO ADVANCE EPIDEMIOLOGY ❖12502

Reuel A. Stallones

School of Public Health, University of Texas, Houston, Texas 77025

INTRODUCTION

This discussion is specific to epidemiology. That is, it neither presents recent advances in our knowledge of coronary heart disease or Bolivian hemorrhagic fever, nor does it deal directly with strategies for matching in case/comparison studies. I have, instead, chosen to comment on a few very general matters that I believe to be important in the development of epidemiological theory and in advancing epidemiological practice. The time is propitious for these reflections. In 1976, swine influenza, Legionnaire's disease, and Guillain-Barre syndrome generated a glare of publicity, which our field had not seen since 1954; epidemiological rules for living have been formulated and rather more widely disseminated than adopted; and the recently departed Secretary of Health, Education, and Welfare mentioned epidemiology in an extraordinary proportion of his public addresses.

Prior to 1940, those epidemiologists with a penchant for generalization wrote almost entirely about infectious disease phenomena. Frost sought to discover and codify the laws that governed epidemics (1, 2), and others studied such factors as season (3) and age (4) as general determinants of the frequency of infections. In the 1950s and 1960s, the rapid growth of epidemiological studies of noninfectious conditions was accompanied by a preoccupation with methods and uses of epidemiology (5, 6). During this time, the conceptual basis of retrospective and prospective study designs was clarified (7–10) and statistical methods were tested and refined, coincident with the explosive growth of computer resources that permitted expansion by orders of magnitude of the volume of data that could be processed within even our modest budgets.

Two threads can be traced in the 1970s:

1. A continuing concern for methods, and especially the dissection of risk assessment, that would do credit to a Talmudic scholar and that threat-

69

0163-7525/80/0510-0069$01.00

ens at times to bury all that is good and beautiful in epidemiology under an avalanche of mathematical trivia and neologisms.
2. Increasing interest in the nature of epidemiology, its rational foundations, and its history.

In this chapter, the latter set of concerns is divided, somewhat arbitrarily, into four interrelated topics: the territory of epidemiology, concepts of causation, classification of disease, and epidemiological theory.

THE TERRITORY OF EPIDEMIOLOGY

A useful way to characterize biomedical research is to locate disciplines along a scale of biological organization (Figure 1). Although the scale is a continuum, the research emphases tend to be discontinuous, and, with increasing specialization, the tendency toward fragmentation is enhanced. Knowledge of the molecular basis of disease has contributed little to disease prevention, but neither does knowledge of the patterns of diseases in communities contribute to advances in therapeutics. Nevertheless, the spectrum of biomedical research efforts stretches along a continuum, which should be an integrating force, not a divisive one, and ultimately the knowledge accrued by different subspecialities must all fit together without internal contradictions. The focus of integration is the individual, and the totality of biomedical research should be coherent, with different disciplines sustaining and supporting each other.

Epidemiologists have aired publicly a concern for definitions of their field, which is unusual among the biomedical disciplines and which is, at times, curiously defensive. In 1942 an editorial entitled "What and who is an epidemiologist?" appeared in the *American Journal of Public Health* and elicited a spate of responses (11). Bolduan's statement that "the epidemiologist should, of course, be a physician and have had training in laboratory work and statistical methods" (12) expressed the modal view, although

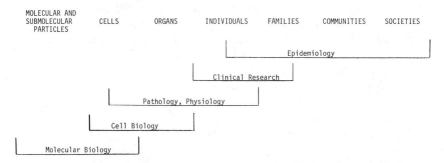

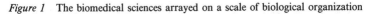

Figure 1   The biomedical sciences arrayed on a scale of biological organization

Lumsden's injunction that "he avoids needless or obfuscating high mathematics and formulae" (13) echoed the opinion of several that the epidemiologist should not be so adept in statistics as to do harm to himself. Not surprisingly, the respondents were thinking almost solely of people working with infectious diseases, although by 1942 the handwriting on the wall should have been plain enough. The proportion of the respondents we would today recognize as epidemiologists is no higher than that in a current roster of the American Epidemiological Society. Although all textbooks and a regrettably high proportion of articles in the field begin with a definition of epidemiology, little more was published on definitions specifically until some comments by Terris (14) in 1962 evoked responses of greater or lesser (15) profundity. In 1978, an article by David Lilienfeld (16) stimulated another modest outpouring of ruminations (17–19). The plainest conclusion to be drawn from them is that the length of the definition is inversely related to the age of the epidemiologist. The territory of epidemiology, insofar as it is defined by the dissection of definitions (16, 20), is presently generally agreed to be the concern for the occurrence of disease (and, by inference, health) in groups of people. The unfortunate use of the term epidemiology for a gaggle of peripheral activities has been supplanted by the more popular perversion of the term ecology. Because epidemiology is very properly a subset of the field of human ecology, we may not have gained much, but the respite is welcome.

The most significant feature of the history of human disease in the twentieth century has been the rapid decline of most infections in urban, industrial societies, and the concomitant increase in importance of noninfectious conditions. By mid-century, as epidemiologists began to concern themselves increasingly with noninfectious diseases, an unfortunate schism developed, based on the presumption that a new kind of epidemiology had been created, based on the principle of multifactorial causation, based on misperception (21). Gradually an ecumenical tolerance has developed and, though the rift may not be healed, the monistic nature of the central core of epidemiology seems to be more widely accepted than it was a couple of decades ago. The denial of that nature makes no sense in a world in which kuru and Lassa fever, and possibly some cancers, are due to infections. Whatever lingering doubt may persist over this issue should have been laid to rest by Barrett-Connor's trenchant contribution (22).

I embrace as a matter of faith that only one epidemiology exists. However, I believe that three significant classes of applications of epidemiology can be identified. The same tool can be employed in different ways, more or less successfully, as in using the small blade of a pocket knife to take out a screw, lance a blister, clip an item from a newspaper, or carve a sacred image.

The Epidemiology of Specific Diseases

The vast majority of epidemiological research has been devoted to studies of diseases taken one at a time. Students in epidemiology are commonly advised that the first step in the investigation of an outbreak is to confirm the diagnosis, and most epidemiologists pursue single diseases with the determination of a well trained bloodhound following a singular scent through a sea of enticing odors. The successes of the past are ample evidence that this approach is more meritorious than meretricious and, with no shortage of interesting and unresolved problems, most epidemiological effort will continue to be expended on studies of specific diseases.

Evaluation of Medical Care

THE EVALUATION OF PROGRAMS AND SYSTEMS   Health services research is a misnomer for the evaluation of medical care systems and programs, which deal almost exclusively with the treatment of sick people rather than with health. Gradually, an appreciation has grown that medical care programs, agencies, and systems should be evaluated by what they accomplish rather than by what they do, and accomplishments in medical care must have something to do with the health and disease status of clients, subscribers, and communities, thus placing the evaluation firmly in the camp of epidemiology. Two conferences (at least) have been devoted to this: one, a meeting of the International Epidemiological Society in Primosten in 1971 (23), and one sponsored by the Health Resources Agency of the Department of Health, Education, and Welfare in 1975 (24). In addition, Henderson (25) has argued persuasively for recognition of the utility of epidemiology in this arena, but the argument at this time is based more on promise than on solid accomplishment.

THE EVALUATION OF THERAPIES   *Controlled trials*   The most powerful means to evaluate therapy is the random allocation, double-blind, clinical trial. When a preventive measure is studied, the research seems clearly to qualify as experimental epidemiology, but the evaluation of a new drug for the treatment of existing disease is a direct application of statistical experimental design in clinical practice. Often enough, the epidemiologist's role in this is to serve as interpreter in the dialogue between statistician and clinician.

Quantitative medicine   So many constraints surround the conduct of controlled trials that most therapeutic modalities have not been and will not be assessed by the most rigorous methods available. An alternative is to apply epidemiological precepts in a systems analytic approach to the evaluation of treatment without intervening in an experimental way.

Ecologically Based Epidemiology

No necessary requirement exists that epidemiological studies must begin with a defined disease. Walter Rogan (casual communication) has suggested that some aspects of epidemiological research are better pursued by first defining an environmental exposure and studying the effects on health that arise from it. This is a close analogue of the strategy adopted by academician Pavlovskii (26) for the control of infectious diseases in opening for settlement new territories in the USSR. The concept of an ecologically oriented epidemiological approach is only a short additional step along this path. To pursue these researches, we must characterize communities simultaneously by both physical and social circumstances (Darwin Labarthe, in a casual communication has proposed the term *demotype* for the latter classification), measure individual traits, and relate all of these not just to single diseases, but to the overall morbidity and mortality patterns of the communities (27).

CONCEPTS OF CAUSATION

Epidemiological research on infectious diseases deals extensively with social and physical environmental phenomena and a large assortment of individual traits, but the presence of a microbiological agent in the equation, retrievable on culture or leaving tracks of its passage in the serum of infected persons, provides a base of reference against which the importance of other variables can be validated. Without an etiological checkpoint, epidemiologists working with the major noninfectious diseases began seriously to consider definitions of causation that extended beyond the concept of specific etiology (28, 8).

As a biological phenomenon, disease in an individual may be expected to have biologically understandable causes. Even where social factors impinge on a person so as to contribute to his illness, we usually believe there is a conversion of the stress into some physiological or biochemical strain (29). On the other hand, a community is a social organization; thus, the distribution of disease in communities is a social phenomenon, and as such may be expected to have social causes. Cause must therefore be understood to operate in two modes: in one case to produce the illness of an individual, and in the other, to produce the pattern of illness in a population.

The expanded view of causation of disease holds that the antecedents of illness are many and that they are interrelated in complex ways. Perhaps an etiologic factor can be identified as a necessary cause and perhaps not;

in either case, risk of disease can be altered by intervention at multiple entry points. Further, some intervention strategies that may not relate directly to specific etiologic factors can be more effective than some that do; indeed, effective disease control is quite feasible without detailed knowledge of those specific etiologies.

The evolution of epidemiological thought has proceeded from very general to very specific concepts, and we are now beginning to reexplore some of the more general concepts.

Unfavorable Environment Causes Disease

The widely accepted interpretation of the writings of Hippocrates, that unfavorable environment causes disease, had little utility. The unfavorable environment was often conceived of in cosmic, astrological, or theological terms, which did not readily lead to effective disease prevention. In the eighteenth and nineteenth centuries, the unfavorable environments were visibly and olfactorily evident as miasmata and effluvia. Regrettably, the concept was applied inappropriately to explain yellow fever and cholera, and it lost all credibility as the microbiological advances provided appropriate explanations. Now, more than a hundred years later, the miasmata and effluvia of urban and industrial environments are again being invoked as environmental causes of disease.

Specific Environmental Hazards Cause Specific Diseases

Ramazzini was perhaps the earliest, most renowned expositor of the principle of specificity in unfavorable environments in workplaces. This construct was fully robust and is fully applicable today.

Specific Microorganisms Cause Specific Diseases

The microbiological era produced such powerful techniques and such powerful ideas that other concepts were, for a time, almost entirely discarded. However, epidemiologists working with infectious diseases learned early that differing disease frequencies could not be explained solely by variations in exposure to an etiological agent, and that differences in susceptibility were an equally important component. The recognition that physical and social environmental factors affect the specific etiological agents, the likelihood of exposure, and the degree of susceptibility of exposed persons destroyed any notion that the distribution of disease in a population could be accounted for by a simple one agent, one disease model.

The Web of Causation

As elegantly propounded by MacMahon et al (30), the antecedents of disease are conceived as arrayed in complex, interacting series, with or without a final common pathway or specifically definable etiological agent. This formulation was virtually imposed by the conduct of epidemiological research on diseases for which no specific etiological agent was known. Data derived from these studies revealed clusters of variables more or less strongly associated with a disease and more or less associated with each other, and frequently the biological structure did not provide a useful guide as to how they should be ordered. The struggle to sort this out has been carefully traced by Evans (31) from the difficulties faced by the bacteriologists in the late 1800s, through the "virologist's dilemma," to the wailing wall of chronic disease research. A number of people have proposed criteria for judging the causal significance of characteristics associated with disease (28, 32–34), and the debate continues (35, 36). Partly because our biological underpinnings are insecure, some have sought truth through analysis (mathematical, not Freudian), a violation of the Ashley-Perry Statistical Axiom Number 5.[1] The problem is clear, and clearly will not be resolved easily: the most complicated models are simplistic by comparison with the social and biological realities, and the judgments required are too subtle to be reduced to a set of rules or a mathematical expression.

Regression of Disease on Multiple Variables

Analysis of data on the relation of coronary heart disease to a number of characteristics of the study subjects by Truitt et al (38) marked the beginning of a rapid increase in the use of multiple regression models in epidemiology.

This approach may be considered to be a logical mathematical formulation of the web of causation concept. Without question, these kinds of analysis have been of great value in helping epidemiologists to bring a semblance of order to messy heaps of data. However, the limitations of the model are severe:

1. The equations explain variance in the dependent variable. The temptation to interpret an explanation of variance as an explanation of the disease is difficult to resist, has not always been resisted, and may sometimes lead to grievous error.
2. The equations accept very well the measured characteristics of individuals as independent variables. However, linking environmental and social variables with individual characteristics is difficult and this model does not help. Therefore, the mathematical expression incorporates only a fraction of the information available for a disease.

[1]"The product of an arithmetical computation is the answer to an equation; it is not the solution to a problem" (37).

3. The model implies that when blood pressure, serum cholesterol, and cigarette smoking are found to be associated with coronary heart disease, a deficit of one of these may be compensated for by adding some defined amount more of either of the others. Somehow, this does not make biological sense.

Constellation of Causes and Effects

Whatever constructs we may devise must be understood to represent our biased views of what a representation of reality should be. Because it is not the reality, the value of the model depends upon its utility, and utility depends upon the purpose for which the model is used. Rothman has spoken of a constellation of component causes (35), but I think his concept is closely akin to the web of causation model, in which the causes converge upon an effect. If the purpose is more global than studying one disease at a time, then the multiple regression/web of causation model is inadequate. An approach that holds promise is to consider the interdependence of a number of diseases, characteristics of individuals, and environmental and social variables as elements in a constellation which is n-dimensional, and within which directed pathways are incidental to the complex as a whole (27).

CLASSIFICATION OF DISEASE

Len Syme once said to me, "The trouble with you epidemiologists is that too many of you are doctors." If we understand that in his sociologically imprecise way he meant physicians when he said doctors, the implication of his statement is that physicians have been conditioned to think in certain channels and this may stifle creativity. The extensive training, the intense programming, and the incidental education that comprise curricula in medicine leave us deeply imprinted and reluctant to accept that most biomedical research is irrelevant to the solution of community health problems. We are equally disinclined to recognize that our discipline has little contribution to make to unraveling the mysteries of disease progression.

One effect of this conditioning is that in the conduct of epidemiological research, we have tended to cling to a system of disease classification (39) that was developed by and for practitioners of clinical medicine, which, although it is strongly oriented toward etiologic doctrines, does not take account of the social and environmental causes of disease distributions. A second-order classification scheme has long been in use in infectious disease epidemiology that has utility in relation to disease prevention, although this use is rarely presented explicitly as the justification for the system. In this scheme, diseases are grouped according to portal of entry, portal of exit, and mode of transmission. For teaching purposes, I have used a general illustration of these ideas, as shown in Figure 2. In this formulation, an etiologically defined entity, such as hepatitis A, is represented in several epidemiologic rubrics—water-borne, food-borne, and perhaps a respiratory disease acquired by inhalation. This may be anathema to a microbiologist or a clinican, but clearly a preoccupation with preventive approaches established a requirement for this kind of grouping.

John Cassel and I discussed casually over many years the attractiveness of treating noninfectious diseases in an analogous fashion. We may think, for example, of diseases of modern industrial societies, diseases that accompany certain kinds of mental or emotional stress, or diseases that follow sensory overload. Just as purification of water may reduce the frequency of a number of water-borne diseases of diverse etiology, so also preventive measures based on an epidemiological classification of noninfectious disease may have nonspecific beneficial effects crossing over standard classification rubrics. To use such a classification, we must ignore or at least put in a subordinate position such cherished concepts as classification by organ system or by underlying pathologic process.

Clinical definitions of disease, as represented in the *International Classification of Diseases* (ICD), have been presented so authoritatively that questioning them borders on heresy. However, a review of the changes that have occurred in the classification system since 1900 is a positive inducement to become a heretic. Long ago, Roy Acheson (40) proposed that the epidemiologic characteristics of angina pectoris, especially the sex ratio, set it apart from other manifestations of ischemic heart disease, and I have stated (27) that ischemic heart disease must be a complex of at least three entities in order for the epidemiological data to make sense. The eighth revision of the ICD has sorted ischemic heart disease mortality into two major categories, acute myocardial infarction and chronic ischemic heart disease. Since 1968, these two rubrics show distinctly different time trends and age/sex distributions. The point is clearly established that epidemiological characteristics provide a basis for grouping and differentiating diseases that is supplementary to and as valid as those derived from pathology and clinical medicine.

EPIDEMIOLOGICAL THEORY

Although a more appropriate classification scheme represents a genuinely epidemiologic approach to a more advanced stage of generalization than is represented by accumulation of disease-specific data, it still does not constitute epidemiologic theory applicable to the field as a whole.

One of the genuinely perceptive statements about epidemiology was that of Wade Hampton Frost in his introduction to *Snow on Cholera* (41).

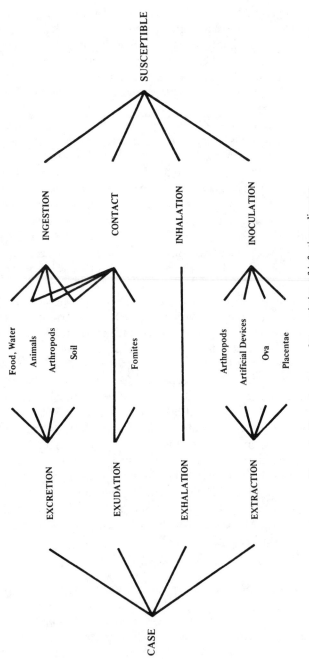

Figure 2   General scheme of transmission of infectious diseases.

Epidemiology at any given time is more than simply the accumulation of facts. It includes their arrangement into orderly chains of inference which extend more or less beyond the bounds of direct observation. Such of these chains as are well and truly laid guide investigation to the facts of the future; those that are ill made fetter progress.

By implication, the arrangement of facts into orderly chains of inference connotes the development of epidemiological theory. Even Frost, however, with his profound appreciation for and insight into the field, was inclined to limit his theorizing to specific infectious disease entities and viewed with suspicion the notion that epidemiology had utility in understanding noninfectious diseases (42). In a World Health Organization (WHO) monograph on mental illness, Donald Reid (43) presented some very general epidemiological concepts with charming lucidity. Nevertheless, epidemiologists generally have been empiricists, not theoreticians, and a quick check of the indices of four recent textbooks in epidemiology showed that not one had an index entry under "Theory." Theorizing has been designated speculation, derogated and discouraged; thus, our information stores are disorderly piles of often unrelated observations classified mostly by disease according to a system of classification that was designed for diagnostic or therapeutic rather than preventive purposes.

The names of several renowned philosophers of science have cropped up in recent writings on epidemiology (44–47). Because the philosophy of science seems largely devoted to attempts to rationalize what scientists have done and how they did it, it is, in epidemiological terms, a retrospective rather than a prospective study, with the limitations on inference that those terms imply. However, that we have colleagues reading in the philosophy of science is heart-warming, and that we have colleagues who are willing to assume "that epidemiology is a fully-fledged science" (47) is exhilarating. This kind of introspection may serve as an antidote to the excessive pragmatism that has marked our field.

One scientific discipline is distinguished from another by three components: the body of knowledge accumulated by the discipline, the methods of study whereby this knowledge was collected, and the theory guiding its collection. Neither the body of knowledge nor the methods are necessarily unique to a discipline, for knowledge referable to one field may be assembled from a variety of disciplines, and methods may have broad applicability. Theory, however, is more likely to be unique, and thus is the most distinctive feature of a discipline.

Knowledge is fluid, comprised of facts that are added and deleted continually as new truths are discovered and old truths are shown to be untrue. Methods change, but less readily, and once a method is found useful it will serve to uncover many facts. Theory changes least rapidly. Indeed, the stability of a theory is a measure of its success. The volume of these components of a discipline is also sharply ordered; few theories control many methods, the application of which may generate enormous numbers of bits of information.

I believe that we have a central axiom, not subject to proof, but upon which epidemiology is based, and without which no epidemiology is possible.

Axiom: Disease does not distribute randomly in human populations.
Corollary 1: Nonrandom aggregations of human disease are manifested along axes of measurement of time, of space, of individual personal characteristics, and of certain community characteristics.
Corollary 2: Variations in the frequency of human disease occur in response to variations in the intensity of exposure to etiologic agents or other more remote causes, or to variations in the susceptibility of individuals to the operation of those causes.

Unlike content statements, these statements appear to be substantially invariant. Unlike methods, they are peculiarly and uniquely referable to epidemiology, they are not limited to any special kind of epidemiology, and therefore they meet the qualifications for certification as bona fide epidemiologic theories.

If epidemiologic research has inescapably been based on the central axiom and has been possible only because the axiom has prevailed, the value of stating it explicitly may be questioned. The value rests in constructing a framework into which theories borrowed from biological, mathematical, physical, and behavioral sciences can be fitted while still allowing us to recognize that which is uniquely epidemiological.

SUMMARY

Epidemiology represents the recognition that the patterns of occurrence of disease and disability in human communities are determined by forces that can be identified and measured, that these forces include but are not limited to medical concepts of etiology, and that modification of these forces is the most effective way to prevent disease. This establishes a territory of especial beauty at the intersection of the biomedical and social sciences—a subset of human ecology which is especially focussed on human health and disease. To advance our field we need to extend further our explorations of epidemiological theory.

Literature Cited

1. Frost, W. H. 1976. Some conceptions of epidemics in general. *Am. J. Epidemiol.* 103:141–51
2. Sartwell, P. E. 1976. Memoir on the Reed-Frost epidemic theory. *Am. J. Epidemiol.* 103:138–40
3. Aycock, W. L., Lutman, G. E., Foley, G. E. 1945. Seasonal prevalence as a principle in epidemiology. *Am. J. Med. Sci.* 209:395–411
4. Godfrey, E. S. 1928. The age distribution of communicable disease according to size of community. *Am. J. Public Health* 18:616–31
5. Morris, J. N. 1955. Uses of epidemiology. *Br. Med. J.* 2(4936):395–401
6. Lilienfeld, A. M. 1960. The distribution of disease in the population. *J. Chronic Dis.* 11:471–83
7. White, C., Bailar, J. C. III. 1956. Retrospective and prospective methods of studying association in medicine. *Am. J. Public Health* 46:35–44
8. Lilienfeld, A. M. 1957. Epidemiological methods and inferences in studies of noninfectious diseases. *Public Health Rep.* 72:51–60
9. Cornfield, J., Haenszel, W. 1960. Some aspects of retrospective studies. *J. Chronic Dis.* 11:523–34
10. Stallones, R. A. 1966. Prospective epidemiologic studies of cerebrovascular disease. In *Cerebrovascular Disease Epidemiology-A Workshop*, pp. 51–56. Public Health Monogr. No. 76. PHS Publ. No. 1441. Washington: GPO
11. Editorial. 1942. What and who is an epidemiologist? *Am. J. Public Health* 32:414–15
12. Bolduan, C. F. 1942. Letter to the editor. *Am. J. Public Health* 32:1280
13. Lumsden, L. L. 1942. Letter to the editor. *Am. J. Public Health* 32:1040–42
14. Terris, M. 1962. The scope and methods of epidemiology. *Am. J. Public Health* 52:1371–76
15. Stallones, R. A. 1963. Epidemi(olog)²y. Letter to the editor. *Am. J. Public Health* 53:82–84
16. Lilienfeld, D. E. 1978. Definitions of epidemiology. *Am. J. Epidemiol.* 107:87–90
17. Frerichs, R. R., Neutra, R. 1978. Letter to the editor. *Am. J. Epidemiol.* 108:74–75
18. Abramson, J. H. 1979. Letter to the editor. *Am. J. Epidemiol.* 109:99–102
19. Rich, H. 1979. Letter to the editor. *Am. J. Epidemiol.* 109:102
20. Evans, A. S. 1979. Letter to the editor. *Am. J. Epidemiol.* 109:379–82

21. Sartwell, P. E. 1955. Some approaches to the epidemiologic study of chronic disease. *Am. J. Public Health* 45:609–14
22. Barrett-Connor, E. 1979. Infectious and chronic disease epidemiology: Separate and unequal? *Am. J. Epidemiol.* 109:245–49
23. Davies, A. M, ed. 1973. *Uses of Epidemiology in Planning Health Services: Proceedings of the Sixth International Scientific Meeting.* Belgrade: Savremana Administraciya. 1064 pp.
24. White, K. L., Henderson, M., eds. 1976. *Epidemiology as a Fundamental Science: Its Uses in Health Services Planning, Administration, and Evaluation.* New York: Oxford Univ. Press. 235 pp.
25. Henderson, M. 1976. The engagement of epidemiologists in health services research. *Am. J. Epidemiol.* 103:127–37
26. Pavlovskii, E. N. 1966. *Natural Nidality of Transmissible Diseases, with Special Reference to the Landscape Epidemiology of Zooanthroponoses.* Urbana: Univ. Illinois Press. 261 pp.
27. Stallones, R. A. 1973. Epidemiologist as environmentalist. *Int. J. Health Serv.* 3:29–33
28. Yerushalmy, J., Palmer, C. E. 1959. On the methodology of investigations of etiologic factors in chronic diseases. *J. Chronic Dis.* 10:27–40
29. Cassel, J. 1974. Psychosocial processes and "stress:" Theoretical formulations. *Int. J. Health Serv.* 4:471–82
30. MacMahon, B., Pugh, T. F., Ipsen, J. 1960. *Epidemiologic Methods*, pp. 18–21. Boston: Little, Brown
31. Evans, A. S. 1978. Causation and disease: A chronological journey. *Am. J. Epidemiol.* 108:249–58
32. Lilienfeld, A. M. 1959. "On the methodology of investigations of etiologic factors in chronic disease"—Some comments. *J. Chronic Dis.* 10:41–46
33. Sartwell, P. E. 1960. "On the methodology of investigations of etiologic factors in chronic disease"—Further comments. *J. Chronic Dis.* 11:61–63
34. Stallones, R. A. 1964. In *Smoking and Health. Report of the Advisory Committee to the Surgeon General of the Public Health Service*, p. 20. PHS Publication No. 1103. Washington: GPO
35. Rothman, K. J. 1976. Causes. *Am. J. Epidemiol.* 104:587–92
36. Koopman, J. 1977. Causal models and sources of interaction. *Am. J. Epidemiol.* 106:439–44

37. Dickson, P. 1978. *The Official Rules,* p. A5. New York: Delacorte
38. Truett, J., Cornfield, J., Kannel, W. 1967. A multivariate analysis of the risk of coronary heart disease in Framingham. *J. Chronic Dis.* 20:511–24
39. Moriyama, I. 1960. The classification of disease—a fundamental problem. *J. Chronic Dis.* 11:462–70
40. Acheson, R. M. 1962. The etiology of coronary heart disease: A review from the epidemiological standpoint. *Yale J. Biol. Med.* 35:143–70
41. Frost, W. H. 1965. Introduction. *Snow on Cholera,* pp. ix–xxi. New York: Hafner
42. Frost, W. H. 1941. Epidemiology. In *Collected Papers of Wade Hampton Frost,* ed. K. F. Maxcy, pp. 493–542.
New York: Commonwealth Fund
43. Reid, D. 1960. The epidemiological approach. In *Epidemiological Methods in the Study of Mental Disorders.* Public Health Pap. #2, pp. 8–16. Geneva: WHO
44. Buck, C. 1975. Popper's philosophy for epidemiologists. *Int. J. Epidemiol.* 4:159–68
45. Davies, A. M. 1975. Comments on "Popper's philosophy for epidemiologists' by Carol Buck. *Int. J. Epidemiol.* 4:169–71
46. Jacobsen, M. 1976. Against Popperized epidemiology. *Int. J. Epidemiol.* 5:9–11
47. Marmot, M. 1976. Facts, opinions, and affairs du coeur. *Am. J. Epidemiol.* 103:519–26

Ann. Rev. Public Health 1980. 1:83–94

PUBLIC HEALTH NURSING: ❖12503
The Nurse's Role in
Community-Based Practice

Rheba de Tornyay

School of Nursing, University of Washington, Seattle, Washington 98195

The term *public health nursing* has been largely replaced by *community health nursing* by the profession of nursing because for many people the term *public health* refers to the activities of those who work for government bodies in the delivery of health care to various populations. Today many nongovernmental groups are involved in delivering health care and community health nurses work in a wide variety of governmental and community settings—from migrant agricultural workers' camps to ambulatory clinics located in all types of hospitals—and, for these reasons, the term *community health* is more descriptive for nurses than public health.

Changes in the health care needs of society have created a demand for changes in health care services as well. One result has been the expansion of the nurse's role in the delivery of care. In keeping with the broad goal of public health practice, community health nursing has as its objective the improvement of the health of the total community. Practice therefore tends to be focused on community groups, particularly those groups that are at risk because of specific problems, such as disadvantaged preschool children, high risk pregnant women, or people suffering from specific long-term health problems.

Community health nursing has focused for much of its history on case-finding and health maintenance, as well as on health teaching and counseling activities. The community health nurse's responsibilities have included 1. administrating personal health services, 2. supervising other nursing personnel in providing such services, 3. teaching people and providing information about health, 4. recording and analyzing health data for

0163-7525/80/0510-0083$01.00

individuals and groups, 5. coordinating activities and resources in the community, 6. helping to maintain a healthful environment, and 7. assessing the health needs of the community (1). Community health nursing emphasizes continuous (as opposed to acute) nursing that is designed essentially for the maintenance of health and the prevention of disease.

The designation *nurse practitioner* has become a commonly used term to describe a nurse who has received training in the specific areas of (*a*) taking a systematic health history from a patient, (*b*) performing a physical examination to determine the patient's health status, and (*c*) managing certain stabilized problems such as hypertension or diabetes, usually with the help of a protocol developed jointly with a physician.

As health departments in the United States have become increasingly involved in the diagnosis and treatment of disease as well as in its prevention, the role of the nurses working within these agencies has changed (2). Although traditionally the emphasis of community health nursing has been on the maintenance of health, today the emphasis is shifting to the provision of primary care to individuals or groups of people. This is happening at least in part because health insurance carriers in their current reimbursement policies recognize diagnostic and treatment procedures but not health maintenance activities. As a rule, patients cannot be reimbursed by third party payers for home nursing visits, which were at one time the major means of getting the health of an entire family assessed. On the other hand, reimbursement is obtainable for skilled home nursing for an illness.

Many community health nurses are prepared to make physical assessments and are functioning in clinic settings as substitutes for more expensive physicians. There is the danger that medical or disease-oriented care will displace the health-promoting care now typifying community health nursing services. In many agencies, except for routine immunizations, the nurse is currently spending considerably less time on primary prevention, an activity that used to be the hallmark of the public health nurse of the past. About 12% of the actual health care problems are those related to curing disease, whereas 88% of the problems people encounter are those related to care: education for health, periodic health examinations, advice on diet and nutrition, and care to prevent long-term health problems from becoming acute (3).

In the past, public health nurses were distinct from other nurses because of the settings in which they practiced, but during the last two decades nurses in other types of practice also have been moving into the community. For example, pediatric services have been offered in schools, churches, and recreation centers (4). To be consistent with the practices of other health disciplines, and because of the rapid development of new knowledge, the profession of nursing has divided its practice into specialty areas. The generalized area of practice within community health nursing is now be-coming a specialty in much the same way that the general practice of medicine is developing a new specialty called *family practice*. As with medicine, nursing has found a new term for this old practitioner who uses many of the traditional nursing skills, but who also has acquired some new skills. The term *community nurse practitioner* or *family nurse practitioner* is being used more frequently to designate the nurse who works with indi-viduals and families, giving out-of-institution care. Archer & Fleshman (5) have developed a useful classification system to describe the major functions of community nurse practitioners. The four most appropriate for this review are the responsibilities of the community health nurse (*a*) in long-term care, (*b*) in primary care, (*c*) in working with specific population groups, and (*d*) in providing a range of services for people living in a specific area.

RESPONSIBILITIES OF THE COMMUNITY HEALTH NURSE IN LONG-TERM CARE

At one time the diagnostic category in which the nurse most often worked was the control of tuberculosis and other infectious diseases. Although patients are now less often hospitalized for tuberculosis, tuberculosis re-mains a substantial health problem. Unless the objectives of adequate and consistent ambulatory care help the patient to remain on the recommended self-care regimen (including the taking of prescribed medications and re-turning for regular follow-up care), out-of-institutional care will be safe and effective for neither the patient nor society. In the early 1970s the Miami Veterans Administration Hospital started a nurse-managed intermittent therapy clinic for patients with tuberculosis who required extra instruction and attention in order to remain on the therapeutic regimen (6). The goals for this program included preventing the need to rehospitalize the patient, keeping the patient noninfectious, and retaining the patient in treatment as long as it was medically indicated. The nursing care was coordinated by the community health nurse and included teaching the patient about the dis-ease, as well as obtaining the necessary information for the health depart-ment's communicable disease records. The pilot study at the Miami Veterans Administration Hospital, consisting of 15 patients who were seen twice a week by nurses in nurse-managed clinics over an average period of six and one half months, provided initial evidence that the nurse-managed clinics were highly effective. During the two-year period of the pilot study, none of the 15 patients were rehospitalized for tuberculosis and none had sputum specimens that were positive for the bacillus after discharge from the hospital. Eleven patients completed the prescribed regimen and were transferred to the regular follow-up clinic, one was lost to follow-up, one died from an unrelated condition, and two continued in the clinic. This small but important study gives some evidence that nurses are able to monitor vital signs, give antituberculosis drugs and observe for side effects, keep the tuberculosis registry, and refer the patient for medical care when indicated. Most important, patients so managed appear to remain with the treatment and so to benefit themselves as well as society.

Studies comparing the care given to patients with diabetes mellitus by nurse practitioners with those managed traditionally by physicians support the notion that nurses offer more than medical services. Stein (7) observed the care given to 23 female patients with maturity-onset diabetes mellitus. The management of the 12 patients who made up the experimental group was supervised by a nurse practitioner; that of the remaining 11 patients was supervised by a clinic physician in the traditional way. After a six-month period there was no significant difference in patient morbidity or mortality and only minor differences in specific measurements of the course of the disease. However, the patients in the experimental group had a significantly better understanding of the disease than did the others. In another study (8), patients assigned to a nurse for continuing care required fewer subsequent hospitalizations than did those managed in the traditional ambulatory setting.

Investigators who have studied the effects of care by nurse practitioners on patient management with other long-term health problems have found the same results. Runyan (9) studied the processes of patients with diabetes, hypertension, or cardiac disease who had been cared for by nurse practitioners. Comparing them with a group of patients attending traditional hospital outpatient clinics, he found that their diastolic blood pressures and blood glucose levels were significantly lower than those given traditional treatment, and that they spent 50% fewer days in the hospital.

The community health nurse practitioner usually becomes involved with the patient after the medical diagnosis has been made and assists the patient to cope with the physical, emotional, and social problems caused by the disease. The management of chronic health problems requires the patient to be motivated toward self-care in such areas as diet modification, weight control, and regular exercise; and in discontinuing harmful habits, such as the use of tobacco, alcohol, and drugs that are not prescribed. Many nurse clinics include group activities among the patients, thereby making use of the effectiveness of the self-help groups, which are often sponsored by lay organizations that believe that people who experience and share certain health problems have the capacity to manage their illnesses more effectively than can professional experts. Such practices will undoubtedly become more prevalent as their successes are documented.

Home care of people with stabilized long-term health problems is increasing because of the emphasis on cost containment by health agencies and because of the desire for improved quality of life by those who suffer from such health problems. Home health care is provided by community health nurses who assess the needs of the patient and family, prescribe the necessary nursing care, and supervise the care given by home health aides. In addition, the community health nurse's expertise regarding community agencies provides coordination of health and social activities as well as counseling and teaching for the patient and family.

RESPONSIBILITIES OF THE COMMUNITY HEALTH NURSE IN PRIMARY CARE

There are as many definitions of primary care as there are speakers and writers on the subject. A succinct, all-encompassing definition upon which everyone agrees has not yet been devised. For the purpose of this review, however, the definition accepted by the American Academy of Nursing is used (10). This definition makes explicit two dimensions in primary care: (a) the person's initial contact with the health delivery system in any given episode of illness, which leads to a decision of what must be done to solve the problem, and (b) the added responsibility for the continuum of care, including the maintenance of health, the evaluation and management of conditions, and referral of the patient to other health personnel or agencies. The provision of primary care is a complex process involving the determination of the basic health services to be provided by a variety of health professionals.

The background and interests of community nurses are particularly relevant to the needs of patients for primary care (11). A fairly comprehensive study in the state of Virginia (12) of the reasons that patients seek the care of family physicians showed that physicians are often asked to serve in roles other than that of the curer of disease. People who are troubled, in pain, or are disabled want to see someone with whom to share their troubles. They are lonely, so they go to the clinic, the doctor's office, or the emergency room of the hospital. They are often really seeking sympathy, reassurance, and encouragement. Furthermore, many of the patients in the Virginia study sought care for health supervision and health maintenance, an observation also made in another study of patient's needs (13).

All of these services, as beneficial as they are for the patient, have led to the escalation of health care costs by clogging the delivery system with the result that people who really need the physician's time are not able to be seen as quickly as they should be. The medical management of the more commonly occurring problems that are brought to the primary care practitioner may not be complex, but as long as there is the capacity within the health delivery system to differentiate between uncomplicated problems causing the patient discomfort and the problems that are potentially serious, care can be offered to those with uncomplicated problems that is less expensive, more accessible, and more satisfying to these patients.

Ideally, primary health care should include all of the health maintenance activities that are included in traditional community health nursing. For example, family planning, counseling, well-child supervision, pre- and postnatal follow-up activities, immunizations, and disease detection assessments all should be included in the responsibilities of the health provider who offers primary care.

The literature pertaining to the delivery of primary care tends to focus on individuals, yet considerable attention should be oriented toward family-centered care. In addition to its other basic functions, there is no question that the family constitutes the most important social context within which illness occurs and is resolved. The family constitutes an independent, dependent, and intervening variable as well as a precipitating, predisposing, and contributing factor in the etiology, care, and treatment of both physical and mental illness and as a basic unit of interaction and transaction in health care (14). Although the role of the family as a hereditary link, causal agent, or source of communication of disease has been the subject of a number of studies, the investigation of the family as a clustering of illness is a neglected area of concentrated study and one that community nurse/primary care practitioners with their emphasis on family-centered approaches should focus upon in their practice and research.

Traditionally, community health nursing has focused on the care of the family as a unit within the community. Regardless of the reason for which a person seeks professional help, and regardless of the reason that the community health nurse has contact with a patient or client, these nurses have been prepared to apply wide-ranging casefinding methods or preventive measures as needed.

RESPONSIBILITIES OF THE COMMUNITY HEALTH NURSE IN WORKING WITH SPECIFIC POPULATION GROUPS

For a long time community health nurses have had their attention focused on high risk people: the young, the elderly, and the pregnant. In addition, all people regardless of age are more at risk if they are poor and without access to medical care. One exceedingly important population group that has benefited from increased health services through the Head Start programs is the high risk preschool group. The major goal of Head Start health programs is primary prevention through health promotion programs, through protective practices such as immunizations, and through tooth fluoridation in areas where the water is not fluoridated. Secondary prevention through early diagnosis of abnormalities and disease treatment has also proven successful in these programs.

Expanding on the functions of casefinding and referral to community-agencies, which are responsibilities assumed by all community health nurses, the additional skills of performing physical examinations and giving treatment for the minor illnesses of childhood have facilitated nurses' expanded and more comprehensive care to infants and children. The pediatric nurse practitioner (PNP) has functioned since the early 1970s in health department settings. The lack of physicians within the health department structure and the already established effectiveness of the public health nurse has contributed to the early acceptance of the PNP in this role (15). The PNP is able to establish branch clinics to extend the outreach of the main health care delivery site and has the ability to make an in-depth assessment of the child and the family. These qualities have increased the availability of health care in the more sparsely populated areas.

As a further specialization stemming from the successes of pediatric nurse practitioners, school nurse practitioners have been providing a broad range of health services to school-age children since 1970 when the first program to prepare this type of practitioner was established at the University of Colorado (16). School nurse practitioners are prepared to assess children's health status and to provide them with health care by managing a variety of health problems including the more common pediatric illnesses. They can also 1. provide well-child care with an emphasis on prevention, 2. integrate care through participation in formulating and implementing plans involving the family, school, and community, 3. foster health education through participation with other school personnel in the prevention of disease and maintenance of health, and 4. assist parents to learn about health problems and assume responsibility for maintaining their children's health care.

In Galveston, Texas, improved access to community health care was achieved through two changes in the secondary school health services (17): (a) the upgrading of the educational training of school nurses to include pediatric nurse practitioner training and (b) more efficient management of the school clinics. The latter was accomplished through the employment of a full-time health aide to assist the nurse in collecting data on the three most common complaints—headaches, colds and upper respiratory complaints, and stomachache and other abdominal complaints. In addition to attempting to improve problem identification and access to health care for adolescents, this approach to high school health services educated students to become more competent and involved in their own health care.

One special population with whom community nurse practitioners can make a particularly valuable contribution is that of pregnant teenagers and teenage mothers. Teenage mothers have special needs because often they are inexperienced, immature, impulsive, undirected, and unfocused, having little self-esteem or self-identity. Of most importance, they are struggling with the tasks of adolescence and the tasks of motherhood simultaneously. One demonstration project located at Columbia-Presbyterian Medical Center in New York provided, through the services of pediatric nurse practitioners, well-child care as well as intensive counseling to teenage mothers (18). This project, targeted toward high risk mothers, achieved the reduction of problems connected with inadequate infant feeding and child abuse, as well as the mother's school problems.

Parents constitute another population group often served by community health nurses. Some groups are formed around the usual needs of new parents, others are specicially focused on the special needs of single parents or parents with preschool age children or with teenage children. Also receiving attention are the special problems encountered by parents who have children with developmental disabilities, or with major long-term health problems such as diabetes or cystic fibrosis, or with children who have social adjustment problems caused by long-term illnesses.

Community health nurse practitioners are involved with fertility-related services for women. The success of family planning depends largely on the patient's understanding and acceptance of the methods selected and also on the development of rapport with the patient (19). Nurses are assuming greater responsibility in family planning activities, and although at present they are in short supply, they outnumber available physicians. It is important to stress that these nurses are prepared to make decisions and assist patients in making informed choices, rather than to serve simply as medical technicians or limited physician surrogates.

The community health nurse's responsibilities for the care of the aged includes the teaching of preventive measures, early detection of changes, effective monitoring of chronic illness, and continuity of care. Nurses serving elderly populations do so in clinics, geriatric day centers, single room occupancy residences, and homes for the chronically ill or infirm. They serve as the primary health care contact and maintain a collaborative relationship with a physician or hospital clinic (20). Characteristically, community health nurses act as liaisons between the nursing home and the community, but do not assume decision-making responsibilities within the nursing home.

The role of a gerontological nurse practioner as the primary care provider for many elderly persons is being investigated at the University of Colorado

Medical Center (21). The program evaluation staff has observed instances of the patient advocacy role assumed by nurse practitioners contributing to the improved physical and psychosocial status of persons with chronic illnesses. However, the scarcity of hard data to substantiate these observations requires that they be viewed as tentative and somewhat subjective. There is a great need for the development of instruments to measure improved health status among the elderly in terms of the quality of life in addition to the common medically oriented measures (22). The elderly commonly worry about living arrangements, diminished memory, ability to move about, isolation, poverty, nutrition, and the access to medication supplies. The multiplicity of problems leads to feelings of being overwhelmed by problems and depression. The effectiveness of programs for the elderly should be judged according to their alleviation of these worries.

As the number of nursing home beds increases in the United States, and with the nursing home industry underserved by physicians, registered nurses have been assuming more and more patient care and decision-making responsibilities, often without the benefit of advanced training (23). The gerontological nurse practitioner can serve nursing homes as the planner and evaluator of care of patients, as well as serving as the consultant to the registered nurse or practical nurse who has had limited educational or practice background in the care of the elderly.

In her review of studies published from 1972 through 1976, Highrighter (24) found that the population group most frequently studied to determine specific patient needs were the elderly. It is interesting to note that these studies found fewer unmet serious medical needs than had been expected. Most of the needs of the elderly were for dental, eye, and foot care, and most were for difficulties in coping with day-to-day living problems and for social needs.

RESPONSIBILITIES OF THE COMMUNITY HEALTH NURSE IN PROVIDING SERVICES FOR PERSONS LIVING IN A SPECIFIC AREA

The nurse as a primary care provider for a geographically isolated group of people was first introduced into rural southeastern Kentucky more than 50 years ago by the Frontier Nursing Service (FNS). The aim was to establish and maintain a health care system in medically underserved areas; the nurse-midwife was selected as the most appropriately prepared health care provider for meeting the problems of the rural areas. She was more easily attainable at less cost than was the physician (25). She could manage the common day-to-day health problems encountered by a family and could take care of the mother throughout the childbearing period and later care for the newborn infant. She was prepared in health teaching and in public health. On the whole, this is still true in some sparsely populated areas of the country; mobile units staffed by community health nurses provide clinic care, particularly to preschool children (26).

Recruiting health professionals into smaller and more geographically distant areas continues to be a major problem in health delivery. With the legislation allowing direct reimbursement for nurse practitioners who serve rural areas, predictably more nurse practitioners will practice in such areas. At least one leader in community health nursing (27) insists that more emphasis must be placed on teaching self-care to clients than on continuing to rely on health professionals to give most of the health care. Self-care has been defined as a process whereby a person can effectively provide for his or her own health promotion, prevention of illness, disease detection, and treatment (28). Such care can be provided through the knowledge that many people now possess and with the addition of new skills that can be taught to populations at risk. The practice of self-care is a return to a very old practice and concept: like other aspects of survival and social development, self-care was at one time an individual responsibility.

In addition to the importance of reducing reliance on physicians, the major long-term health problems, particularly the problems caused by the degenerative diseases, require constant self-monitoring. Results of one study (29) suggested that compliance with medical regimens may not be as desirable as is consistently believed by health professionals. In this investigation, patients with compliant, nonquestioning attitudes were shown to be unable to cope with their problems, and this may have had a detrimental effect on recovery. There is, however, an interesting paradox in connection with self-help activities. Although the economic incentive ought to be a major factor in the rationale for increasing a patient's self-care competence, only the health maintenance organizations include education of the patient among their benefits.

Other examples of nurses working in specific geographic areas include (a) the traditional public health district assignments, (b) occupational groupings such as industrial units, in which nurses assume responsibility for the entire population employed, and (c) camp nursing in which nurses contribute to the welfare of the entire population group.

SUMMARY AND CONCLUSIONS

A change in awareness of the community's needs for health care services is forcing changes in how and by whom care is being delivered today. The increasing emphasis on primary care, particularly care provided on an ambulatory basis; the increased awareness of the importance of health maintenance and preventive care, including health assessment, counseling, and education; and increased pressure to contain health care costs have all influenced these changes. Community health nurses have expanded their roles to include the provision of primary care to people at risk by caring for patients with stabilized chronic health problems and helping them to manage their lives as independently as possible.

The focus of community health nursing continues to be on public health, i.e. the provision of health services among people of the community and the encouragement of health-promoting behavior. These populations include the young, the pregnant, the old, those with specific health problems, the poor, the disadvantaged, and the isolated. Williams (30) points out that in order for community health nurses to continue to retain the public health approach, they must concern themselves with the aggregate problems of a given community. She also suggests that the systematic and rigorous study of the community is needed in order to determine the needs of people living within the community, and that the programs within the health agency should be restructured or refocused on the basis of those needs. Community health nurse practitioners not only must meet the needs of patients who seek care, but also must continue to assume responsibility for monitoring, protecting, and fostering the health of a given population group.

The success of community health nursing depends in large measure on the future direction of the American health care delivery system. If, as is so frequently proposed, a greater emphasis on health maintenance and disease prevention to complement our present system of care for acute and episodic conditions really becomes a reality, then community health nursing will flourish in the way in which it was originally intended.

ACKNOWLEDGMENTS

Appreciation is expressed to Betty Pesznecker and Dr. Barbara Horn for their valuable assistance and constructive comments. I also thank Judith Bedell, Alison Ross, and Bernice Freeman for technical assistance.

Literature Cited

1. Miller, M. H., Albers, L. L. 1975. The role of the local health officer—Why not a nurse? *South. Med. J.* 65:534–37
2. Archer, S. E., Fleshman, R. P. 1979. *Community Health Nursing.* N. Scituate, Mass: Duxbury. 646 pp. 2nd ed.
3. Lysaught, J. P. 1972. Distributive health care needs and the occupational health nurse. *Occup. Health Nurs.* 20:8–9
4. Archer, S. E. 1976. Community nurse practitioners: Another assessment. *Nurs. Outlook* 24:499–503
5. Archer, S. E., Fleshman, R. P. 1975. Community health nursing: A typology of practice. *Nurs. Outlook* 23:358–64
6. Peterson, L. D., Green, J. H. 1977. Nurse-managed tuberculosis clinic. *Am. J. Nurs.* 77:433–35
7. Stein, H. H. 1974. The use of a nurse practitioner in the management of patients with diabetes mellitus. *Med. Care* 12:885–90
8. Jordan, J. D., Shipp, J. C. 1971. The primary health care professional was a nurse. *Am. J. Nurs.* 71:922–25

9. Runyan, J. W. 1975. Memphis chronic disease program. *J. Am. Med. Assoc.* 213:264–67

10. American Academy of Nursing. 1977. *Primary Care by Nurses: Sphere of Responsibility and Accountability,* p. 2. Kansas City, Mo: Am. Nurses Assoc. 79 pp.

11. Aiken, L. 1977. Primary care: The challenge for nursing. *Am. J. Nurs.* 77:1828–32

12. Marsland, D. W., Wood, M., Mayo, F. 1976. A data bank for patient care, curriculum, and research in family practice: 526,196 patient problems. *J. Fam. Pract.* 3:25–28

13. Pesznecker, B. L., Draye, M. A. 1978. Family nurse practitioners in primary care: A study of practice and patients. *Am. J. Public Health* 68:977–80

14. Litman, T. J. 1974. The family as a basic unit in health and medical care. *Soc. Sci. Med.* 8:495–519

15. Thorp, R. J. 1975. The use of the pediatric nurse practitioner in comprehensive health care. *Pediatr. Nurs.* 1:33–35

16. Silver, H. K., Igoe, J. B., McAtee, P. R. 1977. School nurse practitioners: A concise descriptive definition of their functions and activities. *J. Sch. Health* 47:589–98

17. Nader, P. R., Conrad, J., Williamson, M., McKevitt, R., Berrey, R. 1978. The high school nurse practitioner. *J. Sch. Health* 48:649–54

18. Brown, C. A. 1978. Teen-age mother's well child clinic. *Pediatr. Nurs.* 4:27–31

19. Manisoff, M., Davis, L. W., Kaminetzky, H. A., Payne, P. 1976. The family planning nurse practitioner: Concepts and results of training. *Am. J. Public Health* 66:62–64

20. Schwartz, D. R. 1978. Public health nursing's responsibilities for the care of the aged. *Bull. NY Acad. Med.* 54:555–60

21. Heppler, J. 1976. Gerontological nurse practitioner: Change agents in the health care delivery systems of the aged. *J. Gerontol. Nurs.* 2:38–40

22. Keith, P. M. 1976. A preliminary investigation of the role of the public health nurse in evaluation of services for the aged. *Am. J. Public Health* 66:379–81

23. Richard, E. C., Miedeman, L. 1977. The nurse practitioner in the nursing home. *J. Nurs. Admin.* 7:11–13

24. Highriter, M. 1977. The status of community health nursing research. *Nurs. Res.* 26:183–92

25. Browne, H. E., Isaacs, G. 1976. The frontier nursing service: The primary care nurse in the community hospital. *Am. J. Obstetr. Gynecol.* 124:14–17

26. McNeil, J., Bergner, L. 1975. Use of mobile unit to provide health care for preschoolers in rural King County, Washington. *Public Health Rep.* 90:344–48

27. Brewer, K. 1978. Three nurses strive to make health planning a reality. *Am. Nurs.* 10(4):12–16

28. Levin, L. S. 1976. The layperson as the primary health care practitioner. *Public Health Rep.* 91:206–10

29. Glogow, E. 1973. The "bad patient" gets better quicker. *Soc. Policy* 4:72–76

30. Williams, C. A. 1977. Community health nursing—What is it? *Nurs. Outlook* 25:250–54

Ann. Rev. Public Health 1980. 1:95–119

STRATEGIES FOR THE REIMBURSEMENT OF SHORT-TERM HOSPITALS

❖12504

C. A. Watts, W. L. Dowling, and W. C. Richardson

Department of Health Services, University of Washington,
Seattle, Washington 98195

INTRODUCTION

The form and amount of payment to suppliers is an important determinant of the output characteristics of any industry. Ordinarily, these payments are market prices that reflect industry demand and supply conditions. In the hospital industry, however, financing arrangements are complicated by the existence of public and private underwriters who purchase hospital services on behalf of their beneficiaries.

Some of these third parties deal only with beneficiaries, leaving the fee-for-service payment mechanism essentially unchanged. Others enter into direct contracts with the institutions, offering various methods of compensation usually based on costs rather than on a predetermined schedule of service-specific charges.

The purpose of this chapter is to contribute to the current debate regarding the impact of these different payment strategies on industry performance. Although most observers agree that the method of provider payment greatly affects the equity and efficiency of resource allocation in this industry, there is less agreement as to how poorly our current methods perform and how we can improve them. As the share of public payment for services increases, the importance of this debate grows. An understanding of the hypothesized impact of alternative reimbursement mechanisms, complemented by empirical tests of these hypotheses, is an essential first step in developing sensible public policy in this area.

This chapter examines present reimbursement mechanisms and assesses their implications for supplier behavior. In addition to the conceptual argu-

95

ments, existing empirical evidence is also discussed. The focus of the discussion is limited in two ways. First, it deals only with reimbursement of short-term general hospitals. Not only do these hospitals account for the largest dollar volume of industry business [$57.7 billion in 1977 (1)], but there is a feeling among many authors that current hospital reimbursement policies may be responsible for the rapid rise in overall health care costs in recent years as well as other industry problems. Second, this chapter does not address the equally important interactions between consumers of hospital services and their third party representatives. Although a full understanding of this complex industry cannot be achieved by looking at only one portion of it, a more complete analysis is well beyond the scope of this chapter.

BACKGROUND

In 1977, total expenditures for health care (including research, construction, and the administrative costs of health insurance firms) amounted to $737 per capita, or 8.8% of the US gross national product (1). Of that total, 40.4% was spent for hospital services, an increase from 31% in 1950. Expenditures for physician services claimed the second largest share at 19.8% of the total, a figure that has remained roughly constant since 1950 (1).

The sources of these funds are revealing. In 1977, 30% of all expenditures for personal health care services came directly from consumers. The federal government, primarily through the Medicare and Medicaid programs, contributed 28%, with an additional 12% coming from state and local governments. Charity and direct industry payments amounted to 2%. The balance of 28% came from private insurance (1).

When the revenues of community hospitals are examined separately, public and private third party payments become more important. According to the American Hospital Association (2), direct consumer payments to hospitals provided 11.9% of the total revenues in 1975, private health insurance companies provided 43.6%, and public funds added 44.5%. These numbers have changed rather dramatically over time. In 1960, nearly 30% of hospital revenue came from direct consumer payments. Another 52.5% came from private insurance contributions. Only 18.8% came from public sources.

The changes in these expenditure shares over time from direct consumer payments toward government and insurance contributions have been accompanied by annual increases in total expenditures per capita far exceeding the experience of other sectors of the economy (3). These increases reflect changes in per capita utilization and even larger changes in the nature and sophistication of the hospital product (4). It is generally agreed that this is a causal relationship (5–8)—indeed, one of the expressed purposes of the Medicare and Medicaid programs was to increase service utilization by target groups (9). In addition, however, the shift in expenditures brought about a shift in the dominant form of reimbursement because of the major differences in the reimbursement policies of the various payers. Thus, a question of substantial policy interest is the extent to which the relationship between expenditure shares and expenditure increases is primarily a function of demand side changes (e.g. changes in the financial incentives facing consumers) and the extent to which it is a function of supply side changes (e.g. changes in the incentives facing providers). That is: What is the contribution of the reimbursement method to changes in average costs and expenditures[1] given a particular set of demand incentives?

Much of the existing research focuses on demand incentives alone (10–16). These studies investigate the effect of deductibles, coinsurance, and other financial restrictions directed at the consumer. Although the robustness of the results varies a great deal, the general conclusion from these studies is that financial incentives facing consumers have a significant impact on both the numbers and types of services purchased. The studies do not, however, examine the interaction between changes in the demand variables and changes in the financial incentives facing suppliers. Thus, the conclusions of those studies in which demand variables were examined across different provider reimbursement modes (which happens even in a single hospital) are biased because adjustments for these supply variations do not appear to have been made (10, 11, 12).

Empirical investigations of the impact of supply incentives have also been undertaken. As with the demand studies, however, few of the attempts have dealt carefully with the interaction between demand and supply variables. The remainder of this chapter focuses on the financial incentives facing suppliers. However, it is important to keep in mind the existence of the demand side of the market and its role in determining system costs.

ALTERNATIVE REIMBURSEMENT PRACTICES

A number of reimbursement arrangements coexist in the hospital industry, with individual institutions typically subject to several forms of payment simultaneously (5, 17).

---

[1]It is important to distinguish between changes in the average cost per unit of hospital service and changes in total expenditures. The latter involves not only average costs per unit, but also the number of units consumed.

Charges

A declining share of hospital services are paid for on the basis of service-specific charges set by the hospital. Patients without insurance coverage (self-pay patients), most commercial insurance carriers, and 27 of the 74 Blue Cross plans across the country (representing 30% of total Blue Cross enrollment) pay charges (18). This reimbursement mechanism is completely analogous to the fee-for-service system in the physician market. Generally, it requires the least amount of interaction between the payer and the provider. A hospital first determines the units of service that are to be priced separately and then sets its charges based on expected volume relative to projected operating costs, bad debts and charity care, depreciation and interest on existing debt, and a margin for expansion and new technology (5). Because most hospitals are organized as nonprofit entities, distribution of earnings is not allowed.

Cost

The remaining 47 Blue Cross plans (representing 70% of total Blue Cross enrollment) and Medicare and Medicaid all base reimbursement on costs incurred in the provision of services to their respective beneficiaries. In recent years, these three groups together have accounted for roughly two-thirds of community hospital revenue (6).

In general, cost reimbursement is based on the retrospectively determined costs of providing service. It is typically paid as an average per diem rate. Periodic payments are made throughout the payment period on the basis of projected costs and volume with an end-of-period settlement to adjust for differences between projected per diem costs and actual costs.

All cost payers begin by excluding costs that are unrelated to patient care such as the costs associated with the gift shop, the cafeteria, and the parking lot. In addition, research costs are typically excluded. Bad debts and the costs of charity care are not covered by Blue Cross plans; Medicare pays only for the bad debts of its own beneficiaries.

In keeping with the wide spectrum of the population they enroll, most Blue Cross plans pay the share of a hospital's total costs calculated on the ratio of Blue Cross patient days to total days, without adjustments to reflect cross-patient differences in actual services received. Alternatively, because Medicare serves a very distinct population (primarily the elderly) whose hospital use patterns differ significantly from the rest of the patient population, the Medicare apportionment formula is more complex. Termed the RCCAC (ratio of charges to charges applied to costs), the Medicare formula calculates the government's share of a hospital's costs by multiplying total costs by the ratio of charges for services rendered to Medicare patients to charges for services rendered to all patients. In addition, because nursing costs are billed separately from the basic room and board charge, Medicare pays an 8.5% nursing differential in recognition of the higher nursing demands of its patients.

Although depreciation of existing plant and equipment and interest payments on borrowed capital are allowable costs, explicit contributions to an internal fund for future capital expenditures (analogous to retained earnings in a for-profit firm) are excluded by all cost payers.[2] Instead, many Blue Cross plans add a plus factor to costs that generally ranges between 2% and 8% (5). Medicare originally added a 2% plus factor to costs, but dropped it early in the Nixon administration (19).

As costs have increased over time, other conditions have been added to the contracts or regulations governing payer-provider relationships. For example, attempts have been made to determine the level of reimbursable costs prior to the period of service delivery. These attempts at cost control and their success are discussed in a later section.

THE INCENTIVES

General Considerations

A study of the predicted or actual effects of alternative reimbursement systems on industry cost and output decisions must begin with the development of a conceptual model of provider behavior. It is from this theoretical framework that testable hypotheses regarding firm response are derived. Without such a framework, empirical observations are difficult to interpret.

A Model of Hospital Behavior

The development of a behavioral model of the hospital industry is somewhat difficult because of the nonprofit status of the majority of industry firms. Few general models of the nonprofit firm exist [Weisbrod (20) provides the best example], although a number of attempts have been made to develop a model specific to the nonprofit hospital (21–27). With two exceptions (25, 27), these models assert that hospitals pursue a set of objectives generally related to growth, technological sophistication, and/or prestige. Pauly & Redisch (25) and Shalit (27) argued, instead, that the fee-for-service physician plays an important if not dominant role in hospital decision-making. The latter model implies that output, pricing, and investment decisions will be made to further the financial and other interests of the profit-making physician.

---

[2]Roughly 8% of all short-term US hospitals are organized as for-profit ventures (2). These institutions are allowed a "reasonable" return on equity capital.

Empirical Tests of the Model

Only some of these models withstand careful conceptual scrutiny and even fewer have been subjected to empirical tests of their validity (see 28 for a critical review of these models). Davis (29) attempted to test a number of hypotheses that purportedly distinguished among the various growth-technology-prestige models. Her results were weak, however, in part because she was unable to develop testable propositions clearly associated with a single model. Pauly (30) attempted to verify his model (25) by testing hypotheses relating to hospital investment decisions. Again the results were weak because of econometric identification problems resulting from the absence of testable hypotheses that were not also consistent with other theories. A series of other authors (31–42) have attempted to investigate hospital behavior by estimating cost functions for these institutions. Most of these studies, however, focused on the relationship between average costs and observed output levels assumed to be exogenously determined.

The strongest evidence regarding the behavior of nonprofit hospitals comes from five additional studies (43–47). Salkever (43) and Hartman & Watts (44) found that community demand variables play an important direct role in the determination of hospital output. Further, the results obtained by Davis (45), Feldstein & Waldman (46), and Hellinger (47) suggest that the pricing decisions of these nonprofit firms respond to changes in market conditions in much the same fashion as those of for-profit organizations. Finally, Etzioni & Doty (48) found a substantial amount of profit-pursuing behavior in nonprofit hospitals.

These results indicate that nonprofit hospitals and for-profit counterparts exhibit reasonably similar responses to changes in their financial environments. This similarity is assumed in the following sections.

Incentives: The Charge-Based Approaches

PROBLEMS   There are two major concerns with the use of charges as a payment mechanism. The arguments supporting these concerns are outlined below, followed by possible counterarguments in each case.

Equity   The first concern arises from the belief that not all purchasers of care pay the full cost of services rendered to them or to their beneficiaries. As a result, the payments made by other purchasers of care must be inflated to cover these deficits. As states begin to review and regulate hospital rates for all payers, the issues involved in cross-subsidization must be resolved to enable rate setters to make appropriate policy decisions.

Generally, there are believed to be two types of cross-subsidization in hospitals: subsidization across payer groups (49) and subsidization across individual charge-paying patients (49, 50). It is argued that when charge-based payment coexists with payment on the basis of incurred costs, costs that are disallowed by the cost payer (e.g. research costs, contributions to a growth and development fund) can be added into the charges billed to other payers. Thus, decisions by Medicare or Blue Cross to exclude a portion of teaching costs or to lower the amount of allowable depreciation expenses need not result in a lower level of hospital costs to the community at large, but only a shift in who pays them.

The struggle over the amount of charity care that must be provided by hospitals participating in the Hill-Burton program provides a recent example of this potential for cross-payer subsidization. In this case, one agency of the Department of Health, Education, and Welfare (DHEW) has defined the amount of free care that hospitals will have to provide to meet their obligations under the Hill-Burton guidelines. At the same time, another agency of DHEW has developed regulations that exclude the cost of providing this care from Medicare and Medicaid reimbursement. Thus, the federal government has forced the hospital without nonpatient care sources of revenue to shift the cost of treating Hill-Burton patients to nongovernment payers. Because the cost-based Blue Cross plans also disallow bad debts and the costs of charity care, these expenses must be built into the charges paid by commercial insurers and self-pay patients.

With respect to subsidization across charge-paying patients[3] it is widely believed (49, 50) that hospitals systematically set prices above costs for some services and use the resulting surpluses to fund deficits from below cost prices on other services. Thus, to the extent that the patients who receive the former services do not also receive the latter, some subsidization across patients occurs.

The arguments against these pricing practices generally focus on the question of equity: Why should different patients (or their third parties) pay different amounts for the same services; or why should different mark ups over cost be paid by consumers of different services? Although the existence and magnitude of cross-subsidization can be examined empirically, the equity concern that it causes is subjective and thus cannot be analyzed for its conceptual validity. It is important to distinguish, however, between true cross-subsidization and the payment of different amounts for different services. That is, if Blue Cross specifies that it is unwilling to contribute to teaching activity but Medicare regulations do not, then presumably a different product is being demanded by the two groups. If, as a result, all teaching

---

[3]Because the Medicare formula uses the ratio of Medicare charges to total charges to determine the federal share of a hospital's costs, the issue of cross-patient subsidization is relevant here as well.

costs are shifted to the Medicare account, this cannot be labeled cross-subsidization. The federal government could also limit its educational contributions by specifying a maximum amount it is willing to pay for teaching or by following Blue Cross and refusing to pay anything for educational activities.

Further, as Posner (50) pointed out, to the extent that hospitals use the surplus from above cost pricing to fund charity care, additional teaching activities, or other collective goods (20), the institution takes on some of the functions of a governmental body. The margin between prices and costs functions as a tax with which the "public goods" are financed. However, the private hospital is unlike the government authority in that it is generally not governed in any way by elected officials who represent the public interest. (An exception would be the hospital districts that have been established in some regions.) Thus, the amount of the "public good" provided, and therefore the level of the "tax" to finance it, is determined by the decision-making body in the hospital, not in a collective arena (50). As a result, there is no assurance that the optimal level of these services will be provided.

There is no question that cross-subsidization can exist in the hospital industry. It can, and probably does, exist in every industry to some extent. Thus, the crucial issue for rate setters is not so much the potential for cross-subsidization, or even its existence, but its observed magnitude. However, the only empirical evidence that exists at the present time is anecdotal. Systematic empirical analysis of this issue has not been undertaken. In addition, cross-subsidization is likely to have been attenuated somewhat in recent years because of increases in insurance coverage and increases in public disclosure, which reduce the provider's desire and ability to cross-subsidize.

The primary determinant of a firm's ability (in any industry) to charge prices above cost on some of its items, or to some of its consumers, is the sensitivity of its total revenue to changes in price. If patients have less costly alternatives from which to choose, it may not be in the hospital's interest, in spite of its ability to raise prices, to do so. Most of the studies of consumer price sensitivity in the health industry (13, 14, 51) do not consider hospital services separately, and so are of limited usefulness in examining cross-subsidization. A few studies examined hospital demand alone (37, 38, 52), but they typically suffered from severe data constraints and multiple econometric difficulties. In addition, the two specific questions that are most relevant to the present question have not been studied empirically: What is the sensitivity to prices of self-pay patients (who are frequently low income)? What is the magnitude of the combined long run response, not only of the patient insured under a charge based contract, but also of the third party underwriter? Given the important role of the third party in determining hospital revenues, its response to price changes is equally critical.

The evidence regarding the latter question is very sparse. Some examples of third party attempts to limit payments to hospitals exist (53–55); however, an Oregon case study reported by Greenberg & Goldberg (56) suggests less price sensitivity. These authors concluded that hospital insurance companies attempting to hold down subscriber costs by monitoring the medical industry's activities were driven out of business by the Oregon chapter of Blue Shield, Oregon Physicians Service (OPS). This was made possible, according to the authors, by the fact that patients who did not agree to pay the higher premiums of the Blue Shield policy were threatened with the withdrawal of services by their physicians (who had established OPS). Uncooperative physicians, in turn, were threatened with loss of medical society membership and hospital admitting privileges. Because of the implied coercive role of the physician in this instance, more evidence is needed before any firm statements can be made regarding the value consumers might place on third party efforts to hold down premiums in this fashion.

However, even the existence of cost-conscious third parties is only a necessary, but not a sufficient, condition for the absence of extensive cross-subsidization. Competition among hospitals for the patients of these third parties is also essential. Competition among hospitals is strongly affected by the ability of new institutions to enter the market. Since the early 1970s, legal barriers to entry in the hospital industry have existed in the form of certificate of need. Although proponents of certificate of need can provide arguments in favor of these controls (57), the reduction of competition within the hospital market is one theoretical effect (58). In fact, these controls appear to have been less than perfectly effective (59, 60).

The conclusion that can be drawn from this evidence, then, is that firm statements about the magnitude of cross-subsidization must await further study.

Operating Margins   The second major concern about the use of charges is the level of overall operating margins. The argument is that if hospitals are allowed to set their own prices, they can establish any mark up they choose and can thus generate whatever funds for future expansion and addition of new technology they desire.

The counterargument here is much the same as in the previous section. Hospitals will charge prices in accordance with market conditions. Only if demand is very insensitive to price changes can hospitals add large mark ups to costs. Further, eliminating internal surpluses will not limit growth as long as hospitals have access to borrowed capital (which can be financed as a cost item) or donated capital. Ginsburg (61) has shown that hospitals do respond to increases in the price of one source of capital funds by switching to another. In addition, certificate of need controls exist to provide an external check on hospital expansion, subject to the qualifications noted above (59, 60). Finally, if purchasers of care (defined to include payers as well as patients) are insensitive to price changes, then charge-based payment systems cannot be singled out for criticism. In this environment, no form of unregulated reimbursement will prevent hospital growth and cost inflation.

The evidence regarding actual levels of operating margins is small. One source (5) estimated operating margins to be in the range of 3 to 4%. However, a number of factors make the relative magnitude of these figures difficult to assess. Although cost payers do allow depreciation and interest charges to be included in reimbursable costs, depreciation is typically based on the historical cost of the asset. Given the rapidly rising construction and equipment costs of the recent past, these payments cannot be expected to fund the full replacement costs of these assets. In addition, philanthropy, which has been an important source of hospital capital, has only held steady in absolute dollars. In terms of its value in this inflated period it has therefore declined as a source of investment funds.

ADVANTAGES   The previous section outlines the problems that have been associated with charge-based reimbursement. There are also advantages.

First, charges are set prior to the period of service based on the hospital's expectations about future costs and volumes. Thus, at least in the short run, the burden of input price increases or other cost-increasing events falls on the institution rather than on the patient or the third party (62). In addition, the consumer can determine in advance what her financial liability will be per billed unit. This is less of an advantage in this particular industry because the number and type of units in the complete episode is highly uncertain a priori and heavily influenced by the attending physician. The fact of the uncertainty with respect to the number and type of services required, however, suggests another advantage to the charge system applied to individual services. Because the hospital is assured of receiving additional revenue for every service that is consumed, it has no incentive to constrain the availability of required services because of financial restrictions. From a quality of care standpoint, this may be an important consideration, especially given the consumer's relative lack of knowledge about appropriate treatment patterns. Of course, an incentive for quality degradation may still occur within individual service categories for which prices have been set.

Further, unlike average total cost reimbursement, payment is at least somewhat related to services received (5). (It is noteworthy that the equity problems involved with cross-subsidization are concerned with charge-based systems in which cross-patient (as opposed to cross-payer) subsidization is much lower than with many cost-based systems.)

Incentives: Incurred Cost-Based Approaches

PROBLEMS   There are many who have assailed cost-based reimbursement (63–65). The spirit of their criticisms is best summarized by Holohan et al [p. 39 in ref. (64)]: " 'Reasonable cost' reimbursement, the predominant method of hospital payment, is highly inflationary and inefficient." The rationale for this criticism is that if hospitals are assured of being reimbursed for all incurred costs, there is little incentive to lower costs through increased efficiency and every incentive to pursue the most sophisticated technology available, the fastest growth desired, and any other objective the hospital's decision-makers may have.

However, as Dowling (6) and the discussion in the previous section point out, the method by which hospitals are paid is far less important in determining system costs than is the sensitivity of purchasers to the amount that is paid. Thus, as Dowling [p. 261 in ref. (6)] has stated: "The prevailing methods of payment have not caused the rapid rise of costs, but they have facilitated the rise by financing the pursuit of other objectives."

Pauly & Drake (66) reported some empirical results that provide at least weak support for the proposition that differences in method of payment alone do not substantially affect costs. These authors examined hospital performance in four midwestern states operating under Blue Cross plans with differing reimbursement methods. Two of the four plans paid on the basis of charges and two paid on the basis of incurred costs. No significant differences appeared on various cost and performance measures across the four states. The conclusions of the study, however, must be qualified to some extent because the authors had to rely on relatively aggregate secondary data sources. In addition, the study hospitals' revenues typically came from many sources. Thus, Blue Cross payments as a proportion of total revenue varied widely across the sample. This characteristic of the hospital industry renders any empirical analysis of the impact of alternative reimbursement strategies very difficult.

Allowable costs   One of the greatest problems in implementing a cost-based reimbursement system is the determination of which costs are allowable and how they are to be measured. Virtually no existing system is without a set of rules detailing which costs will be reimbursed and how allowable costs are to be defined and calculated. The rules differ across payers, as described in an earlier section. These rule differences often raise equity concerns. If Medicare disallows a particular component of capital costs because of a restrictive definition of depreciation, will the hospital simply load those costs onto the bills of other patients?

Monitoring costs   Another problem with this type of payment is the cost of monitoring hospital performance. To assure that payment rules are followed (and to minimize the kind of cost shifting outlined above), most payers engage in at least a minimal amount of cost monitoring. This may extend only to receiving and filing detailed cost reports or periodic audits, or it may be a larger effort. In either case, with several thousands of providers, the costs of these activities can be substantial and must be counted into the cost of conducting business in this fashion.

ADVANTAGES   The use of cost reimbursement contracts is not restricted to the hospital industry (62). Cost contracts are found in development, research, and consulting activities, in construction, defense weaponry, and in many other areas in which the exact characteristics of the product to be purchased are difficult to specify a priori. This form of contracting is chosen because of its flexibility: product specifications can be changed mid-contract without expensive renegotiations of product price. In addition, it provides the maximum incentive for high quality output. The producer is never induced to make quality trade-offs to lower production cost unless explicitly requested to do so by the purchaser. Finally, the burden of upward changes in costs falls on the purchaser. Where cost conditions are uncertain or changing rapidly, the purchaser can "buy" the assurance of access to supply by transferring these risks of doing business to herself.

COST CONTAINMENT EFFORTS

Alarmed by the rapid escalation in total costs during the post-Medicare period, many payers have directed increasing efforts toward developing strategies for containing their financial liabilities without unduly reducing the package of covered services offered to beneficiaries. With the exception of several prospective reimbursement experiments, which are discussed in a later section, these attempts have focused primarily on limiting the "blank check" approach to cost reimbursement. The federal government interceded briefly with the Economic Stabilization Program in the early 1970s, and a number of states have legislated their own mandatory cost containment programs (67). Finally, a new round of controls at the federal level are under active consideration in the Ninety-sixth Congress (68).

Controls on Charges: The Economic Stabilization Program

The Economic Stabilization Program (ESP) was introduced by the federal government in 1971 as an attempt to restrain price increases in the economy generally. In the hospital industry, the exact form of controls changed over the ESP period, leading to some confusion among industry firms (69) and possibly resulting in a reduction in the effectiveness of the program. Generally, the controls took the form of limitations on price increases for hospital services, with average per diem costs serving as prices for cost payers.

THE ARGUMENTS   The conceptual arguments in favor of price controls as a means of cooling inflation are weak. Evidence from other industries consistently indicates that at best they are ineffective in the long run (though costly to administer); at worst they lead to shortages, uncertainty, and black markets (70). When applied to products as complex as hospital services, the former result typically applies because the ability of the firm to escape the controls by redefining the product is practically limitless (71). For example, services previously included in the room and board charge can be split off and billed separately. Procedures that could be performed in one visit can be drawn out over two visits. It is possible that the total costs (including time, transportation, and inconvenience) are actually increased as firms find ways out from under the price lids (71).

Another disadvantage of price controls as a long-term strategy to cost containment is that they address the symptoms, not the problem. To the extent that unit and total cost increases are caused by increasing demand for hospital services (for whatever reason), artificial restrictions on price will not solve the problem because they do not dampen demand. To achieve long term stability of prices and expenditures, some means of controlling pressure from the demand side must be found.

THE EVIDENCE   The ESP program lasted only three years. Good empirical evidence on its effects is not readily available. Of the major studies that have been conducted of this period (4, 69, 72–77), a number address only conceptual issues or make predictions about cost savings using data from other periods; the evidence is somewhat conflicting among the remaining studies. Ginsburg (69) and Lave & Lave (75) concluded that the direct effects of ESP were insignificant. Altman & Eichenholz (72) and Schlenker & McNeil (77) reported significant decreases in the rate of increase of selected hospital prices. The semiprivate room rate price rose 13.3% annually from 1969 to 1971; 5.4% between November 1971 and November 1972 [p. 87 in ref. (77)]. However, the rates of increase of expense per patient day and total hospital expenditures slowed relatively less: from 13.2% in fiscal year 1971 to 12.4% in fiscal year 1972 for expenses per day, and from 13.5% in 1971 to 10.5% in 1972 for total expenditures [p. 87 in ref. (77)]. Schlenker & McNeil (77) noted further that prices had peaked in 1970 and were declining before the beginning of the ESP. Thus, observations of price and cost decreases must be viewed with caution.

Controls on Costs: The Prudent Buyer Approach

The major cost payers, namely Blue Cross plans and the federal government, have tried various mechanisms to contain their outlays by placing restrictions on reimbursable costs.

MEDICARE   The first Medicare attempt to reduce costs was the elimination in 1969 of the original 2% plus factor on total costs (19). The Medicare and Medicaid Amendments of 1972 further modified the payment system (64). Section 223 of those amendments authorized the Secretary of the Department of Health, Education and Welfare to set prospective limits on reasonable costs, based on estimates of the costs necessary in the efficient delivery of patient care. The guidelines are fairly general: Limits can be set for groups of hospitals, for all costs or a subset, and can be established on a per diem, per case, or other method. As a result of this provision, the Secretary has published a set of limits every year since 1974 (78). Though the method of determining the limits has changed somewhat over time, at present the limits are set on routine costs per day (i.e. ancillary service costs are excluded) for each of several groups of hospitals. The groups are formed by cross-classifying hospitals into cells according to bed size, urban or rural location, and area per capita income (78). The dollar value of the limit is calculated by arraying the hospitals in each group by their past year's reported routine per diem cost, finding the cost at the eightieth percentile, and adding to it 10% of the group median cost. An inflation factor is then applied to project this figure into the current reporting period. Hospitals are paid reported costs up to the limit. A hospital whose routine per diem costs exceed this amount receives only the limit per diem. Ancillary costs continue to be reimbursed on a reported cost basis. Fitzmaurice (79) reported that an estimated 11.5% of all hospitals are affected by the limit, although an appeals mechanism is available.

Another limitation on allowable costs for Medicare and Medicaid reimbursement was established by Section 221 of the 1972 Amendments (70). This section, called the 1122 review program, disallows all capital costs associated with certain capital expenditures exceeding $100,000 that do not receive prior approval from a local health planning body. The limitation is aimed at reducing hospital investment under the assumption that reduced industry capacity also means lower operating costs and therefore lower federal outlays for service programs.

BLUE CROSS   The federal 1122 program had a precedent in the private sector. A number of Blue Cross plans across the country had written "conformance clauses" into their hospital reimbursement contracts well before the 1122 program began (80). The conformance clauses conditioned payment of certain capital costs on prior planning agency approval.

In addition to these limitations, various Blue Cross plans have attempted to restrict reimbursable cost through exclusions of expense categories like charity and bad debts, nonpatient care activities, and other specific categories deemed unrelated to Blue Cross subscriber well-being. Blue Cross plans have also entered into prospective reimbursement experiments. These are discussed below.

EFFECTS   This somewhat piecemeal approach to controlling expenditures through the cost reimbursement mechanism has dissatisfied many observers (64). Many have judged it to be ineffective in generating substantial savings or in promoting large increases in system efficiency. Critics also point out the cross-payer equity problems noted earlier.

These criticisms must be viewed with caution. Although it is true that no one has reported significant drops in Medicare expenditures since the implementation of the 223 limits or significant increases in occupancy rates from reduced investment following the 1122 controls, the prudent buyer approach to cost reimbursement has a number of advantages.

Rarely is there an objective that our public policy seeks to pursue without qualification. So it is with cost containment in the hospital industry. Strategies that are more successful in reducing unit costs and total expenditures limit, by definition, the resources that flow to the industry. When this happens, industry firms have no choice, in the absence of gross operating inefficiencies in prior periods, but to respond by reducing the services they produce. There is no evidence of technical inefficiencies in hospitals sufficiently great to withstand significant cutbacks in revenue without cutting services.

Some observers (81, 82) would welcome a trade-off of services for lower costs, but their views would not be shared at every level. The prudent buyer approach to cost-based reimbursement retains the incentives for high quality and ready access without ignoring altogether the issue of expense. In this complex industry in which the precise product to be delivered varies with each patient, the prudent buyer approach provides a payment mechanism that allows the purchaser to broadly specify the kind of output that is desired (e.g. no teaching, no research) and generally the acceptable price range (e.g. no payments will be made above this defined limit), while assuring equitable treatment of the provider and thus the financial health of the industry in the long run. The price of this approach is that some "slippage" will occur. Hospital decision makers will perhaps choose more sophisticated or expensive equipment than might do the job. Patients may get more tests than would be adequate to make the same diagnosis, and they may be discharged a few days later. Capital assets may sit idle a larger percentage of the time. The alternative is to trade-off the quality enhancing incentives for stronger cost-minimizing incentives. The extent to which this is desirable may differ greatly among payers. It is clearly a policy issue well beyond the scope of this chapter.

A Middle Ground: Prospective Reimbursement

An approach that appears to be gaining increasing favor with Blue Cross plans, many state governments, and some federal policy makers is a kind of middle ground between the payment of charges and the reimbursement of incurred costs. The generic term for this approach is prospective reimbursement (sometimes called incentive reimbursement). Its manifestation takes many forms. Basically, it refers to a payment system in which the amount to be reimbursed per unit is determined prior to the service delivery period (as with charges), but it is based on actual, relative, or projected costs (as with cost reimbursement). As a result, it has some of the advantages and disadvantages of each. Like a charge-based system, the provider, not the purchaser, bears the burden of unanticipated cost-increasing factors. Once the payment limit has been determined, the provider's incentive is to stay within the limit. This can be done by increasing efficiency, reducing quality, shifting costs to other payers who do not impose limits, or some combination of all of these. Like a cost-based system, the purchaser pays only for the direct costs of service. Contributions to reserves for future expansion and new technology, to charity care, or to teaching activities are made only if allowed by the payer.

Few other general comments can be made about this approach because the incentives are so dependent on the particular design of the program (63).

PROGRAM DESIGN ISSUES   There are a number of critical program design issues that determine the ability of a prospective reimbursement system to achieve desired results without severe and unwanted side effects. Many conceptual papers have been written discussing these issues in detail (5-7, 53, 63, 64, 67, 70, 79, 83-94). Their conclusions are summarized here.

There are four basic design questions, each with a number of important side issues. What costs should be included in the reimbursement base? For what unit of output should the reimbursement rate or limit be set? How should the rate or limit be determined? How are differences between actual costs and the payment rate shared between the provider and the payer? There are no universally correct answers to these questions because there are no universally accepted objectives. Thus, in the discussion that follows, the important design decisions to be made are cataloged and their expected effects are examined, but no judgments as to the desirability of any particular approach are given.

Allowable costs   The question of which costs to include in the reimbursement base generally focuses on the treatment of four categories: teaching costs, capital costs, contributions to the growth and development fund, and charity and bad debts. The decision for each category must be based primarily on policy judgments and existing complementary constraints such as certificate of need controls. Sometimes, as with the Medicare program, ancillary service costs are not covered by the prospective limit. Because this is the area in which most of the interpatient variation in costs per case occurs, a more uniform (and therefore less expensive) control can typically be applied to the remaining routine costs. However, this also reduces the potential for cost savings. A difficulty in the implementation of payment systems that include ancillary service costs in the prospective rate is the measurement of the diagnostic mix of patients served by each hospital. Because much of the cross-patient variation in the use of ancillary services can be explained by the admitting diagnosis (93), an equitable payment based on average costs across all patients must account in some fashion for interhospital differences in diagnostic mix. At the present time, however, accepted techniques for adequately characterizing this dimension of hospital output are not readily available (93).

Unit of output   The choice of the unit of output upon which to establish the payment rate greatly affects the behavior of the firm and the nature of its product (7, 63, 71, 90, 92). In each case, the hospital can moderate the constraint it faces by substituting uncontrolled product characteristics for controlled product characteristics. Thus, per diem reimbursement encourages increased length of stay with a decrease in intensity of service (i.e. cost) per day. Per case reimbursement encourages an expansion in the number of cases treated and a decrease in average intensity and/or length of stay per case. Total budget reimbursement has no volume increasing incentives unless volume adjustments are allowed.

Payment rate   The question of how to determine the payment rate itself has many components. Rates can be set based on the past performance of each individual hospital or on the past performance of a group of hospitals. The former has the advantage of flexibility and equitable treatment of unlike institutions; the latter allows for performance comparisons to avoid subsidies of inefficient operations. There are two major criticisms of the group approach. First, it may be difficult to find sufficiently similar hospitals for their comparison to be both fair and useful. Further, how is similarity to be defined (7)? How is it to be measured (7, 91, 93, 94)? The second criticism is that comparisons based on observed past performance only identify relative inefficiencies (55). If costs are "too high" in all hospitals, empirical standards are biased. However, in the absence of accepted objective standards of efficiency, empirical standards are all that exist.

A number of approaches have been suggested for turning the individual or group standards into per unit rates. These include the regression approach (55), the negotiated budget approach (86), the percentage of the mean approach (64), and the formula approach (95). The regression approach estimates a cost function for all hospitals or for each group of hospitals. The regression coefficients are then used in conjunction with the hospital's individual values for the independent variables to yield a reimbursement rate for each institution. This approach has the advantage of allowing continuous adjustment for cost-influencing variables, and it is relatively inexpensive to administer. However, this approach has the disadvantage that agreement has not yet been reached on the appropriate form for the regression, especially with regard to the independent variables that should be included.

The negotiated budget approach treats each hospital separately. The rates are determined only secondarily to the approval of the overall budget of the institution based on projected volumes. This is probably the most flexible system; it is also the most expensive to administer. In addition, given the inescapable immersion of the payer or regulator in the specific circumstances of each individual institution in the review process, third party objectivity is difficult to maintain. Because of these factors, a number of modified negotiated budget review systems have been attempted. For example, full scale budget review can take place at several year intervals with payment rates determined by a more aggregate approach in the intervening year. Another modification may be to require detailed budget review for only those institutions whose cost experience is significantly higher than that of similar facilities.

The percentage of the mean approach essentially sets the reimbursement level as some function of the average experience of all hospitals or all similar hospitals. As Lave et al (55) have pointed out, this approach induces hospitals with below average costs to raise costs as well as encouraging high cost hospitals to decrease costs. The resulting upward trend of the group mean over time reduces system savings.

The formula approach projects historical costs into the future by multiplying the share of each cost category (e.g. labor, food, fuel) by the projected local inflation rate for that category during the period in question. This assures that hospitals facing the same markets for purchased inputs are treated equally. However, the inflation projections are costly to obtain and frequently suffer from inaccuracies. In addition, straight pass-throughs of such costs as wage increases weaken the hospital's incentive to negotiate carefully at the bargaining table. Further, rapid price changes or changes in technology alter the share of various categories in total costs. Thus, the share weights must be recalculated periodically.

Surpluses The final question relates to the treatment of surpluses resulting from cost reductions below the reimbursement limit. If the surplus is retained by the hospital, the purchaser gains nothing. If the purchaser reclaims the entire amount, either directly or by reducing the cost base for future years, the hospital's incentive to achieve these efficiencies is lost. Further, if the institution's nonprofit legal status prevents the distribution of these surpluses to owners, and the planning agencies prevent their investment in new plant and equipment, what incentives does the hospital have to earn them at all?

There are obviously more design issues that must be faced in implementing a prospective payment system, and various combinations of the above approaches can be used. The important point is that the incentives inherent in the design parameters must be recognized so that appropriate choices can be made.

EMPIRICAL EVIDENCE   A number of prospective reimbursement programs have been established. Some, like the Indiana program, are run by private organizations (Blue Cross, in this case) and are voluntary. Others, like those in New York, Maryland, Massachusetts, Washington, and New Jersey are run by state governments under legislative authority. The empirical evidence regarding the effects of some of these programs is incomplete, but increasing (54, 95–109). A detailed account of this evidence, because it covers a wide variety of diverse programs, is beyond the scope of this chapter. An evaluation of the results of these published studies would thus require a complete understanding of the detailed design of each program.

In general the evidence is inconclusive. A number of authors have reported estimates of cost savings resulting from the programs. O'Donoghue's (106) estimate for Indiana is $200 million from 1968 to 1973. The Health Care Financing Administration (109) has published a summary of the results of five prospective reimbursement evaluation studies. The studies were conducted on prospective payment systems of different types in Rhode Island, western Pennsylvania, New Jersey, upstate New York, and downstate New York. The estimates of savings per hospital day from the programs ranged from 1% in upstate New York to 4% in downstate New York. When calculated on a per admission basis, the estimates ranged from 2% in upstate New York to 3.1% in Rhode Island. However, in many cases, the statistical significance of the estimated impact is low (98, 109). Further, very few complete analyses of the side effects of the payment systems have been undertaken. O'Donoghue (106), Dowling (98), and Lave et al (55) are exceptions. O'Donoghue (106) found few side effects in Indiana. Dowling (98) reported from New York that hospitals increased the average length of patient stay in response to the per diem control in that state. Lave et al

(55) concluded that western Pennsylvania hospitals, in response to changes in the reimbursement system, altered the diagnostic mix of patients treated. It should be noted, however, that these studies were almost uniformly conducted when the evaluated programs were in their infancy. Further cost savings may accrue over time as program administrators gain experience and as institutions have more time to respond to the new incentives. Thus, additional research is needed to examine the long-term effects of incentive reimbursement.

Estimates of the administrative costs of running the programs typically do not exist. This is becoming an important consideration, especially for the government-sponsored programs. In addition, suppliers incur costs in complying with (or appealing) the restrictions imposed by these programs. The addition of an accountant to allocate department costs as specified or clerical staff to complete required forms are examples. Anecdotal evidence suggests that these costs may be substantial in some cases. Future evaluations of the benefits of prospective payment systems must certainly take these administrative costs into account.

At this point, an overall conclusion as to the desirability and effectiveness of prospective payment systems is premature. Documented experience appears to vary, but little work has been done to examine the relationship between this variation in program success and the design and implementation of the payment system. Further research and experimentation is needed to determine the potential of incentive reimbursement for the improvement of industry performance.

SUMMARY AND CONCLUSION

The form and amount of reimbursement that a purchaser offers to the supplier of a good or service determines the nature of the product received. This chapter has outlined the dominant methods of reimbursement in the hospital industry and examined the special industry features that set these methods, and their accompanying problems, apart from those in other sectors of the economy. The advantages and disadvantages of the two major forms, charge-based reimbursement and incurred cost reimbursement, were discussed. Finally, efforts to constrain expenditures were listed and their effects were examined. Prospective reimbursement, a relatively new payment method that has been used in both private and public settings, was examined. Throughout the discussion, existing empirical evidence was brought to bear on the arguments.

The primary conclusion that can be drawn from the existing research is that no single reimbursement system performs best in all settings or assures the achievement of all objectives. The payment system offers only one constraint; in the delivery of a multi-faceted service, this is simply not enough control for the purchaser to assure that all dimensions of that service are as desired. Each reimbursement alternative carries with it different incentives for the provider. When those incentives induce provider behavior that is contrary to the desires of the purchaser, the purchaser has three options: bear the adverse consequences, change to another method of reimbursement (with other undesirable incentives), or add more constraints. The alternative that best serves the interests of the purchaser differs in each case depending upon what those interests are, what alternative reimbursement methods are available (and the nature of their disadvantages), and the expected ability of additional constraints to reduce the undesired activities.

In the market for hospital services, two important output dimensions are cost and access. A reimbursement system that is most effective at containing the cost of the product may also have the worst side effects on access. Alternatively, the system that most effectively encourages the ready accessibility of high quality output may also result in the highest costs. The relative importance of the two objectives must therefore be established. The optimal reimbursement system in this situation represents a compromise between the competing goals. System costs are likely to be higher when access is of no concern; access will be less when cost is of no concern. However, the reduction (increase) in accessibility (cost) can be lessened by applying secondary constraints to the system rather than relying solely on the reimbursement constraint. Cost ceilings, such as those embodied in Medicare's 223 program, and quality monitors, like Professional Standards Review Organizations, are examples of such side constraints. Further, because the importance of cost containment relative to assured accessibility may differ across payers, there is no reason to suppose that the reimbursement scheme that is appropriate for a Blue Cross plan is also best for Medicare, Medicaid, or other payers.

Finally, many of these decisions hinge upon policy judgments, not on technical ones. Thus, the advice of the expert is essential in some areas and irrelevant in others. When the question relates to the experience of an existing program or to the identification of the likely side effects of an available constraint, the expert's testimony is of utmost value. When the question is one of how much Blue Cross subscribers are willing to pay for increased flexibility in the choice of a provider, or how much does society wish to subsidize the education of medical professionals, expert testimony can come only from consumers. The most appropriate method of extracting this expertise is a challenge that remains.

Literature Cited

1. Gibson, R. M., Fisher, C. R. 1978. National health expenditures, fiscal year 1977. *Soc. Secur. Bull.* 41(7):3–20
2. Am. Hosp. Assoc. 1976. *Hospital Statistics.* Chicago: AHA. 206 pp.
3. Feldstein, P. J. 1977. Forecasts and costs in the hospital sector. *Proc. Health Care in the Am. Econ., 1st, Hilton Head, SC,* 1976, pp. 23–63
4. Scitovsky, A., McCall, N. 1976. *Changes in the Costs of Treatment of Selected Illnesses: 1951–1964–1971.* Res. Dig. Ser. Natl. Cent. Health Serv. Res. Washington DC: GPO. 15 pp.
5. Richardson, W. C. 1979. Financing health services. In *Health Services and Medical Care,* ed. S. J. Williams, P. R. Torrens. New York: Wiley. In press
6. Dowling, W. L. 1977. Hospital reimbursement. See Ref. 3, pp. 256–77
7. Klastorin, T. D., Watts, C. A., Trivedi, V. 1979. *A Study of the Classification of Hospitals for Prospective Reimbursement.* Rep. No. 10, Health Care Financ. Res. Demonstr. Ser. Washington DC: GPO. 125 pp.
8. Phelps, C. E. 1977. Insurance benefits and their impact on health care costs. See Ref. 3, pp. 230–48
9. 42 US Code § 1395. 1976 ed.
10. Acton, J. P. 1976. Demand for health care among the urban poor, with special emphasis on the role of time. In *The Role of Health Insurance in the Health Services Sector,* ed. R. N. Rosett, pp. 165–207. New York: Natl. Bur. Econ. Res. 548 pp.
11. Davis, K., Russell, L. B. 1972. The substitution of hospital outpatient care for inpatient care. *Rev. Econ. Stat.* 54(2):109–20
12. Joseph, H. 1972. Hospital insurance and moral hazard. *J. Hum. Resour.* 7(2):152–61
13. Phelps, C. E., Newhouse, J. P. 1972. Effects of coinsurance: A multivariate analysis. *Soc. Secur. Bull.* 35(6):20–28
14. Russell, L. B. 1973. An econometric model of the Medicare system. *Q. J. Econ.* 87(3):482–89
15. Russell, L. B. 1973. The impact of the extended-care facility benefit on hospital use and reimbursement under Medicare. *J. Hum. Resour.* 8(1):57–72
16. Williams, R. 1966. A comparison of hospital utilization and costs by types of coverage. *Inquiry* 3(3):28–42
17. Klarman, H. E. 1969. Reimbursing the hospital—the difference the third party makes. *J. Risk Ins.* 36(5):553–66

18. Berman, H. J., Weeks, L. E. 1976. *The Financial Management of Hospitals,* pp. 120–28. Ann Arbor: Health Adm. Press. 674 pp. 3rd ed.
19. Comm. on Finance, U.S. Senate 1970. *Medicare and Medicaid: Problems, Issues, and Alternatives,* Rep. of the Staff, 91st Congr.; 1st session. Washington DC: GPO. 323 pp.
20. Weisbrod, B. A. 1977. *The Voluntary Non-Profit Sector,* pp. 51–76. Lexington: Heath. 179 pp.
21. Feldstein, M. S. 1971. *The Rising Cost of Hospital Care.* Washington DC: Inf. Resour. Press. 88 pp.
22. Lee, M. L. 1971. A conspicuous production theory of hospital behavior. *South. Econ. J.* 38(1):48–58
23. Lee, M. L. 1972. Interdependent behavior and resource misallocation in hospital care production. *Rev. Soc. Econ.* 30(1):84–95
24. Newhouse, J. P. 1970. Toward a theory of non-profit institutions: An economic model of a hospital. *Am. Econ. Rev.* 60(2):64–74
25. Pauly, M. V., Redisch, M. 1973. The not-for-profit hospital as a physicians cooperative. *Am. Econ. Rev.* 63(1):87–99
26. Reder, M. V. 1965. Some problems in the economics of hospitals. *Am. Econ. Rev.* 55(2):472–80
27. Shalit, S. S. 1977. A doctor-hospital cartel theory. *J. Bus.* 50:1–21
28. Watts, C. A. 1976. *A managerial discretion model for hospitals.* PhD thesis. Johns Hopkins Univ., Baltimore. 120 pp.
29. Davis, K. 1972. Economic theories of behavior in private, non-profit hospitals. *Econ. Bus. Bull.* 24(2):1–13
30. Pauly, M. V. 1974. Hospital capital investment: The roles of demand, profits, and physicians. *J. Hum. Resour.* 9(1):7–20
31. Baron, D. P. 1974. A study of hospital cost inflation. *J. Hum. Resour.* 9(1):33–49
32. Berry, R. E. 1974. Cost and efficiency in the production of hospital services. *Milbank Mem. Fund Q.* 52(3):291–313
33. Davis, K. 1972. Rising hospital costs: Possible causes and cures. *Bull. NY Acad. Med.* 48(11):1354–71
34. Davis, K. 1974. The role of technology, demand, and labor markets in the determination of hospital cost. In *The Economics of Health and Medical Care,* ed. M. Perlman, pp. 283–301. London: Macmillan. 547 pp.

35. Davis, K. 1973. Theories of hospital inflation: Some empirical evidence. *J. Hum. Resour* 8(2):181–201
36. Evans, R. G. 1971. Behavioral cost functions for hospitals. *Can. J. Econ.* 4(2):198–215
37. Feldstein, M. S. 1974. Econometric studies of health economics. In *Frontiers of Quantitative Economics*, Vol. 2, ed. M. D. Intrilligator, D. A. Kendrick, pp. 377–447. Amsterdam: North-Holland. 580 pp.
38. Feldstein, M. S. 1971. Hospital cost inflation: A study of nonprofit price dynamics. *Am. Econ. Rev.* 61(5):835–72
39. Feldstein, M. S., Schuttinga, J. 1977. Hospital costs in Massachusetts: A methodological study. *Inquiry* 14(1): 22–31
40. Lave, J. R., Lave, L. B. 1970. Estimated cost functions for Pennsylvania hospitals. *Inquiry* 7(2):3–14
41. Lave, J. R., Lave, L. B. 1970. Hospital cost functions. *Am. Econ. Rev.* 60(3): 379–95
42. Lee, M. L., Wallace, R. L. 1973. Problems in estimating multiproduct cost functions: an application to hospitals. *W. Econ. J.* 11:350–63
43. Salkever, D. S. 1972. A microeconomic study of hospital cost inflation. *J. Polit. Econ.* 80(6):1144–66
44. Hartman, R., Watts, C. A. 1978. The determination of average hospital length of stay. *Q. Rev. Econ. Bus.* 18(3): 83–96
45. Davis, K. 1971. Relationship of hospital prices to costs. *Appl. Econ.* 3:115–25
46. Feldstein, P. J., Waldman, S. 1969. The financial position of hospitals in the first two years of Medicare. *Inquiry* 6(1): 19–27
47. Hellinger, F. J. 1975. Hospital charges and Medicare reimbursement. *Inquiry* 7(4):313–19
48. Etzioni, A., Doty, P. 1976. Profit in not-for-profit corporations: The example of health care. *Polit. Sci. Q.* 91(4):433–55
49. Cohen, H. 1974. *Issues in state rate regulation.* Presented at Conf. on Regulation in the Health Industry, Washington DC
50. Posner, R. A. 1971. Taxation by regulation. *Bell J. Econ.* 2(1):22–50
51. Newhouse, J. P., Phelps, C. E. 1974. Price and income elasticities for medical care services. See Ref. 34, pp. 139–61
52. Rafferty, J. A. 1971. Patterns of hospital use: An analysis of short run variations. *J. Polit. Econ.* 79(1):154–65
53. Bauer, K. G. 1973. *Containing Costs of Health Services Through Incentive Reimbursement.* Boston: Harvard Univ. Press
54. Elnicki, R. A. 1975. SSA—Connecticut hospital incentive reimbursement experiment cost evaluation. *Inquiry* 12(1):47–58
55. Lave, J. R., Lave, L. B., Silverman, L. P. 1973. A proposal for incentive reimbursement for hospitals. *Med. Care* 11(2):79–90
56. Goldberg, L. G., Greenberg, W. G. 1977. The effect of physician controlled health insurance. *J. Health Polit. Policy Law* 2(2):48–78
57. Somers, A. R. 1969. *Hospital Regulation: The Dilemma of Public Policy,* pp. 162–91. Princeton: Princeton Univ. Press. 240 pp.
58. Havighurst, C. C. 1973. Regulation of health facilities and services by certificate of need. *Va. Law. Rev.* 59:1143–1242
59. Hellinger, F. J. 1976. The effect of certificate of need legislation on hospital investment. *Inquiry* 8(2):187–93
60. Salkever, D. S., Bice, T. W. 1976. The impact of certificate of need controls on hospital investment. *Health Soc.* 54(2): 185–212
61. Ginsburg, P. B. 1972. Resource allocation in the hospital industry: The role of capital financing. *Soc. Secur. Bull.* 35(10):20–30
62. Goldberg, V. P. 1976. Regulation and administered contracts. *Bell J. Econ.* 7(2):426–88
63. Dowling, W. L. 1974. Prospective reimbursement of hospitals. *Inquiry* 11(3): 163–80
64. Holohan, J., Spitz, B., Pollak, W., Feder, J. 1977. *Altering Medicaid Provider Reimbursement Methods,* pp. 39–102. Washington DC: Urban Inst. 215 pp.
65. McCarthy, C. 1975. Incentive reimbursement as an impetus to cost containment. *Inquiry* 13(4):320–29
66. Pauly, M. V., Drake, D. F. 1970. Effect of third party reimbursement on hospital performance. In *Empirical Studies in Health Economics,* ed. H. E. Klarman, pp. 297–314. Baltimore: Johns Hopkins Univ. Press. 443 pp.
67. Watts, C. A., Updegraff, G. E., Bryant, A., Grayson, H. 1975. *Cost and Price Regulation: Background Discussion and Annotated Bibliography.* Denver: Spectrum Res. 140 pp.
68. Dunn, W., Lefkowitz, B. 1978. The hospital cost containment act of 1977: An analysis of the administration's proposal. In *Hospital Cost Containment,*

ed. M. Zubkoff, I. E. Raskin, pp. 167–216. New York: Prodist. 656 pp.

69. Ginsburg, P. B. 1978. Impact of the economic stabilization program on hospitals: An analysis with aggregate data. See Ref. 68, pp. 293–323

70. O'Donoghue, P. 1974. *Evidence About the Effects of Health Care Regulation,* pp. 47–58. Denver: Spectrum Res. 202 pp.

71. Barzel, Y. 1976. An alternative approach to the analysis of taxation. *J. Polit. Econ.* 84(6):1177–98

72. Altman, S. H., Eichenholz, J. 1973. *Control of Health Care Costs Under the Economic Stabilization Program.* Washington DC: Cost of Living Counc. 41 pp.

73. Elnicki, R. A. 1972. Effect of phase II price controls on hospital services. *Health Serv. Res.* 7(2):106–17

74. Horowitz, L. 1973. Medical care price changes under the economic stabilization program. *Soc. Secur. Bull.* 36(3): 28–34

75. Lave, J. R., Lave, L. B. 1978. Hospital cost function analysis: Implications for cost controls. See Ref. 68, pp. 538–71

76. Lipscomb, J., Raskin, I. E., Eichenholz, J. 1978. The use of marginal cost analysis estimates in hospital cost containment policy. See Ref. 68, pp. 514–37

77. Schlenker, R. E., McNeil, R. 1973. *Phase II and Phase III Controls on the Hospital Sector.* Minneapolis: Interstudy. 49 pp.

78. 43 Fed. Reg. 43558–43564. September 26, 1978

79. Fitzmaurice, J. M. 1976. *An Evaluation of Alternative Systems of Establishing Hospital Reimbursement Limits Under Medicare.* Washington DC: Heath Care Financ. Admin.

80. Watts, C. A., Updegraff, G. E. 1975. *Regulation of Capital Expenditures: Background Discussion and Annotated Bibliography.* Denver: Spectrum Res. 111 pp.

81. Somers, A. R. 1977. Comments on Feldstein's presentation. See Ref. 3, pp. 68–78

82. Carlson, R. 1975. *The End of Medicine.* New York: Wiley. 290 pp.

83. Chassin, M. R. 1978. The containment of hospital costs: A strategic assessment. *Med. Care* 16: Suppl. 10, pp. 36–45

84. Hardwick, C. P., Wolfe, H. 1970. Incentive reimbursement. *Med. Care* 8(3):173–88

85. McCann, W. F. 1973. Regulating costs —the cost ceiling approach. In *Regulat-*

ing the Hospital, a Report of the 1972 National Forum on Hospital and Health Affairs, pp. 55–65. Durham: Duke Univ. Press. 133 pp.

86. McGavin, E. P. 1973. Regulating costs —the budget review approach. See Ref. 85 pp. 29–41

87. Prussin, J. A., Wood, J. C. 1975. Private third party reimbursement—cost containment mechanisms. *Top. Health Care Financ.* 2(1):47–64

88. Rafferty, J. 1971. A comment on incentive reimbursement. *Med. Care* 9(4): 518–20

89. Shuman, L. J., Wolfe, H., Hardwick, C. P. 1972. Predictive hospital reimbursement and evaluation model. *Inquiry* 9(2):17–33

90. Worthington, P. N. 1977. Prospective reimbursement rates for hospitals—by unit of service versus type of case. *Q. Rev. Econ. Bus.* 17:65–72

91. Berry, R. E. 1973. On grouping hospitals for economic analysis. *Inquiry* 10(4):5–12

92. Cohen, H. A. 1973. Cost functions of hospitals diagnostic procedures: A possible argument for diagnostic centres. *J. Econ. Bus.* 25(2):83–88

93. Fetter, R., Thompson, J., Mills, R. 1976. A system for cost and reimbursement control in hospitals. *Yale J. Biol. Med.* 49:123–36

94. Ro, K. K., Auster, R. 1969. An output approach to incentive reimbursement for hospitals. *Health Serv. Res.* 4(3): 177–78

95. Berry, R. E. 1976. Prospective rate reimbursement and cost: Formula reimbursement in New York. *Inquiry* 13(3): 289–301

96. Bauer, K. G. 1976. Hospital rate setting —this way to salvation? See Ref. 68, pp. 324–69

97. Cohen, H. A. 1978. Experiences of a state cost control commission. See Ref. 68, pp. 401–28

98. Dowling, W. L. 1976. Prospective reimbursement in downstate New York and its impact on hospitals—a summary. *Center for Health Services Research Discussion Paper No. 3.* Univ. Washington, Seattle

99. May, D. 1975. A report on prospective reimbursement in Connecticut. *Hosp. Prog.* 56(9):93–96

100. Hall, C. P., Henemier, S. M., Raphaelson, A. H. 1977. Some issues in limiting hospital cost reimbursement: A Maryland experience. *J. Risk Ins.* 44(2): 267–87

101. Hardwick, C. P., Wolfe, H. 1972. Evaluation of an incentive reimbursement experiment. *Med. Care* 10(2):109–17
102. Hellinger, F. J. 1977. Communication: Re-examining the Rhode Island experience with prospective reimbursement. *Inquiry* 14(2):189–92
103. Hellinger, F. J. 1978. An empirical analysis of several prospective reimbursement systems. See Ref. 68, pp. 370–400
104. Hellinger, F. J. 1976. Prospective reimbursement through budget review: New Jersey, Rhode Island, and Western Pennsylvania. *Inquiry* 13(3):309–20
105. Hersch, J. 1973. *A Case Study of Cost Containment: The State of New York.*

Washington DC: DHEW
106. O'Donoghue, P. 1978. *Controlling Hospital Costs: The Revealing Case of Indiana.* Denver: Policy Cent. 146 pp.
107. Worthington, P. N. 1976. Prospective reimbursement of hospitals to promote efficiency: New Jersey. *Inquiry* 13(3): 302–8
108. Zimmerman, H., Buechner, J., Thornberry, H. 1977. Prospective reimbursement in Rhode Island: Additional perspectives. *Inquiry* 14(1):3–16
109. Health Care Financ. Adm. 1977. *Research in Health Care Financing.* HEW Publ. No. (SSA) 77–11901. Washington DC: GPO

Ann. Rev. Public Health 1980. 1:121–36

PUBLIC HEALTH AND INDIVIDUAL LIBERTY

♦12505

Dan E. Beauchamp

Department of Health Administration, School of Public Health, University of North Carolina, Chapel Hill, North Carolina 27514

INTRODUCTION

The focus of this article is upon the growing tensions between the goals of protecting the public health and individual liberty. This issue is especially acute in the present period in which the limits of medicine in effecting substantial future improvements of the health of the public are widely discussed. The term "lifestyle" has entered the vocabulary of health policy.

The document that precipitated this shift in attention was undoubtedly Canada's *New Perspectives on the Health of Canadians* (1). Few policy documents in the field of health have been as influential or as widely quoted. Within the past five years a flood of editorials, articles, and books have proclaimed the new gospel. Leon Kass captured the spirit of the time in the title of his widely read article, "Regarding the End of Medicine and the Pursuit of Health" (2).

This new attention to lifestyle risks has contributed to a growing skepticism about the appropriateness and feasibility of a more activist public role in enhancing the public's health. Some feel that, aside from increased health education (3, 4), the government can or should do little to regulate or change the lifestyles of the American public. Because lifestyles are individual problems (so the argument goes), the legitimacy of governmental policy is questionable and its effectiveness weak. Aaron Wildavsky stated the position in this way (4):

> We are not talking about peripheral or infrequent aspects of human behavior. We are talking about some of the most deeply rooted and often experienced aspects of human life—what one eats, how often and how much; ... whether one smokes or drinks and how much; even the whole question of human personality. ... To oversee these decisions would require a larger bureaucracy than anyone has yet conceived and methods of surveillance bigger than big brother.

121

0163-7525/80/0510-0121$01.00

Tampering with the lifestyles of the public may seem patently paternalistic. As the authors of the *New Perspective on the Health of Canadians* remarked, there is in Canada a widespread sentiment that individuals should be free to "choose their own poison" (1). It is likely that this viewpoint is at least as prevalent in the US.

Even the right to health care now seems a potential casualty of the argument that medicine doesn't matter very much (2, 5, 6). Can equality be a goal of health care policy if so much depends on individual lifestyles? Perhaps the most articulate spokesman for this point of view is Leon Kass. Kass argues that there really is no way in which we can clearly speak of health as a right because health cannot be given by one to another (2). Health is a product of living wisely—the reward of individual duty and virtue (2).

The lifestyle controversy is a serious challenge for public health. If, as a community and a society, we are not justified in accepting reasonable governmental restrictions on lifestyle risks, a future in which early death and serious disability are sharply reduced may be beyond our grasp.

PUBLIC HEALTH AND PATERNALISM: THE DILEMMA OF VOLUNTARY RISKS

Perhaps the clearest recent treatments of paternalism in the philosophical literature are Gerald Dworkin's (7, 8). According to Dworkin, paternalism is "the interference with a person's liberty of action justified by reasons referring exclusively to the welfare, good, happiness, needs, interests or values of the person being coerced" (7). Paternalism is the restriction of the liberty of a class of individuals to confer a benefit on that same class of individuals (8). Dworkin's definitions strive to capture the essence of paternalism: the provision of benefits for the individuals' own good—benefits that individuals might not prefer (7, 8). A third criterion, which Dworkin discusses obliquely, is that individuals might obtain these benefits if they acted otherwise. Dworkin provides an illustrative list of policies that he defines as paternalistic (7, 8):

> Laws requiring motorcyclists to wear safety helmets when operating their machines; laws forbidding persons from swimming at a public beach when lifeguards are not on duty; laws regulating the use of certain drugs which may have harmful consequences to the user but do not lead to anti-social conduct; laws compelling people to spend a specified fraction of their income on the purchase of retirement annuities. . . .

As Feinberg notes, because there is a presumption for liberty in our society, limiting liberty has to be justified (9). Limiting the liberty of a class of individuals to confer a benefit on that same class is deemed suspect. Presumably, the individuals whose liberty is restricted may not prefer these benefits, as they could act otherwise (7, 8). We should limit liberty only to prevent harms to others or harms to some important public interest. This distinction has been made unforgettable in a famous quotation from John Stuart Mill's essay, *On Liberty* (10).

> The only purpose for which power can be rightfully exercised over any member of a civilized community, against his will, is to prevent harm to others. His own good, either physical or moral, is not sufficient warrant. He cannot rightfully be compelled to do or forbear because it will be better for him to do so, because it will make him happier, because, in the opinions of others, to do so would be wise or even right. These are good reasons for remonstrating with him, or reasoning with him, or persuading him, or entreating him, but not for compelling him or visiting him with any evil in case he do otherwise. To justify that, the conduct from which it is desired to deter him must be calculated to produce evil to some one else. The only part of the conduct of any one for which he is amenable to society is that which concerns others. In the part which merely concerns himself, his independence is, of right, absolute. Over himself, over his own body and mind, the individual is sovereign.

As Feinberg (9), Dworkin (7, 8), and others (9) have argued, both tradition and common sense make us unwilling to reject all forms of paternalism (6). The consensus appears to be that, indeed, we have come to accept at least weak (9) forms of paternalism, although we seem wary of expanding these specific instances beyond a short and familiar list. John Knowles, for example, listed governmental measures that he deemed acceptable to protect the health of the public: heavy taxation on alcohol and tobacco are at the head of the list (11). The *1977–1981 Forward Plan* of HEW gave prominent attention to prevention measures, including a number of limits to voluntary risks, such as taxation on alcohol and tobacco, the labeling of alcoholic beverages, restriction on advertising for a wide number of harmful products, etc (12). White singles out restrictions on drugs, diet, and automobile operation (13).

Richard Bonnie argues that the measures advocated exemplify the "new paternalism" (14). Bonnie sees many of these policies as justified because they provide substantial aggregate savings in lives and serious disability, yet they involve only minimal restrictions on individual choice (14). In the case of drugs (including alcohol), he mentions three permissible forms of "weak paternalism": (*a*) altering the conditions of availability of harmful substances, (*b*) deterring individual behavior through (mild) punishment (e.g. fines for smoking in public places), (*c*) symbolizing the posture of the government toward the behavior, and (*d*) influencing the content of messages in the mass media (14).

Thus, although there is concern and anxiety in public health about the appropriate scope and role of government regarding limits to voluntary risks, some argue that some forms of "weak paternalism" are justified (7–9, 11, 13, 14). Typically, these expansions of the government's power are

justified on the bases of the desired health consequences, historical precedent, and because they do not involve serious restriction of the public's
liberty. These authors do not so much attempt to resolve the dilemma of
paternalism as to argue that mild doses will not be so hard to take [but see
Etzioni (15) for a discussion of social influences over personal lifestyles].

Nevertheless, objections to paternalism, even in a weak form, remain
substantial and widespread. A recent monograph on ethical dilemmas in
lifestyle interventions found widespread concern by health professionals
and philosophers over the coercion involved in even weak paternalism,
including some forms of persuasion and community organization (3). It
seems likely that the controversy and quasi-legitimacy surrounding public
limits over self-regarding and voluntary risks will increase rather than
diminish.

Burdens on Society

The major alternative for a justifying principle to limit voluntary risks that
avoids paternalism is based on the utilitarian tradition. This alternative
points out the costs or secondary harms to others of voluntary risk-taking
(14, 16). These secondary harms or costs (economic burdens, usually) are
largely indirect in effect. Thus, the argument is made that we restrict
smokers' rights and privileges by taxation not to prevent harm to them, but
rather to prevent the burden or cost to society of excess morbidity or loss
of production. In the case of motorcycle helmet legislation, many courts
have adopted the *public ward* theory, arguing that the state is justified in
adopting these measures in order to reduce the cost of emergency services
and hospital costs, as well as the risk that crash victims who were not
wearing helmets will become wards of the state (14, 15, 16).

Clearly, John Kaplan points out, Mill would not find these arguments
very convincing because the notion of indirect or secondary harms is not
only vague, it is subject to limitless expansion (16). [The Hawaii court (14)
acknowledged this point in the motorcycle helmet issue.]

An extreme extension of this particular line of reasoning can be found
in a recent article in the *American Journal of Public Health* in which the
authors point out the cost of obesity to the nation's fuel bills (17). The
overweight, according to the authors, consume a substantial fraction of the
nation's fossil fuel because of the excess food they consume. This excess
consumption is quite costly to the society because as much as one fourth
of the nation's food bill is based on fuel costs (farm machinery, transportation, processing, etc) (17).

These economic justifications for saving lives are reminiscent of a slogan
attributed by Sartre to Polish public health officials: "Tuberculosis slows
down production" (18). To argue that we are not concerned with crippling

diseases or early death per se but rather the avoidance of the burdens these misfortunes place on the rest of us would help to create a climate of callousness and disregard for the value of life and health. Michael Halberstam has charged that these economic arguments "blame the sick" for society's medical bills (19). But others, such as Leon Kass, would retort that our drive for a "right to health" is based on a "no-fault" principle (2). Individuals are left free to pursue unhealthy lifestyles and to present society with the bill for increased medical costs, disability benefits, or benefits to dependents (2).

Tom Beauchamp suggests cost-benefit or utilitarian principles for justifying some limits to voluntary risks (20). This approach has the virtue of consistently following through on Mill's basic utilitarianism, for as Dworkin (7, 8) and Kaplan (16) point out, Mill was rarely "utilitarian" in his thoughts about paternalism. Mill in his essay *On Liberty* almost always defended self-regarding behavior categorically, setting a high boundary around the personal realm (10). Beauchamp suggests that "cost-benefit analysis can be employed to make explicit the tradeoffs between . . . lives lost and money expended to save them . . ." (20).

We have reviewed two contrasting sets of justifying principles for limiting —at least minimally—voluntary risks: weak paternalism and the indirect costs or burdens to the larger society. The disadvantage of the first is that it leaves unanswered the charge of paternalism. The second option makes the major justification for intervention not the prevention of illness or early death, but rather economic savings. Either option may fill many public health officials with some unease.

There is a third option, however, that is open—one that disavows paternalism (even weak paternalism) and the economic argument (although the costs of illness and early death can still remain an important secondary argument for legitimating reasonable restrictions to voluntary risks). This third option is based on the tradition of social justice (21, 22).

PUBLIC HEALTH AND SOCIAL JUSTICE

Traditionally, philosophers have paid relatively little attention to the problem of public health when considering the issue of social justice. The reasons are varied but there is one that needs highlighting.

Justice is broadly concerned with the distribution of benefits and burdens in society (9, 23). This distribution is to be accomplished in accordance with some basic principle: rights, needs, and desert are the leading candidates. Historically, the term "social justice" has been used by those who seek to alter or redistribute the burdens and benefits within society according to the principle of need. These benefits are often secured through the protection of rights or legislative entitlements.

The search by philosophers for a fair or just principle of allocation has led to an important distinction—the distinction between the principle of aggregation and that of distribution. Aggregation refers only to the total amount of good enjoyed by a particular group, whereas distribution refers to the share of that good or benefit that different members of the group have for themselves (23, 24). Aggregative principles are usually associated with utilitarianism, which is that political philosophy that seeks to maximize the total amount of happiness or utility for a society (23, 24).

Social justice, on the other hand, is typically concerned with the distribution or shares of a good in society. In fact, the major criticism of the aggregation principle is that it cares "not a whit" for how the aggregate good that is amassed (such as happiness) is distributed in the population (25).

Public health does not neatly fall into either of these categories. Although public health produces aggregate benefits (reduction of early death and disability), these benefits are not necessarily converted into other, more general benefits (such as happiness or dollars). Instead, the goals of public health (saving lives, reducing disability) are evaluated against an optimal or ideal community or societal standard that other societies have reached or that is otherwise deemed achievable. Public health is not concerned with shares because its policies are "collective goods" that tend to benefit the entire community like other collective goods (defense, fire, and police protection) (26). It is the level of that collective protection (the rates) that is the crucial standard for evaluation, and this level or standard is the measure of justice obtaining in the community.

Further, public health typically distributes benefits in the form of what Fried terms "statistical lives" (27). It is impossible to say who specifically (e.g. named individuals) receives the benefits of lowered infant mortality rates or lowered rates of liver cirrhosis or coronary disease. These are aggregate gains to the entire community.

Self and Other in Social Justice

In both the paternalist and the burden to society options, the fundamental idea that individuals should normally be able to determine their own good is retained. This is the core notion behind the idea of the self and the central objection to paternalistic interventions. In the burden to society argument, this point is never challenged, but rather the claim is made that one man's good has become another man's shackles in higher taxes and insurance premiums (11).

It is interesting to see that in the social justice perspective this fundamental idea about the self undergoes a slight but crucial modification. Here we are following the contract tradition of social justice, a tradition brilliantly updated by John Rawls (25), and drawing particularly on his ideas of the "original position" and the "veil of ignorance" (25). The original position is a position outside and prior to society from which persons view the world without knowing whether they will turn out to be male, female, white, black, rich, poor, sick, healthy, etc. Furthermore, those in the original position do not know their own particular good or plan of life. They can only know "primary goods," or goods which are necessary if everyone's plan of life has a reasonable chance of completion. Ignorance of their own particular good or plan of life leads individuals to agree that fairness demands the provision of those primary goods "individuals would want whatever else they would want" (25). Primary goods would likely include maximum liberty, protection against poverty, ignorance, serious disability, racial discrimination, etc.

The interesting point about the original position is what happens to the idea that individuals should remain free to determine their own good, or the basic idea of the self. The original position forces individuals to consider the interests of others and to recognize that there are certain basic protections that are just and fair, e.g. in the interest of everyone taken together (28). But oddly, the condition in which individuals do not know their own particular good forces a reconsideration of the unqualified claim that individuals should be free to shape their own plans. This freedom would likely be considered a primary good but its protection would be hedged by the provision of those other primary goods that are necessary for the completion of everyone's plans. Thus, the parties would insist that justice and fairness demand the freedom to pursue one's own plans as a primary good, but would, out of justice and fairness, also consent to reasonable restrictions to this freedom when this is required to provide primary goods that are the necessary means to the completion of everyone's plans.[1] Rawls devotes little serious attention to the impact of the original position on the issue of paternalism. The problem is that the original position and the veil of ignorance expose both the self and other to the same disinterested moral gaze, forcing the consideration of serious and fundamental harms to everyone's interest. In that position of disinterest, deaths in airline crashes because of

---

[1]Rawls equivocates on this point. He asserts that the universe of moral obligations would still remain obligations to others because "in the original position the parties assume that in society they are rational and able to manage their own affairs. Therefore they do not acknowledge any duties to self, since this is unnecessary to further their own good" [p. 248 in ref. (25)]. Rawls later states, "It is also rational for them to protect themselves against their own irrational inclinations by consenting to a scheme of penalties that may give them a sufficient motive to avoid foolish actions and by accepting certain impositions designed to undo the unfortunate consequences of their imprudent behavior" [p. 249 in ref. (25)].

faulty airline safety practices would not be considered a categorically more serious harm than deaths in automotive crashes because of the absence of mandatory seatbelt laws. This point is discussed further below.

The central point is that in the social justice perspective, the categories of self and others cannot serve to automatically define the boundaries of the moral community. (In Rawl's world the moral community consists only of enforceable obligations to others.) The view here is that the moral community is the project of assuring a decent minimum for human welfare. This project would include accepting reasonable limitations to self-regarding risks, as long as these restrictions promised important gains in reducing the risk of early death and yet avoided serious harms to the basic interests of privacy, autonomy, basic political liberties, or the provision of other primary goods. The acceptance of limits to voluntary risks would be justified, however, not in terms of obligations to self or with reference to narrow or specific benefits for the regulated group, but rather in the broader terms of public health and human welfare as a project for building the just society or community. In the just community or society the risk of premature death (and associated serious disability) would be lowered as much as possible in precisely the same way that protections are provided against poverty, old age, unemployment, and racial discrimination. To see how these ideas may be given more substance, let us examine more closely how members in the original position (or persons who take an objective, disinterested moral point of view) would approach the issue of death as a harm.

THE HARM OF EARLY DEATH

Those in the original position would know that death itself, although perhaps the most serious harm confronting human beings, is itself not capable of eradication. What is susceptible to change is premature death. But what constitutes a premature death? How would those in the original position come to an agreement on this crucial issue?

It is not likely that the members would choose the goal of prolonging life (added years at the end of life such as increasing the life expectancy for those who survive to age 70 or 75). Such a goal would demand a technology and a scientific revolution not in hand or in sight. It is far more likely that premature death would be seen as early death, death before some period widely regarded as the defining point of a ripe life. For the American society, such a boundary might well be the ages 65 or 70 (29). Thus, although death after this age would still remain a harm, death before that time would be regarded as an even more serious harm and one from which citizens deserve basic protection.

For the sake of discussion, let us assume that early death would be defined as death before age 65. It seems plausible that those in the original position would see policies to reduce or minimize the risk of early death as a primary good—one enjoying equal status with the other primary goods of the just community and in the interests of everybody taken together. The evidence that other societies do in fact enjoy much lower risks of early death while still retaining the basic political liberties and other key social goods would only strengthen the case. Refusal to secure this protection would be almost unthinkable. Why would the participants be any more eager to live with high rates of early death than high rates of unemployment, poverty, or violation of civil liberties?

To dramatize this situation, let us consider the present American society and the problem of early death as it would appear to members in the original position. We are fortunate to have James Vaupel's definitive analysis of a problem he calls "the American tragedy" (29). As Vaupel points out, the US ranks 26 among all nations in survival rates at age 65, behind the leaders, Sweden and Norway, and "all other major developed countries and behind Bulgaria, Puerto Rico and Hong Kong" [p. 86 in ref. (29)]. The US ranks just above Finland, which has the highest rates of heart disease in the world. Nevertheless, life expectancy at age 65 for Americans is almost exactly the same as for Swedes; the disparity truly lies in early deaths or deaths before age 65.

To the participants in the original position, over one quarter of all who enter the American society would die before age 65 [given the survival rates used in ref. (29)]. One third of all males would die before age 65 and one half of all black males would fail to reach 65. If the participants were to examine Sweden, however, better than 4 out of 5 males would survive to age 65. Females in the US would experience roughly the same survival rates as Swedish males, whereas almost 9 out of 10 Swedish women could expect to live to age 65.

There is little doubt that those in the original position would find this disparity truly alarming, especially if there were evidence that Sweden was prosperous, democratic, and otherwise not paying exorbitantly for its much lower rates of early death. Although the participants may concede that achieving Sweden's rates of early death might be more difficult in the US, it is still likely that those in the original position would regard the rates of early death in the US as intolerable.[2] As Vaupel argues [p. 82 in ref. (29)], this level of risk would mean that in the US today the risk of early death (25%) is more grave than the risk of poverty (12%).

[2]Vaupel provides dramatic evidence of the too long ignored tragedy of early death in America, arguing that "there is a tremendous inequality in life-chances between the early and late dead" (29). Although he does suggest that Americans should consider eliminating this tragedy as a gift to the future, he stops without developing an argument regarding the kinds of obligations and limits this injustice creates. In fact, he seems to reject governmental limits over self-regarding risks.

We now come to a crucial point in the argument. If the participants agree that this primary good ought be provided (early death ought be minimized) and that this goal necessitates some limits over self-regarding behavior, would these limits be paternalistic as Rawls seems to think (25)?

The answer is surely no. The central idea behind paternalism is the state limiting the freedom of individuals to make their own plans. But we have seen how the idea of social justice would result in individuals consenting to reasonable limits to this freedom in order to secure those primary goods that are the necessary means for the completion of everyone's plans.

But the objection may still be raised that this protection—at least in the case of policy to avert early death—is paternalistic because it provides benefits that individuals could obtain if they acted otherwise. As Kass argues, if individuals would act more wisely, the harm of early death could be dramatically reduced (2). But from the viewpoint of the original position, this line of reasoning would seem wrong if not absurd. The participants in the original position would not refuse to consider reducing the very serious harm of early death simply because the individuals involved could have acted otherwise. They would only refuse to eliminate the harm of early death when those restrictions on lifestyle risks incurred a more serious harm, such as a violation of fundamental liberty, privacy, or autonomy.

The virtue of choosing the goal of minimizing the harm of early death is that it moves the justifying principle away from reasons referring exclusively to the interests of the regulated group (7, 8). The focus is upon the broader societal goal of reducing the harm of early death. This shift helps to move the issue away from what individuals might do if they acted more wisely toward a goal that members of society would regard as urgent and justified. By focusing on the harm itself, a future with a high rate of early death would be as unjust as a future without social security or protection against poverty.

The parties probably would develop other criteria governing the selection of policies to minimize early death, choosing to focus on the most serious and widespread threats such as occupational hazards, highway safety, handguns, automobiles, smoking, use of alcohol and drugs rather than risks such as mountain climbing, skiing, skydiving, and hang-gliding.

Further, it is likely that the participants would stipulate that priority be given to risks and hazards in which there is an important commercial or industrial interest—an interest that actively promotes and encourages the widespread adoption and acceptance of risk-bearing activities. The participants would do so for two reasons: 1. As Etzioni argues (15), commercial interests promoting the hazardous activity dilute the purely voluntary aspect of these activities, thus increasing the legitimacy of intervention. 2. The fact that such institutions encourage these activities and risks offers public avenues for regulation and control that avoid the harm of invasion of privacy and the precedent of established tradition. As Kaplan (16) and Bonnie (14) argue, these are important assets for a social policy that seeks to influence self-regarding behavior or lifestyles.

Finally, the participants would attempt to clearly articulate a set of limits for policies to save lives, especially in cases that involve influencing life-styles. These limits are discussed in more detail below.

SOCIAL JUSTICE IN THE CONTEMPORARY SOCIETY

Using the criteria developed in the last section it is possible to turn to concrete cases and to approach the topic of social justice and the harm of early death in the contemporary society. For purposes of discussion, the case of policy for alcohol and tobacco will be considered.

The attainment of social justice in the contemporary society is a struggle that is conducted amid the swirl of competing and conflicting interests: commercial interests, consumer interests, minority interests, individual in-terests (privacy, autonomy), and the interest of the health and safety of the public. The conflicts between these interests grow most evident as the goals of social justice (in our case the reduction in rates of early death) are pressed.

The goal of public health in the contemporary society from Rawl's origi-nal position would be to dramatize the urgent priority of minimizing early death and to elevate this interest as a primary social goal and central achievement of the just community. This goal cannot be achieved without an adjustment of the benefits and advantages enjoyed by other important interests in society (industry, the consuming public, etc). As Anthony Downs has observed, many of our most serious problems in American society (racism, unemployment, poverty) are rooted in advantages and benefits enjoyed by the most influential and the most numerous (30). The essential challenge to public health in its shared struggle for the just com-munity is to work for a future as free as possible from early death.

This perspective on social justice goes beyond the search for the abstract distributive principles, anticipating realistically and without sentimentality the resistance of key groups to the burdens of dramatically reducing early death. Protecting the health and safety of workers, achieving higher levels of highway safety, and effecting even reasonable restrictions on tobacco and alcohol consumption will be accomplished only by altering institutional arrangements and existing distributions of property and power. Those who stand to lose or suffer inconveniences if this realignment is brought about do not remain passive. Because "one man's prize is another man's loss"

(31), attempts to realize social justice lead to wars and skirmishes over distribution (32). This conflict and involvement of a wide group of interests is yet more evidence that policies to reduce early death (including limits to voluntary risks) involve far more than restrictions on a class of individuals to benefit that same class of individuals (8).

Policy for Alcohol and Tobacco

It is clear that the parties in the original position would give high priority to attempts to discourage the use of tobacco and the heavy use of alcohol for the reason that these hazards contribute substantially to early deaths— perhaps 15 to 20% of the approximately 700,000 early deaths (29) each year.[3] The parties would also focus on these two commodities because of the important interests involved in advertising, promoting, and otherwise encouraging the use of these commodities, a situation that creates a case of voluntary behavior that at the least is clearly influenced. Likewise, these two commodities offer opportunities for public regulation (affecting the conditions of availability, legal prohibitions against certain uses, and taxation) that avoid invasions of privacy; there is compelling if not overwhelming evidence that these restrictions would have an impact, at least for alcohol (35, 36) (although in this paper the effectiveness of specific interventions is not the central issue).

The form of justification in regulating these hazards is crucial. The issue of the harm of early death should be placed again and again before the public. This harm and injustice must constantly be raised so that the entire community can determine for itself whether the current levels of early death are acceptable and fair, and if not, whether a collective response is justified. In other words, a central goal of developing policy for alcohol and tobacco (and related lifestyle risks) is to allow for the formation of consensus. If we defend regulatory policy for these substances only in terms of protecting the interests of the persons being regulated, we run the risk that the fundamental issue of early death will be buried under familiar clichés about individual freedom and individual responsibility. The issues of individual freedom and responsibility must be weighed against the harm of early death, not used to prevent the harm of early death from being recognized.

Shifting the justifying principles behind these policies would help to avoid the charge of moralism: public health officials could no longer be accused of conducting holy wars against tobacco or alcohol, regulating these com-

---

[3]This estimate assumes that roughly 50,000 to 65,000 early deaths are due to cirrhosis, highway crashes, and other causes that are alcohol-related (33). Statistics on early deaths due to smoking are hard to come by but the assumption that roughly the same magnitude of deaths (50,000 to 65,000), or 15 to 20% of the 325,000 excess deaths attributed to smoking (34), are early deaths does not seem unreasonable.

modities on moral grounds. Rather, tobacco and alcohol would be singled out because of their significant contribution to what Vaupel terms our national tragedy of early death (29).

Paradoxically, focusing on early death would also help to avoid the charge that public health officials seek a zero risk society and attack all risk-bearing activity from nuclear power to skateboarding or hang-gliding. Selecting the goal of minimizing early death would clarify the aims and purposes of public health campaigns and establish a goal that, though ambitious, is certainly not reckless or utopian. Centering on early death avoids the charge that policies regulating the hazards of the workplace, the highways, the marketplace, and a few key lifestyle risks promise the "freedom of the zoo" (37), as prosperous societies exist in which much lower rates of early death obtain without a loss of basic freedoms (Sweden and Norway are the leading examples) (29). There is evidence that major segments of the US population enjoy much higher survival rates than do others (29): It can hardly be argued that women and whites enjoy the "freedom of the zoo."

The central goal and standard used by public health is a community or societal goal derived from consideration of the issue of justice and fairness when the interests of all are surveyed from a detached, objective standpoint (the original position). Of course, the goal of minimizing early death is a long-term one and no consideration has been given here to the problem of establishing interim objectives that would be fair and acceptable. In establishing such a goal or standard, consideration should be given to historical trends and to the experience of comparable societies whose record is distinctively better, as well as to the testimony of citizens, experts, advocates, and opponents.

LIMITS TO PUBLIC HEALTH

Although the problem of early death is a serious problem for our society, its elimination is not the only goal of the just community. Equality and justice give rise to other values and protections that constitute important limits to public health and collective action. I will list, without elaboration, the most crucial of these limits (see 22):

1. the broad injunction against public health measures that unreasonably and coercively interfere with the fundamental rights of privacy of individual citizens
2. the injunction against pursuing the goals of public health at the expense of other primary goods such as basic education, elimination of poverty, and, especially, basic political liberties

3. the injunction against the undue emphasis on controlling some public health hazards to the exclusion of others, especially when the control of others may achieve more dramatic results in terms of minimizing disability or early death
4. the injunction against measures that increase, over the long run, the risks of death and disability.
5. the injunction to consider the problems of "redistributive justice," or the special problems of achieving a transition from one model of justice to another. A corollary of this injunction would be that when two or more policy options promise roughly equivalent results, that option should be chosen that is least disruptive of other social or economic values. This suggests that, whereas the focus of discussion has been on governmental measures to reduce risks, education should occupy an important role in the campaign to eliminate early death. This educational focus would not be simply on encouraging changes in individual behavior but would seek to mobilize support and legitimacy for the project of minimizing early death in American society.

CONCLUSION

This essay, in exploring the current debate about lifestyle risks and the question of paternalism, scrutinizes and finds wanting the options of "weak paternalism" and "burdens on society" (secondary harms) as justifying principles for governmental intervention. A third alternative, drawn from the tradition of social justice, is offered as justifying selected and limited restrictions of lifestyle risks. This alternative casts the issue of paternalism in a new light, suggesting the need to submit our assumptions about paternalism to closer scrutiny instead of searching for increasingly ingenious ways of fitting self-regarding behavior into other-regarding categories.

What has been argued is actually quite simple. From the standpoint of the original position and the perspective of social justice, the central issue is not to first decide whether some harm is a wrong or an injustice by determining whether it is self-inflicted. The central question is one of reducing serious harms outright while at the same time avoiding the creation of greater harms. This mode of thinking turns the traditional philosophical approach upside down, but it follows more closely the way we think about public health problems in everyday life. The crucial debate in society centers on whether some problem or condition is indeed a serious harm. Once this is decided, we then ask if this harm can be minimized while protecting the other vital interests in society, including the interests of privacy, autonomy, and individual liberty. Of course, we do not decide whether a condition is a serious problem or harm without considering the question of self-regarding versus other-regarding behaviors; still, the primary issue is whether the harm itself is so serious as to merit a collective response.

The argument here should help to focus the current debate about lifestyle risks in proper perspective. Lifestyle risks are not the only culprits in the problem of early death. This country can make dramatic progress in minimizing early death through more stringent protection of the environment, the workplace, and our modes of transportation. Also, eliminating the great disparities of income and other social advantages between the classes and races would help to close the gap for those groups who bear such a heavy burden. The struggle to minimize early death clearly complements and supports the other goals of social justice: economic equality and justice, full employment, a prosperous economy, and a protected environment.

It is often noted that public health is centrally concerned with the community approach (38). Although the term "community" has various meanings, one meaning is important above all else: the strengthening of community through meeting the needs of all its members, i.e. building the community through the doing of justice. If the ideal of community is to have a redemptive meaning, it must be seen as a project in search of justice. There can be no true community when the demands of justice are ignored.

The obvious truth that many, if not most, lifestyle hazards are powerfully influenced by market forces and societal and cultural constraints (15, 21, 22) has been discussed only in passing. It seemed necessary, instead, to face the hard question: Even if there is a substantial voluntary component in most lifestyle risks (and there surely is), do the demands of justice and community require their reasonable restriction? The answer here is in the affirmative.

Literature Cited

1. Gov. of Canada/Minist. Natl. Health Welfare. 1974. *A New Perspective on the Health of Canadians.* Ottawa: Minist. Natl. Health Welfare. 76 pp.
2. Kass, L. 1975. Regarding the end of medicine and the pursuit of health. *Public Interest* 40:11–42
3. Meenan, R. F. 1976. Improving the public's health—Some further reflections. *N. Engl. J. Med.* 294:45–47
4. Faden, R., Faden, A., eds. 1978. Ethical issues in public health policy: Health education and lifestyle interventions. Health Educ. Monogr. 6(2)
5. Wildavsky, A. 1976. Can health be planned? *Davis Lect., Cent. for Health Admin. Stud.* Univ. of Chicago, Chicago, Ill.
6. Brown, L. 1978. The scope and limits of equality as a normative guide to federal

health care policy. *Public Policy* 26:481–532
7. Dworkin, G. 1972. Paternalism. *Monist* 56:64–84
8. Dworkin, G. 1971. Paternalism. In *Morality and the Law,* ed. R. A. Wasserstrom, pp. 107–206. Belmont, Calif: Wadsworth. 149 pp.
9. Feinberg, J. 1973. *Social Philosophy,* pp. 45–52. Englewood Cliffs, NJ: Prentice-Hall. 126 pp.
10. Mill, J. S. 1859. *On Liberty,* p. 13, ed. C. V. Shields. Indianapolis: Bobbs-Merrill, 1977 ed. 141 pp.
11. Knowles, J. 1978. The responsibility of the individual. In *Doing Better and Feeling Worse,* ed. J. Knowles, pp. 57–80. New York: Norton. 278 pp.
12. US Dept. Health, Educ., Welfare, Public Health Serv. 1975. *Forward Plan for*

Health: FY 1977–81, pp. 100–3. Washington DC: US DHEW. 259 pp.

13. White, L. S. 1975. How to improve the public's health. *N. Engl. J. Med.* 293:773–74

14. Bonnie, R. 1978. Discouraging unhealthy personal choices: Reflections on new directions in substance abuse policy. *J. Drug Issues* 8:199–219

15. Etzioni, A. 1978. Individual will and social conditions: Toward an effective health maintenance policy. *Ann. Am. Acad. Polit. Soc. Sci.* 437:62–73

16. Kaplan, J. 1971. The role of the law in drug control. *Duke Law J.* 1971:1065–1104

17. Hannon, B. M., Lohman, T. G. 1978. The energy cost of overweight in the United States. *Am. J. Public Health* 68:765–67

18. Miranda, J. 1977. *Being and the Messiah,* p. 36. Maryknoll, NY: Orbis. 245 pp.

19. *Washington Post.* Dec. 17, 1978

20. Beauchamp, T. L. 1978. The regulation of hazards and hazardous behavior. *Health Educ. Monogr.* 6:242–57

21. Beauchamp, D. E. 1976. Public health as social justice. *Inquiry* 13:3–14

22. Beauchamp, D. E. 1976. Exploring new ethics for public health: Developing a fair alcohol policy. *J. Health Polit. Policy and Law* 1:338–54

23. Miller, D. 1976. *Social Justice,* pp. 17–153. Oxford: Clarendon. 367 pp.

24. Barry, B. 1963. *Political Argument,* Chap. 3. New York: Humanities. 364 pp.

25. Rawls, J. 1971. *A Theory of Justice* pp. 3–192, 249. Cambridge: Harvard Univ. Press. 607 pp.

26. Olson, M. 1965. *The Logic of Collective Action* pp. 14–15. Cambridge: Harvard Univ. Press. 176 pp.

27. Fried, C. 1970. *An Anatomy of Values,* pp. 207–36. Cambridge: Harvard Univ. Press. 265 pp.

28. Baier, K. 1965. *The Moral Point of View.* New York: Random. 165 pp.

29. Vaupel, J. V. 1976. Early death: An American tragedy. *Law Contemp. Probl.* 40:73–121

30. Downs, A. 1972. Up and down with ecology—The issue-attention cycle. *Public Interest* 20:38–50

31. Klein, R. In Lekachman, R. 1979. Looking for the left. *Harper's* April, pp. 21–23

32. Lekachman, R. 1979. See Ref. 31, p. 22

33. Natl. Inst. Alcohol Abuse and Alcoholism/Alcohol, Drug Abuse, and Mental Health Admin./Public Health Serv. 1978. *Third Special Report to the U.S. Congress on Alcohol and Health,* p. 10. Washington DC: GPO. 98 pp.

34. Public Health Service/Dept. Health, Education, and Welfare 1979. *Smoking and Health: A Report of the Surgeon General,* Chap. 2. Washington DC: GPO

35. Bruun, K., Edwards, G., Lumio, M., Mäkelä, K., Pan, L., Popham, R. E., Room, R., Schmidt, W., Skog, O.-L., Sulkunen, P., Österberg, E. 1975. *Alcohol Control Policies in Public Health Perspective.* Helsinki: Finnish Found. Alcohol Studies. 106 pp.

36. Popham, R., Schmidt, W., deLint, J. 1976. The effects of legal restraint on drinking. In *The Social Aspects of Alcoholism, The Biology of Alcoholism,* ed. B. Kissin, H. Begleiter, 4:579–625. New York: Plenum. 643 pp.

37. Fuchs, V. 1974. *Who Shall Live?,* p. 26. New York: Basic. 168 pp.

38. McGavran, E. 1953. What is public health? *Can. J. Public Health* 44:441–51

Ann. Rev. Public Health 1980. 1:137–61

HEALTH PLANNING   ❖12506
AND REGULATION EFFECTS
ON HOSPITAL COSTS

Thomas W. Bice

Department of Health Services, School of Public Health & Community
Medicine, University of Washington, Seattle, Washington 98195

INTRODUCTION

Although one may assume that health planning and regulation are topics
that naturally should be discussed together, that assumption is only recently
and partially true in the United States. Until the middle of this century,
these activities developed largely independently and under different auspices (1–5). The growth of federal involvement in the health sector following World War II set in motion trends that led to a convergence of planning
and regulatory activities, but their merging within a single organizational
structure did not occur until the late 1960s, and then only partially.

The principal causes of this joining of health planning and regulation
were the rapidly increasing expenditures for medical services and the en-
larging roles of governments as purchasers of care that followed the introduction of Medicare and Medicaid. By the late 1960s, it had become
apparent that health care cost inflation was rooted in systemic features of
the health services industry that could not be remedied by voluntary planning. In consequence, several states and later the federal government
created regulatory authorities to be implemented by networks of areawide
and state planning agencies and subsequently established other authorities
and programs alongside these. Whether health planning and regulation will
continue to converge and, as some propose, eventually be combined in a
unitary planning and regulatory structure remains to be seen. Presently,
however, the various programs established to control health care costs are
proceeding along separate and sometimes conflicting courses (6, 7).

0163-7525/80/0510-0137$01.00

In this chapter we employ the theme of cost containment to focus our discussion of health planning and regulation. While recognizing that health planning and regulatory efforts are directed toward other ends as well as toward controlling costs, this approach was dictated by the need to be selective and the overriding prominence of cost containment as an objective of public policy. Additionally, we concentrate on the effects of planning and regulation on hospitals. Hospital facilities have been the principal concern of health planning (1); because expenditures for hospital services are the largest component of spending for health care and have grown more rapidly than others over the past decade (8), they are the major targets of current cost containment efforts. Finally, our review is confined primarily to research on outcomes of planning and regulation. Vast literatures have accumulated on planning and regulation in the health services industry that address histories, administrative structures, and political environments. Although we allude to these matters, they are not treated systematically.

The chapter begins with an overview of the purposes and processes of the two most significant, federally sponsored health planning programs that preceded the current system. Following this, we review the experiences of the three most widespread types of regulation aimed at moderating hospital costs, namely, (*a*) capital expenditures and services controls, (*b*) utilization review, and (*c*) hospital rate setting. In the concluding section we discuss the implications of current knowledge for public policy and future research.

HEALTH PLANNING

Despite the fact that health planning has been pursued in the United States by agencies organized for that purpose since the early 1960s, little is known about its accomplishments. The paucity of outcome-oriented research in this area is, perhaps, to be expected in view of the history and structure of planning in this country. Effective planning presumes the existence of reasonably well-articulated objectives that are amenable to expression in measurable terms, methods of making rational choices among alternative courses of action, and means of persuading the objects of planning to act in accordance with plans (9). Health planning programs sponsored by the federal government have typically failed to bring all three into concert. Lacking clearcut outcome criteria with which to evaluate performance and being unsure as to what constitutes an exemplary agency, researchers have concentrated for the most part on describing processes. Although such studies cannot provide unequivocal evidence as to effectiveness, they strongly suggest that health planning per se has had little demonstrable impact on the structure and operations of our health services industry.

The Hill-Burton Program

The first major federal involvement in health planning followed the enactment of the Hospital Survey and Construction Act of 1946 (P. L. 79–725), popularly known as the Hill-Burton program. This two-part act initially provided states with matching funds to support facilities planning and construction of nonprofit hospitals in areas lacking adequate medical facilities and services. Over its two decades of operation, the authorizing legislation was amended several times to make subsidies available to the industry for other purposes as well (10).

Although the principal intent of the Hill-Burton program was to eliminate shortages of medical services in the nation's rural and economically depressed regions, its original sponsors conceived of it as a model federal grant-in-aid program in which planning would play a crucial role (1). Funds were to be allocated on the basis of needs for services indentified through periodic surveys of hospitals and documented in state plans. Federal subsidies were allotted to states using a formula that operationalized need in terms of hospital bed-to-population ratios and per capita income that, in accordance with the intent of the program, favored rural and poorer regions. Although similar formulas were employed by state Hill-Burton agencies in disbursing funds within their jurisdictions, Klarman (1) has noted that considerable discretion was exercised in determining which regions and institutions received assistance.

The formula approach to defining need and the program's exclusive attention throughout most of its existence greatly circumscribed planners' abilities to effect broader reforms. Formuli did not take into account how services were to be coordinated within local communities or how they would be operated to attain optimal efficiency. Urged by spokesmen of the hospital industry, in 1962 Congress authorized appropriations to support statewide and regional health facilities planning councils, charging them with the responsibilities of identifying community needs and developing plans for meeting them. Over the five years that such subsidies were in effect, support was provided to 10 statewide and 72 areawide councils (11). Constituted as voluntary agencies with memberships drawn from representatives of health care institutions, professionals, and the general public, these councils were given no formal authority over the operations or financing of provider organizations.

Palmiere's (11, 12) study of these agencies suggests that they typically lacked the resources necessary to develop comprehensive community plans and, indeed, rarely defined their missions that broadly. Of the 77 councils he reviewed, only 46 met the criteria for inclusion in the study; namely, that the council be in operation with at least one full-time staff member for at least one year prior to mid-1967. Fewer than half of those that qualified had four or more employees. From reviews of councils' origins and stated purposes, Palmiere (11) concluded that most agencies had been created in response to specific problems and subsequently served primarily to advance the interests of their institutional members. Accordingly, agencies emphasized coordination and integration of institutionally based services and gave high priority to determining how capital funds would be divided among hospitals. In the author's words, "Efficiency in the use of resources by health care organizations was emphasized much more than the effectiveness of those organizations in the solution of health problems of the population" [p. 1236 in ref. (11)].

Analyses of the Hill-Burton program by Lave & Lave (10) reveal that it was successful in accomplishing its principal objective of increasing supplies of hospital beds in rural and economically depressed regions. The formuli used to distribute subsidies, however, virtually guaranteed that result. Beyond this, little is known about the effect of planning during this period. Only two studies investigated the question, but both employed designs that preclude drawing firm conclusions. One study examined changes from 1948 to 1968 in indicators of the structure and use of hospitals, before and after the introduction of planning study in 45 communities that had planning councils (12). The other study compared four metropolitan areas in which planning had been pursued for five or more years with other similar areas in which no planning agencies existed (2, 12). Neither study found consistent differences that could be confidently ascribed to planning.

Comprehensive Health Planning

With the enactment of the Partnership for Health Act of 1966 (P.L. 89–749), the locus of health planning shifted from health planning councils to comprehensive health planning (CHP) agencies. Like their predecessors, CHP agencies were voluntary bodies without formal authority to implement plans. Reflecting the consumer movement of the times, governing boards of the statewide and areawide agencies created by this program were required to include consumer majorities. Further, the purposes of planning were broadened from the earlier concentration on facilities to cover all aspects of health and health care, including the environment. Over the ensuing decade, statewide CHP agencies were established in all states and 162 areawide agencies were established in local areas.

An exchange between Congressman Symington and the then Undersecretary for Health of the US Department of Health, Education, and Welfare (DHEW) at a 1974 Congressional hearing illustrates what was known about the effects of comprehensive health planning nearly a decade after its inception [p. 454 in ref. (13)]:

Mr. Symington: Wasn't one of the purposes [of Section 314] to achieve efficiency and save health costs through planning?

Mr. Carlucci: Yes, sir.

Mr. Symington: Do you have any idea how much you saved by spending that money that might otherwise have been illogically spent?

Mr. Carlucci: I am frank to admit that I do not think that I can give you such a figure, Mr. Symington, because we are getting into what otherwise would have been spent. You are getting into the cost effectiveness of a planning function which is certainly very hard, very difficult to calculate.

In fact, no comparative studies had been done of the impacts of the CHP program on hospital costs or any other outcome.

Again, however, research on the planning process suggests that most CHP agencies were unable to develop plans. An investigation of 163 CHP agencies by the US General Accounting Office (14), for instance, found that fewer than half had estimates of current needs for inpatient or ambulatory services, and still fewer could document estimates for future requirements in their communities. A study by Lewin & Associates, Inc. (15) confirmed this impression. Most of the 36 areawide planning agencies they reviewed in 1974 relied upon Hill-Burton plans for hospital bed standards, although they were regarded as inadequate and often out of date, and standards for determining needs for special services and equipment were virtually nonexistent. MacStravic's (16) analyses of data from a 1973 assessment of the CHP program by the US Department of Health, Education, and Welfare (17) shows that, on the average, state and areawide CHP agencies satisfied fewer than 6 of 17 criteria for health plan development and implementation. The author observed that low scores on this agency function may have reflected the relatively low priority attached to producing written plans as compared with the development of effective planning processes.

In sum, the fragmentary and largely inconclusive evidence about the effects of health planning before the creation of the current program indicates that it probably did little to thwart forces that contribute to cost inflation. One may justifiably argue that such a criterion is inappropriate inasmuch as these earlier efforts were not directed exclusively or even primarily at cost-containment objectives. Certainly, hindsight has its advantages. Nevertheless, health planning has been guided since its inception by notions of a regionalized health services system as its model of efficiency (1, 18). Had substantial progress been attained toward realizing that ideal, it probably would have been reflected in features of the health services industry that are currently implicated in rising expenditures for medical services.

The Current Program

The current program mandated by the National Health Planning and Resources Development Act of 1974 (P.L. 93–641) replaces areawide CHP agencies with Health Systems Agencies, state CHP bodies with State Health Planning and Resources Development Agencies, and establishes intermediate State Health Coordinating Councils and a National Health Planning Council. Features of this program promise to remedy several of the fundamental deficiencies that have heretofore characterized health planning (19). The statute and subsequently issued administrative regulations define the objectives of health planning more precisely than has been done before, assign specific functions to each of the agencies involved, specify the types of plans that agencies must produce, and establish means for the promulgation of national guidelines and standards. Moreover, planning agencies have been thrust directly into the business of cost containment by virtue of their roles in reviewing and approving uses of federal subsidies and, more importantly, in implementing capital expenditures and services controls.

As these reforms have yet to be fully implemented, attention is once again directed primarily to the processes and conflicts that accompany the creation of new structures and procedures (20, 21). Undoubtedly, however, the program will soon be judged largely in terms of its record in controlling costs through its newly acquired regulatory authorities.

REGULATION

Capital Expenditures and Services Controls

Historically, hospitals have faced strong pressures encouraging growth and improvement of services with few obstacles preventing the pursuit of those ends. Community groups, lay trustees, hospital management, and staff physicians have wanted their hospitals to provide full ranges of services with up-to-date facilities and equipment; our nation's insurance schemes and tax and subsidy policies have provided hospitals resources to employ more or less at their discretion (22). As a result, it is believed that the nation has an overabundance of facilities and services (23) and that, unless deterred by external forces, hospitals will continue to add to the superfluity and rising costs.

Uncontrolled growth and improvements in styles of services have been linked to rising costs by several arguments. 1. Most directly, expansion and modernization of facilities and purchases of equipment involve substantial outlays (8). 2. When not fully utilized, fixed expenses associated with re-sources contribute to increased unit costs. 3. If the availability of services stimulates their use, as has been shown in several studies (24, 25), expansion of facilities and offerings of new services may result in unnecessary utiliza-tion and, therefore, unnecessary expenditures for medical services.

These and related rationales (26) have prompted the federal and state governments to adopt capital expenditures and services (CES) controls. Basically, this form of regulation attempts to limit health care institutions' capital expenditures and offerings of new services to those that are certified as needed in their communities (27, 28). Institutions subject to these controls must submit their plans for designated types and amounts of expenditures and changes of services to areawide planning agencies and state agencies. Each conducts independent reviews and the state agency, with advice from the local planning body, decides whether to issue a certificate allowing the applicant to proceed.

The types of sanctions imposed distinguish two types of CES controls:

1. Financial controls attempt to deter institutions from engaging in un-authorized projects by threatening to withhold payments of costs associated with interest on loans and depreciation. Such an approach has been used since the 1960s by several Blue Cross plans. In areas in which Blue Cross contracts include so-called conformance clauses, member hospitals must submit their plans for capital investments to areawide health planning agencies for review and approval. The 1972 Section 1122 amendment to the Social Security Act created a similar federally sponsored program. In states that have chosen to implement Section 1122 reviews, financial sanctions are levied by the Medicare and Medicaid programs.

2. Legal restrictions are imposed through state certificate-of-need (CON) programs. These are generally more stringent than financial controls in two respects. First, penalties are potentially more severe inasmuch as institu-tions that engage in unauthorized projects are subject to legal actions by the state. Further, these controls cover all designated types of institutions and expenditures regardless of their source of funds. Under financial controls, hospitals could conceivably pursue disapproved projects using funds from charitable contributions or other sources to offset financial penalties im-posed by third parties. CON laws cover this avenue of escape.

The first CON program was enacted by New York State in 1964, and by 1972 about half the states had adopted some form of CON regulation (29). In that year the Section 1122 program was enacted, slowing the adoption of CON laws. Presently, all states impose either one or both of these types of regulation, and provisions of the current planning act make the availabil-ity of funds from various federal health programs contingent upon states having acceptable CON programs by 1980.

Although the growth of CES regulation occasioned considerable debate and speculation as to its likely effectiveness and possible deleterious side effects (30, 31), little research has been done on the subject until recently. No studies of earlier Blue Cross conformance programs have appeared in the general literature, and most available studies of CON and Section 1122 programs are based on early experiences.

Two general approaches have been used to assess the effects of CES regulation. 1. The descriptive approach enumerates the types and costs of applications submitted to reviewing agencies and considers disapprovals as evidence of success. 2. The analytical approach attempts to determine the patterns of capital investment that would be expected in the absence of controls and measures the impacts of regulation in terms of departures of observed patterns from these expectations. For reasons discussed below, the latter is the better method for assessing effects.

DESCRIPTIVE STUDIES   Bicknell & Walsh (32) summarized the first 19 months of CES review in Massachusetts following the enactment of the state's CON law. During that period 209 applications were acted upon. More than 5000 additional short-term and 7000 long-term hospital beds were requested, of which 20% and 25%, respectively, were denied. In general, applications for modernization and improvements of services that did not involve increases of bed capacity were denied less often. From these data and observations about the review process, the authors concluded that CON controls were an effective, albeit limited, counterforce to unnecessary growth.

In 1974 Lewin & Associates, Inc. (15) undertook an assessment of the processes and outcomes of CES regulation in 36 planning areas of 20 states. Although the project was concerned primarily with the Section 1122 program, the inclusion of nine states with CON controls, either in addition to or instead of a Section 1122 program, allowed the authors to comment on both types of CES regulation.

Noting that more than 90% of all completed reviews resulted in approvals, the investigators concluded that CES controls were largely ineffective in controlling capital expenditures. Analyses of determinations on various types of proposals showed that agencies approved more than 90% of all proposed additions of long-term care and psychiatric beds and nearly 70% of all bed additions requested by acute care hospitals. As a result, more than three-quarters of the areas approved levels of hospital capacity in excess of those established as needed in their communities. Rates of approval of applications for selected new equipment and services were higher still: Only about 5% of such requests were denied.

From a more recent national study, the American Health Planning Association (33) attributes greater effectiveness to CES controls. The association collected information on all applications submitted to 166 of the nation's 204 Health Systems Agencies over the two-year period ending in August of 1978. In addition to tabulating disapproved applications, the investigators counted as successes applications that were withdrawn before definitive decisions were taken, as well as those that were discouraged by "unofficial" actions by planning agencies and therefore never reached the formal application stage.

Using this broader definition of success, the study showed that from 1976 to 1978 more than 40% of the beds that hospitals either officially proposed or considered building were denied or discouraged by CES agencies. In dollars, this represented a savings of more than $559 million. Higher rates of approval were observed for proposals involving equipment purchases. About 80% of the proposed $516 million were allowed. Taking into consideration all types of expenditures proposed by hospitals, the study concluded that nearly 20% of the more than $7.0 billion proposed expenditures were averted by CES regulation.

Although these descriptive studies provide useful information about agencies' preferences and activities, they cannot yield unequivocal evidence about the impacts of CES regulation on hospitals' investment behavior. Such studies must make assumptions about the direct effects that regulatory programs have on institutions' investment plans, concerning which there is no empirical information. Some observers argue that the mere presence of this form of regulation deters hospitals from proposing unnecessary projects (32). If so, descriptive studies will underestimate the effects of regulation. Others advance the opposite view, namely, that regulation encourages institutions to attempt to preempt competitors' bids for scarce opportunities to grow or improve services (34). If this so-called franchising effect predominates, one would expect to observe more proposals and, necessarily, more denials. In this case, estimates of savings attributable to CES controls would be overly generous. Furthermore, as CES controls do not cover all types of capital expenditures, regulated institutions may seek to avoid regulation by investing in projects that are exempted from review. Such activity is missed by tallies of official and unofficial agency actions and also leads to inflated estimates of success.

ANALYTIC STUDIES   Rothenberg (35) attempted to assess the effects of New York's CON program by comparing growth in hospital beds before and after the introduction of controls. Using the state's 25 counties as units of analysis, she found that, overall, hospital capacity grew less rapidly during the five years after regulation came into effect than during the five previous years. From the discovery that growth among counties was positively associated with the numbers of nonconforming beds in 1965, the author concluded that CON controls encouraged expansion of facilities in areas of greatest need. However, the finding that growth in beds was highest in areas that experienced losses of population is both counterintuitive and at odds with the conclusion that beds were added where they were needed most.

Limitations of the research design of this study preclude drawing firm conclusions. The implicit use of the preCON period to derive expected growth patterns assumes that expansion occurs linearly with time. One might expect, however, that equilibrating tendencies would result in slower growth in counties that expanded their supplies in earlier periods, and vice versa. If this occurs, estimates of effects of regulation will be confounded with preexisting trends. Results from analyses reported by the author cannot rule out this possibility.

Hellinger (36) attempted to determine the impact of early CON programs on overall hospital investment. Using 1973 levels of total plant assets in place in hospitals and states as units of analysis, he found no evidence of an effect. Other analyses suggested, however, that hospitals may have increased investments before the introduction of controls in anticipation of not being able to do so later. The regression approach employed in this study makes drawing firm conclusions problematic, however. The inclusion of a lagged plant assets variable among the independent variables in the investment equations posed estimation difficulties. This may have accounted for the fact that virtually all other factors, including the indicator of CON regulation, had no detectable effects on the level of hospital investment in 1973.

In the most extensive study of the impacts of CES regulation concluded to date, Salkever & Bice (37, 38) found that CON controls in force in the late 1960s and early 1970s had no appreciable effect on per capita expenditures for hospital services. With states as units of analysis and employing regression analyses to control effects of other determinants of changes in investment from 1968 to 1972, these investigators discovered that, although CON controls did not alter total amounts of investment, they may have altered its composition. Specifically, the patterns of coefficients showed that states with CON programs typically experienced slower growth in hospital beds than states that had no CES controls, and that growth of plant assets per bed was higher in regulated states than in the unregulated states. From these findings the authors reasoned that stringent control of bed growth induced hospitals to invest in the less tightly controlled means of upgrading styles of services such as modernization of plant and the purchase of new equipment. The lower growth of beds in CON states was found to lower overall use of hospital services, thereby tending to diminish per capita expenditures; increases in plant assets per bed were associated with rising per diem rates and, therefore, higher per capita costs. Effects of these competing influences on total per capita expenditures for hospital services were approximately offsetting, resulting in no savings attributable to CON regulation.

Other studies have focussed on the impacts of CON regulation on hospitals' purchases of special equipment and offerings of sophisticated services. Cromwell and his colleagues (39) studied the percentages of hospitals in states that offered 10 specialized services in 1973. Using regression analyses in which the presence of a CON program was measured by a dummy variable, the investigators found that CON coefficients were significantly negative in only three equations. The authors concluded that CON controls deterred the diffusion of these three types of services but had no effect on the other seven.

Russell (40) investigated the levels of four specialized services among hospitals in 1975 and the rapidity with which hospitals adopted three others over the 1965 to 1974 period. With individual hospitals as units of analysis, she employed regression analyses to examine effects of hospitals' structures, market characteristics, and regulatory environments on their adoption of new technologies. Among the latter characteristics was an indicator of CON regulation that classified hospitals as being in states that had no CON controls as of 1974 versus others that enacted programs early (1965–1969) and late (1970–1974). In all four analyses of levels of special services in 1975, dummy variables for early adopting states were negatively signed and two were statistically significant. One coefficient was significantly negative for the late adopting states. These findings suggest that programs operating in early adopting states may have controlled the diffusion of these technologies.

Analyses of the timing of adoption of four special services showed no consistent pattern. Hospitals in states in which CON regulation was in force as of 1969 tended to adopt the services somewhat later than hospitals in states that had no investment control program in 1974. However, hospitals in states that introduced CON controls between 1970 and 1974 tended to adopt the services earlier than the hospitals in the unregulated states.

The studies by Cromwell et al (39) and Russell (40) of effects of CON regulation on levels of services and facilities in place at particular times hint that controls may have deterred the diffusion of at least some types of services. However, because both studies used cross-sectional data for periods in which services had already diffused widely, such an interpretation may be erroneous. The approaches used cannot dismiss the possibility that the estimated effects of CON controls simply reflect preexisting trends.

SUMMARY   Studies of CES regulation suggest that these controls have had no appreciable influence on health care costs. Descriptive studies have shown that CES agencies may be becoming more effective in deterring hospitals from engaging in unnecessary expansions of capacity, but it is less clear whether tendencies to add new equipment and services have been thwarted. Because of the inherent weaknesses of the descriptive approach, however, such studies cannot yield conclusive evidence as to the effects of regulation on either health care institutions' overall investment patterns or populations' expenditures for medical services.

The few existing analytical studies of CES regulation also suggest that controls have slowed bed growth, but findings pertaining to their impacts on offerings of new services are inconclusive. Furthermore, as all available studies focussed on periods in which CES programs were in their infancies and were the only major controls on hospitals aimed at moderating costs, their conclusions may no longer pertain. CES agencies may have improved with experience, and the introduction of other regulatory efforts may have reinforced or complemented those of CES regulators. At present, however, no evidence has been produced documenting such improvements.

Utilization Review

Most insurance organizations attempt to limit the moral hazard of insurance by explicitly itemizing types of losses that are covered by their policies and by acting for or with the insured as prudent buyers. In so doing, insurers maintain control over their outlays and premium prices. The health insurance industry and government subsidy programs have not strenuously exercised these practices (41). Rather, they have provided increasingly broad medical benefits while allowing patients and their physicians to choose the services that are consumed by the insured and paid for by the insurers. With strong encouragement from the medical profession, private insurers and government agencies have historically abdicated prudent buyer responsibilities to the medical profession (41, 42).

Following the introduction of Medicare and Medicaid, the adverse consequences of these arrangements became apparent to public officials. Legislation that created these programs sought to control unnecessary use of inpatient services by requiring participating hospitals and physicians to establish internal peer review committees. However, a 1970 report by the staff of the Senate Finance Committee (43) found these efforts to be woefully deficient, and Congress responded by enacting the Professional Services Review Organizations (PSRO) program (P.L. 92–603). Although the intent of this legislation was initially confused by its presumption that poor quality medical care and unnecessary use of medical services were synonymous (44), recent events have clearly shown that PSRO was expected to contain costs (45).

The PSRO program attempts to control unnecessary medical costs by limiting the medical services consumed by beneficiaries of federal insurance programs to those that are certified as medically necessary. These determinations are made by physician members of local PSROs, which are required to develop and enforce normative standards of medical practice. The principal technique employed by PSROs is concurrent review of hospitalized patients. This involves certifying the appropriateness of admissions shortly after patients enter hospitals and periodically reviewing the necessity of stays that continue past established norms.

Basically similar approaches have been in force in prototypical PSRO programs since the 1950s, and in the late 1960s several states adopted utilization review as a means to eliminate unnecessary use of hospitals by Medicaid enrollees. Although there is as yet little evidence as to the effectiveness of utilization review within the context of the PSRO program, a body of experience has accumulated from earlier programs.

EVIDENCE   One of the earliest continuing efforts to control unnecessary use of medical services is the utilization review program of the San Joaquin (California) Medical Care Foundation (46). Established in the 1950s, the foundation developed a physician reimbursement scheme that has served as a model for current independent practice associations and foundation-type health maintenance organizations and a method of peer review that is credited with influencing the procedures adopted by other peer review programs. In the late 1960s the foundation entered into a contractual arrangement with the state in which it agreed to serve as the intermediary for Medi-Cal (Medicaid) recipients. Accordingly, the foundation's utilization controls were extended to the Medi-Cal population.

Holahan (46) studied the effects of the program on the use of a variety of medical services by Medi-Cal enrollees, including admission rates, total hospital days, expenditures for hospitals services, and surgical rates. Using data from a statewide sample of Medi-Cal records for 1969 and 1970, several regression analyses were performed in which Medi-Cal beneficiaries in the foundation's jurisdiction were identified by a dummy variable. These analyses revealed that, with other factors controlled, admission rates, total hospital days, and costs of hospital services in the area served by the foundation were not significantly different from those of other parts of California. Surgical rates in the San Joaquin Region appeared to be higher than elsewhere, however.

Several assessments of utilization review have employed simpler interrupted time series designs and aggregate experimental control group approaches. The former approach compares indicators of hospital use after the introduction of controls to earlier experience; the latter compares indicators of utilization among patients subject to utilization controls to others who are not. Both approaches have produced only suggestive results, owing to difficulties in ruling out alternative explanations of findings. The most problematic in this regard has been the problem of noncomparable control groups, which is especially troublesome in studies that inadequately adjust for differences in prevalences of diagnostic and other conditions between experimental and control periods and groups.

One such study was reported by Flashner and his associates (47) based on a before-after assessment of the Illinois Hospital Admission Surveillance Program. This utilization review effort was one of the few that required physicians to receive approvals for elective hospitalizations of Medicaid patients before admission as well as for continuing stays. Flashner et al (47) noted that average lengths of hospital stays dropped from 7.2 days before the introduction of the program to 6.2 days during the following six months and attributed this difference to utilization review. Davidson et al (48), however, observed that other changes coincident with the inception of the review program could have caused this difference.

Similar problems plagued Brian's (49, 50) efforts to isolate the effects of utilization review in California. Utilization controls have been in effect in the state's Medi-Cal program since the late 1960s. The first phase required all stays beyond eight days to be reviewed and approved by consultant physicians employed by the counties and the state (49). In 1970, this approach was replaced by one that imposed both preadmission and continuing stay reviews of nonemergency cases and continuing stay reviews of emergency admissions.

From analyses of statewide hospital utilization by Medi-Cal recipients during the nine months following the introduction of the second stage controls Brian (49) concluded that the controls brought about lower rates of hospital admissions and shorter average stays than was observed under the earlier program. Data from the year before the newer controls were established were employed to estimate expected admission rates and average stays. Comparisons of expectations with observed data showed that admission rates were about 11% less than expected, and average stays were about 2 to 4% less.

The program administered in Sacramento differed from that of the rest of California in that it did not require prior authorizations of nonemergency admissions. Further, reviews were conducted, not by government-employed physicians, but by physician members of the Medical Care Foundation of Sacramento (50). Using basically the same approach as described above, Brian (50) compared indicators of hospital utilization by Medi-Cal patients subject to the Sacramento plan reviews to those of other selected California areas. These comparisons revealed that the expected average monthly days of care exceeded observed days in all areas studied and that the greatest relative decline occurred in the Sacramento region. The relative decline of average lengths of stay in Sacramento was greater than that of the two comparison areas, and the relative reduction of the admission rate exceeded that of one of the control sites.

Brian [p. 880 in ref. (59)] concluded from his two studies that "the mere establishment of any peer-review activity will eliminate some of the marginal admissions," and "a local-medical society utilization control program can be at least as effective in controlling unnecessary hospital utilization as a government-operated program." An extensive critique of these studies, however, questions the validity of the conclusions. Sayetta (51) noted that average lengths of stays of Medi-Cal patients had been declining throughout California during the two years before the inception of the second stage of reviews. Hence, the comparisons of later periods to expected rates based on only one year's prior experience may have overstated the effects of controls. Furthermore, Sayetta's (51) comparisons of demographic and other characteristics of the Sacramento region with comparison areas showed that they differed in ways that could have accounted for the observed differences in relative utilization. Important among these were the considerably higher levels of hospital use in the Sacramento region both before the after the introduction of new controls. These findings suggest that excess utilization may have been more effectively controlled in the comparison areas.

In 1972, a pilot program was begun in which Medicare beneficiaries in the Sacramento area came under the foundation's review program. A study of this project by Bluestone & Baugh (52) shows that during its first two years, hospital utilization declined from levels that prevailed in 1971 and that these declines were larger than those observed in five other regions of California.

The state of Massachusetts introduced in 1973 a program modelled on the Sacramento approach. From a before-and-after study using Blue Cross patients as controls, Fulchiero and her colleagues (53) concluded that the program reduced average stays of Medicaid patients. The study examined average stays and total days of hospital care consumed in 57 of the state's 125 hospitals over two six-month periods before the program was introduced and five six-month intervals after it had become fully operational, omitting the intervening year. The investigators developed a predicted mean length of stay by adjusting for age and sex differences between the Medicaid and Blue Cross patient populations during the entire study period. Observed lengths of stay were then expressed as percentages of expected lengths of stay.

Average lengths of stay were lower in each interval of the postperiod than before the introduction of controls for both the Medicaid and Blue Cross populations. However, differences between the average ratios of observed to predicted stays before and after the program was launched were larger in the Medicaid population. These greater declines in average stays among

Medicaid patients were consistent across the state's five PSRO areas and for nine of the ten most common diagnostic groups. From these findings the authors concluded that the review program was successful in eliminating unnecessary utilization.

Weaknesses in the study's design suggest caution in accepting the author's estimates of savings attributable of utilization review. The data clearly show that average stays decreased among Medicaid patients following the introduction of controls. However, data presented by the authors [p. 576 in ref. (53)] show that the age and diagnosis adjusted average stays were declining at a still higher rate during the year before controls were established. Moreover, average stays of Blue Cross patients paralleled those of Medicaid patients, albeit at consistently lower levels, throughout the postperiod. The investigators suggest [p. 578 in ref. (53)] that this may be due to unintended effects of utilization controls on nonMedicaid patients. If so, the Blue Cross population is not an appropriate comparison group. The dissimilarities between lengths of stays of the two groups during the preperiod and throughout the postperiod also raise questions about the authors' conclusions. In both periods aggregate stays and stays for at least seven of the ten most common diagnoses were considerably higher among Medicaid patients. These differences may be due to extraordinary amounts of unnecessary utilization by Medicaid patients in Massachusetts, insufficient adjustment of patient characteristics, or some combination of these. Whatever the explanation, the fact that eight of the ten postperiod, condition-specific average stays of Medicaid patients exceeded those of Blue Cross patients diminishes the force of the argument that utilization controls were effective in reducing unnecessary hospital stays.

Three other studies attempted in various ways to control for patients' diagnostic conditions and other characteristics associated with hospital use. These studies, like Holahan's (46), provide stronger tests of the effect of utilization controls on hospital use.

One such study was done by Brook and his colleagues (54). In September of 1971, the New Mexico Experimental Medical Review Organization established a statewide utilization review program covering all Medicaid enrollees. Brook et al (54) assessed the effects of this program by analyzing the hospital utilization of two cohorts of Medicaid recipients during the four years following its inception. From aggregate time series and regression analyses they concluded that utilization review had no discernible effects on admission rates per 100 Medicaid enrollees, average lengths of stay, or total hospital days billed to Medicaid. Further exploration of their data revealed that the probability of being hospitalized actually increased over the course of the experiment.

Lave & Leinhardt (55) took advantage of a natural experiment to assess the effects of utilization review in Allegheny County, Pennsylvania. In 1973, the state offered hospitals the opportunity to participate in its predischarge utilization review program for Medicaid patients as an alternative to being subject to the possibility of retroactive denials of payment. Half of the county's 28 hospitals elected to participate. The study compared the experiences of participating hospitals with those of nonparticipating institutions over a three-year period, examining four four-month periods before the program was introduced and four after. Hospital utilization by Medicaid recipients and Blue Cross beneficiaries were examined in terms of overall and preoperative average lengths of stay, average lengths of stay adjusted for case-mixes, and the percentages of patients who were discharged within the target stay established at admission. Using hospitals as units of analysis and employing regression techniques, the investigators found no effects that could be ascribed to utilization review. Average lengths of stay declined for both categories of patients in both experimental and control hospitals, and use by Medicaid patients decreased more than that of Blue Cross beneficiaries. Taking other factors into account, however, declines in average stays and other indicators of utilization did not differ among participating and nonparticipating hospitals.

Another study of Allegheny County hospitals was done by Clendenning and her colleagues (56). Although their approach differs from that employed by Lave & Leinhardt (55), the conclusions agree. No consistent evidence of effects of utilization review was found. The project compared average lengths of stays of patients with the ten most common diagnoses in 11 participating hospitals and in matched control hospitals. The authors reasoned that an effective utilization control program would result in a lowering of average stays in participating hospitals to levels significantly below those of nonparticipating hospitals. Employing these criteria, they found that, for all diagnostic groups pooled, utilization review appeared to reduce stays. However, analyses of the disaggregated diagnostic groups showed that this was true only for maternity cases. With these removed, the authors found no significant reductions in hospital stay attributable to utilization review.

The most extensive study of the effects of utilization review published to date was carried out by the US Department of Health, Education, and Welfare (57). Pursuant to Congressional mandates to assess the status and accomplishments of the PSRO program, DHEW launched a two-year study that culminated in 1977 in an 11-volume report. Dobson et al (58) have summarized the methods and principal findings of this project.

Using PSRO areas of units of analysis, the study compared hospital utilization from 1974 to 1976 by Medicare beneficiaries in 18 areas with active PSROs to the corresponding experiences in 26 areas in which PSROs had yet to attain active status. Three indicators of utilization were used: hospital admissions per 1000 Medicare enrollees, average lengths of stay, and total days of inpatient care per 1000 Medicare enrollees. Overall, analyses revealed no aggregate effects that could be attributed to active PSROs, and other special studies produced mixed results. Use of hospital services by Medicare beneficiaries were examined from 1972 to 1975 in Colorado (where a prototypical statewide PSRO had been active since 1974) and compared with the pooled experience of Kansas and Nebraska. These comparisons showed that total days of hospital care declined in Colorado, principally due to decreases in average length of stays. However, similar decreases were observed in Kansas and Nebraska. Other analyses of stays in 92 hospitals with active PSRO programs and 46 control hospitals showed slight declines in average stays among Medicare patients in the regulated institutions, but about equal magnitudes of increases were observed among Medicaid patients.

SUMMARY   Research on effects of utilization review indicates that these controls may have contributed slightly to lowering average hospital stays in some of the areas in which they have been employed. However, there is no conclusive evidence that they lower per capita use of hospitals or eliminate unnecessary costs.

Researchers who have employed simpler comparative designs have concluded that these controls have contributed to lowering utilization. However, in nearly all instances these conclusions are questionable on methodological grounds. Moreover, none of the studies that have used extensive adjustments to rule out confounding effects have found evidence that utilization review has consistently influenced hospital use.

Rate Controls

The conventional practice of retroactively reimbursing hospitals' costs has long been considered a major source of rising expenditures for inpatient services. By virtually guaranteeing payment of all allowable costs, it has not only failed to reward efficiency, but may have encouraged inefficient practices.

Since the late 1950s, insurers and the federal and state governments have explored several avenues by which to reward hospitals for economic operation. Some of the earliest attempts involved incentive reimbursement schemes that focussed on selected departments within hospitals, principally those providing ancillary and support services (59–62). More recently, the press of mounting hospital costs has prompted insureres and several states to extend rate controls over hospitals' total operations. Rate setting is presently in force in at least parts of 28 states and covers all hospitals in 15. Moreover, cost-containment legislation currently being debated in Congress would, in effect, blanket the nation with hospital rate controls.

Although the particular objectives and administrative features of rate setting vary (6, 63), its general purpose is to encourage efficiency in the use of medical and administrative resources by requiring hospitals to operate within prospectively determined budgets. These budgets are typically set by establishing expected costs per unit of service and projected volumes of utilization, which together give total expected expenses (6, 64).

Because most programs have used average daily costs as the unit for establishing budgets, all of the studies of the impacts of rate setting have focussed on per diem rates or the closely related per admission rates as outcomes.

EVIDENCE   One of the first efforts to control hospital costs by prospective reimbursement was sponsored by Blue Cross of Western Pennsylvania. Beginning in 1950, hospitals in a 28-county region that includes Pittsburgh were categorized into three groups on the basis of the economic characteristics of their areas. Ceiling per diem rates were set for each of these groups at 10% above the average rate, and hospitals were reimbursed for incurred costs subject to their groups' ceiling constraints (65). Grouping procedures were modified in 1966 to take account of hospitals' teaching programs in addition to geographical factors, which resulted in nine reimbursement classes.

Lave and her associates (66) reasoned that this reimbursement scheme provided perverse incentives to hospitals operating below ceilings and may have unduly penalized those operating above them. Because of these, they further hypothesized that the scheme would not effectively control hospital costs. To test these hypotheses, they analyzed changes in average per diem costs from 1966 to 1968, adjusting for case-mix and other patient population and hospital characteristics. Findings supported all three hypotheses. A negative coefficient in their equation for the effect on per diem costs in 1966 suggested that hospitals' costs moved toward their group mean. Lower cost hospitals raised their rates, whereas higher cost institutions lowered theirs. Further analyses showed that hospitals whose costs were higher at the outset of the study were put under possibly unfair pressures to lower costs. The study showed that estimates of changes in hospitals' per diem costs attributable to case-mix differences were negatively associated with indicators of pure cost increases, a fact that the authors interpreted as indicating that high cost hospitals with patients requiring more expensive treatment were forced to compensate for circumstances beyond their control. Finally, comparisons of Pittsburgh hospitals with institutions in other urban areas of the country suggested that the western Pennsylvania scheme had no discernible effect on per diem costs.

In 1971, the Blue Cross plan offered hospitals in western Pennsylvania the option of participating in a modified reimbursement scheme. Five small hospitals opted to do so, one of them a long-term care facility (65, 67). The experimental program established a somewhat higher ceiling at 12% of the groups' averages and required individual hospitals to submit budgets from which prospective rates would be set. Unlike the prevailing system, the optional scheme provided incentives to economize by allowing hospitals that operated under their negotiated budgets to retain half of their savings.

Hellinger (65, 67) has summarized findings of an assessment of this experiment in which the five participating hospitals were compared with a group of ten similar western Pennsylvania hospitals from 1970 to 1974. Over this four-year period the experimental hospitals experienced somewhat lower growth in total inpatient costs and in per diem rates. Most of these differences were due to lower increases in costs of hotel functions (e.g. food services, laundry) in the experimental hospitals; increases in the costs of medical departments did not differ among experimental and control hospitals.

The budget review approach to prospective reimbursement was established in 1960 by Indiana Blue Cross and the state's hospital association. Although the program is voluntary, Blue Cross contracts require participation, and other commercial insurers and the Medicare and Medicaid programs base their reimbursement on rates established by the budget review committee. Hence, all Indiana hospitals participate.

A recent evaluation of this program compared changes in the average cost per admission in Indiana hospitals to that of matched hospitals in four other midwestern states (68). Findings showed that from 1968 to 1973 average costs rose 19% less in Indiana, and from 1958 to 1976 the annual differences between average costs in Indiana hospitals and their controls widened. From analyses of components of hospitals' costs O'Donoghue (68) concluded that savings had been realized across all departments.

Mandatory controls on hospitals' daily rates were first imposed in New York State. In 1969, the state adopted a formula-based approach that sets individual hospitals' rates for Medicaid patients on the basis of inflationary trends, subject to ceilings derived from average per diem costs of groups of hospitals. The state government's program operates along a basically similar scheme as those administered by the state's two Blue Cross plans (65).

Dowling et al (69) assessed the impacts of these controls in the downstate region. Estimating cost functions of hospitals in this area and of a control group of hospitals from other urban areas, the authors concluded that rate controls lowered the 1974 average cost per patient day by 4 to 6% and the cost per patient stay by 2 to 5%. Hellinger's (67) reanalysis of these data yielded a higher estimate of the effect of prospective reimbursement on costs of average patient stays. Because the cost function specification employed by Dowling et al (69) included an indicator of utilization, whereas Hellinger's (67) did not, the lower estimate is probably more accurate. Dowling et al (69) noted that average stays declined more in New York than else-where; hence, lower utilization would have decreased average admission costs.

An assessment of rate controls in upstate New York (70) compared the experience of 63 experimental hospitals with that of 56 controls from Michigan, Ohio, and Wisconsin. Unlike the downstate study, this investigation found no significant changes in average costs that could be attributed to the prospective reimbursement scheme.

Similar studies of rate setting in Rhode Island and New Jersey produced negative conclusions. A budget review system was established in Rhode Island by the Blue Cross plan in 1972 and discontinued a year later. With data from 12 Rhode Island hospitals and matched controls from Massachusetts, Hellinger (65) estimated costs functions from 1969 to 1972. Results showed that rate setting in combination with the Economic Stabilization Program had a negative impact on average per diem and per stay costs in Rhode Island. However, the main effects of rate controls were not significant.

In 1970, New Jersey's insurance commission gave hospitals the option of accepting prospectively determined rates or continuing with the then prevailing system in which ceilings were based on hospitals' cost in base years. By 1972 all hospitals had elected the prospective budgeting scheme, which at that time was jointly administered by the state and an arm of the hospital association.

Using pooled data on New Jersey hospitals from 1969 to 1973, Hellinger (65) estimated a series of cost equations. Estimated changes in average costs per day due to rate controls were small but negative; analyses of costs per stay suggested that rate controls may have contributed to increases in costs.

SUMMARY   Findings from several assessments of hospital rate setting programs present a mixed picture of their effects on hospital costs. Some suggest that these controls have brought about lower average per diem and per stay costs, whereas others find no effect.

Because most studies of rate controls have assessed relatively new programs, inconcsistent and negative findings are perhaps to be expected. In this regard, the notably successful achievements of Indiana's efforts over the past two decades may be indeed revealing (68). On the other hand, they may be the result of a unique combination of historical events that are not reproducible elsewhere.

CONCLUSIONS

Available evidence suggests that, as of the early 1970s, health planning and regulation had little influence on forces that have been implicated in rising hospital costs. The implications of current knowledge for health policy are not altogether clear, however, and indeed can be invoked in support of two diametrically opposed positions. On the one hand, the largely negative experience of earlier efforts can be attributed to the limited authorities and inadequate resources given to planning and regulation. From this perspective, the solution is to improve planning and regulation, which usually implies extending their authorities to larger spheres of activities and decisions (71, 72). On the contrary, critics of health planning and regulation see the evidence as being consistent with the largely negative experience of other industries (30) and observe that the root causes of rising expenditures for medical services are located in fundamental organizational and financial features of the health services industry (41, 73, 74). Hence, they argue that several of the concerns to which current planning and regulatory efforts are addressed can be remedied by broader reforms that will strengthen market forces.

Current knowledge about effects of planning and regulation on health care costs is too narrow a base for firm policy decisions in another perhaps more important respect. Although this chapter has singled out cost containment as one objective of planning and regulation, it is by no means the only one. We are finding in some instances that the pursuit of other socially desirable ends through the same planning and regulatory structures that are expected to control costs has led to internal contradictions. Health planners, for instance, are supposed to improve the accessibility, acceptability, continuity, and quality of health services in their communities; PSROs are charged with encouraging high quality. A broader assessment of planning and regulatory activities is thus required to determine whether their impacts on these matters offset their effectiveness in containing costs.

The frequently voiced criticism that planning and regulation have been fragmented and piecemeal applies equally to research in this area. Studies of effects of planning CES controls, utilization review, and rate setting have proceeded largely independently of one another, with each type concentrating on specific outcomes associated with particular programs. Assessments of CES controls have concentrated on investments and purchasing of equipment; studies of utilization review have examined admission rates and average lengths of hospital stays; investigators of rate setting programs have focussed on average per diem and per stay costs. Such approaches were sensible first steps in an environment in which new programs were being adopted, sometimes experimentally, with the expectation that they would deal with explicitly defined portions of the cost containment problem.

However, as planning and regulatory programs have diffused, the program by program approach to evaluating their impacts is no longer an adequate or even feasible strategy. The simultaneous existence of various planning and regulatory programs in many parts of the country has altered the environments within which each functions. Hence, studies of effects of, say, rate setting on per diem costs must take account of the possible confounding impacts of CES control programs on capital decisions that, in turn, affect the intensity and costs of services. Possibilities of such interaction effects multiply as additional regulatory efforts are considered.

Furthermore, the practice of concentrating on particular components of total health care expenditures fails to take account of the organic nature of the health care cost problem. Although important, the lowering of capital investments or per diem costs and lengths of hospital stays are not ultimate objectives. Rather, planning and regulation should be assessed in terms of how they affect, independently or jointly, the types of services that are available to and used by defined populations and the total costs they entail.

Literature Cited

1. Klarman, H. E. 1977. Planning for facilities. In *Regionalization and Health Policy*, ed. E. Ginzberg, pp. 25–36. Washington DC: Health Resour. Adm., U.S. Dep. Health, Educ., Welfare. 192 pp.
2. May, J. J. 1967. *Health Planning—Its Past and Potential.* Chicago: Cent. for Health Adm. Stud., Univ. Chicago
3. Shryock, R. H. 1967. *Medical Licensing in America, 1650–1965.* Baltimore: Johns Hopkins Univ. Press
4. Somers, A. R. 1969. *Hospital Regulation: The Dilemma of Public Policy.* Princeton: Princeton Univ. Press. 240 pp.
5. Thompson, P. 1977. Voluntary regional planning. See Ref. 1, pp. 123–28
6. Bauer, K. G. 1978. Hospital rate setting —this way to salvation? In *Hospital Cost Containment: Selected Notes for Future Policy*, ed. M. Zubkoff, I. E. Raskin, R. S. Hanft, pp. 349–69. New York: Prodist. 656 pp.
7. Budetti, P. P. 1978. HSAs and PSROs: Can the odd couple learn to live together? *Am. J. Health Plann.* 3(1):1–6
8. Gibson, R. M. 1979. National health expenditures, 1978. *Health Care Financ. Rev.* 1(1):1–36
9. Bice, T. W., Eichhorn, R. L. 1975. Evaluation of public health programs. In *Handbook of Evaluation Research*, ed. M. Guttentag, E. L. Struening, 2:605–20. Beverly Hills: Sage. 736 pp.
10. Lave, J. R., Lave, L. B. 1974. *The Hospital Construction Act: An Evaluation of the Hill-Burton Program, 1948–1973.* Washington DC: Am. Enterp. Inst. Public Policy Res. 77 pp.
11. Palmiere, D. 1972. Lessons learned from the experience of health facilities planning councils. *Am. J. Public Health* 62(9):1235–38
12. May, J. J. 1974. The planning and licensing agencies. In *Regulating Health Facilities Construction*, ed. C. C. Havighurst, pp. 47–68. Washington DC: Am. Enterp. Inst. Public Policy Res. 314 pp.
13. Subcomm. on Public Health and Environ., Comm. on Interstate and Foreign Commerce, House of Representatives. 1974. 93rd Congress, 2nd Session. *National Health Policy and Health Resources Development.* Washington DC: GPO. 996 pp.
14. Comptroller General of the U.S. 1974. *Comprehensive Health Planning as Carried Out by States and Areawide Agencies in Three States.* Washington DC: GPO
15. Lewin & Assoc., Inc. 1975. *Evaluation of the Efficiency and Effectiveness of the Section 1122 Review Process: Part I.* Washington DC: Lewin & Assoc., Inc. 182 pp.
16. MacStravic, R. E. 1977. Size and performance of planning agencies. *Health Serv. Res.* 12(2):163–73
17. Div. Compr. Health Plann. 1974. *Interim Analysis of Comprehensive Health Planning Agency Assessments.* Washington DC: Health Resour. Adm., U.S. Dep. Health, Educ., Welfare. 28 pp.
18. Pearson, D. A. 1976. The concept of regionalized personal health services in the United States. In The *Regionalization of Personal Health Services*, ed. E.

W. Saward, pp. 3–51. New York: Prodist. 305 pp.

19. Klarman, H. E. 1978. Health planning:
Progress, prospects, and issues. *Health
Soc.* 56(1):78–112

20. Altman, D. 1978. The politics of health
care regulation: The case of the National Health Planning and Resources
Development Act. *J. Health Polit. Policy Law* 9(4):560–80

21. Gantz, L. H. 1977. Legal aspects of
health facilities regulation. In *Health
Regulation: Certificate of Need and
1122,* ed. H. H. Hyman, pp. 75–104.
Germantown, Md: Aspen Syst. 185 pp.

22. Wolkstein, I. 1978. The impact of legislation on capital development for health
facilities. In *Health Care Capital: Competition and Control,* ed. G. K.
McLeod, M. Perlman, pp. 7–32. Cambridge, Mass: Ballinger. 411 pp.

23. Inst. Med. 1976. *Controlling the Supply
of Hospital Beds.* Washington DC:
NAS

24. Berry, R. E. 1974. Cost and efficiency in
the production of hospital services. *Milbank Mem. Fund Q.* 52(3):291–313

25. Feldstein, M. S. 1971. Hospital cost inflation: A study of nonprofit price dynamics. *Am. Econ. Rev.* 61(5):835–72

26. Salkever, D. S., Bice, T. W. 1978. Certificate-of-need legislation and hospital
costs. See Ref. 6, pp. 429–60

27. Med. in the Public Interest, Inc. 1978.
*Certificate of Need: An Expanding Reg-
ulatory Concept.* Washington DC: Med.
in the Public Interest, Inc. 940 pp.

28. Hyman, H. H. 1977. Introduction to
key issues in regulation of health facilities and services. See Ref. 21, pp. 1–26

29. Curran, W. J. 1974. A national survey
and analysis of state certificate-of-need
laws for health facilities. See Ref. 12, pp.
85–112

30. Havighurst, C. C. 1973. Regulation of
health facilities and services by certificate of need. *Va. Law Rev.* 59:1143–
1242

31. Posner, R. A. 1974. Certificates of need
for health care facilities: A dissenting
view. See Ref. 12, pp. 113–42

32. Bicknell, W., Walsh, D. 1975. Certificate of need: The Massachusetts experience. *N. Engl. J. Med.* 292:1054–61

33. Am. Health Plann. Assoc. 1979. *Second
Rep. on 1978 Survey of Health Plann.
Agencies.* Mimeo. 54 pp.

34. Evans, R. G. 1977. Letter to the editor.
N. Engl. J. Med. 297:732

35. Rothenberg, E. 1976. *Regulation and
Expansion of Health Facilities: The Cer-

tificate of Need Experience in New York.*
New York: Praeger

36. Hellinger, F. J. 1976. The effect of certificate-of-need legislation on hospital
investment. *Inquiry* 13(2):187–93

37. Salkever, D. S., Bice, T. W. 1976. The
impact of certificate-of-need controls on
hospital investment. *Health Soc.* 54(2):
185–212

38. Salkever, D. S., Bice, T. W. 1979. *Hospital Certificate-of-Need Controls: Impact
on Investment, Costs, and Use.* Washington DC: Am. Enterp. Inst. Public
Policy Res. 103 pp.

39. Cromwell, J., Ginsburg, P., Hamilton,
D., Summer, M. 1975. *Incentives and
Decisions Underlying Hospitals' Adop-
tion and Utilization of Major Capital
Equipment.* Cambridge, Mass: Abt As-
soc.

40. Russell, L. B. 1978. *Technology in Hos-
pitals: Medical Advances and Their
Diffusion.* Washington DC: Brookings
Inst. 230 pp.

41. Havighurst, C. C., Hackbarth, G. M.
1979. Private cost containment. *N.
Engl. J. Med.* 300(23):1298–1305

42. Goldberg, L. G., Greenberg, W. G.
1977. The effect of physician controlled
health insurance. *J. Health Polit. Policy
Law* 2(2):48–78

43. Staff of the Comm. on Finance, U.S.
Senate. 1970. *Medicare and Medicaid:
Problems, Issues, and Alternatives.*
Washington DC: GPO. 323 pp.

44. Blumstein, J. F. 1978. The role of
PSROs in hospital cost containment.
See Ref. 6, pp. 461–88

45. Iglehart, J. K. 1978. PSROs reinstated
in FY 1979 budget after Califano's plea.
Hosp. Prog. 59(2):17–18

46. Holahan, J. 1977. Foundations for medical care: An empirical investigation of
the delivery of health services to a
Medicaid population. *Inquiry* 14(4):
352–68

47. Flashner, B. A., Reed, S., White, R.,
Norris, J. 1972. The hospital admission
and surveillance program in Illinois. *J.
Am. Med. Assoc.* 221(10):1153–58

48. Davidson, S. M., Wacker, R. C., Klein,
D. H. 1973. Professional Standards Re-
view Organizations: A critique. *J. Am.
Med. Assoc.* 226(9):1106–08

49. Brian, E. W. 1972. Government control
of hospital utilization: A California experience. *N. Engl. J. Med.* 286(25):
1340–44

50. Brian, E. 1973. Foundation for medical
care control of hospital utilization:
CHAP—a PSRO prototype. *N. Engl. J.
Med.* 228(17):878–82

51. Sayetta, R. B. 1976. Critique of an earlier study of the Sacramento Medical Care Foundation's certified hospital admission program (CHAP). *Med. Care* 14(1):80–92

52. Bluestone, M., Baugh, D. K. 1978. *An Evaluation of a Medicare Concurrent Utilization Review Project: The Sacramento Certified Hospital Admission Program.* Washington DC: Off. of Res. and Stat. Soc. Secur. Adm., U.S. Dep. Health, Educ., Welfare. 22 pp.

53. Fulchiero, A., Miller, S., Foley, C. R., Ballantine, H. T. Jr., Amorosino, C. S. Jr. 1978. Can PSROs be cost effective? *N. Engl. J. Med.* 299(11):574–80

54. Brook, R. H., Williams, K. N., Rolph, J. E. 1978. *Controlling the Use and Cost of Medical Services: The New Mexico Experimental Medical Care Review Organization—A Four-Year Case Study.* Santa Monica: Rand Corp. 76 pp.

55. Lave, J. R., Leinhardt, S. 1976. An evaluation of a hospital stay regulatory mechanism. *Am. J. Public Health* 66(10):959–67

56. Clendenning, M. K., Wolfe, H., Shuman, L. J., Huber, G. A. 1976. The effect of a target date based utilization review program on length of stay. *Med. Care* 14(9):751–64

57. Off. of Plann., Eval., and Legis. 1978. *Professional Standards Review Organizations: Program Evaluation—Executive Summary.* Washington DC: Health Serv. Adm., U.S. Dep. of Health, Educ., Welfare. 155 pp.

58. Dobson, A., Greer, J. G., Carlson, R. H., Davis, F. A., Kucken, L. E., Steinhardt, B. J., Ferry, T. P., Adler, G. S. 1978. PSROs: Their current status and their impact to date. *Inquiry* 15(2):113–28

59. Chassin, M. R. 1978. The containment of hospital costs: A strategic assessment. *Med. Care* 16(10): Suppl. 55 pp.

60. Elnicki, R. A. 1975. SSA-Connecticut hospital incentive reimbursement experiment cost evaluation. *Inquiry* 12(1):47–58

61. Hardwick, C. P., Wolfe, H. 1972. Evaluation of an incentive reimbursement experiment. *Med. Care* 10(2):109–17

62. McCarthy, C. 1975. Incentive reimbursement as an impetus to cost containment. *Inquiry* 12(4):320–29

63. Health Care Financ. Adm. 1978. *Abstracts of State-Legislated Hospital Cost Containment Programs.* Washington DC: U.S. Dep. Health, Educ., Welfare

64. Dowling, W. L. 1974. Prospective reimbursement of hospitals. *Inquiry* 11(3):163–80

65. Hellinger, F. J. 1976. Prospective reimbursement through budget review: New Jersey, Rhode Island, and Western Pennsylvania. *Inquiry* 13(3):309–20

66. Lave, J. R., Lave, L. B., Silverman, L. P. 1973. A proposal for incentive reimbursement for hospitals. *Med. Care* 11(2):79–90

67. Hellinger, F. J. 1978. An empirical analysis of several prospective reimbursement systems. See Ref. 6, pp. 370–400

68. O'Donoghue, P. 1978. *Controlling Hospital Costs: The Revealing Case of Indiana.* Denver: Policy Cent., Inc. 146 pp.

69. Dowling, W., House, P. J., Lehman, J. M., Meade, G. L., Teague, N., Trivedi, V. M., Watts, C. A. 1976. *Prospective Reimbursement in Downstate New York and Its Impacts on Hospitals—A Summary.* Seattle: Cent. for Health Serv. Res., Dep. Health Serv., Univ. Washington. 93 pp.

70. Abt Associates, Inc. 1976. *Analysis of Prospective Payment Systems for Upstate New York.* Cambridge, Mass: Abt Assoc., Inc. 192 pp.

71. Blum, H. L. 1976. *Expanding Health Care Horizons: From a General Systems Concept of Health to a National Health Policy.* Oakland: Third Party Assoc. 217 pp.

72. Joe, T., Needleman, J., Lewin, L. S. 1976. Health care capital financing: Regulation, the market, and public policy. See Ref. 22, pp. 63–80

73. Enthoven, A. C. 1978. Competition of alternative delivery systems. In *Competition in the Health Care Sector: Past, Present, and Future,* ed. W. Greenberg, pp. 322–51. Washington DC: Fed. Trade Comm. 478 pp.

74. Feldstein, M. S. 1977. The high cost of hospitals—and what to do about it. *Public Interest* 48:40–54

Ann. Rev. Public Health 1980. 1:163–225

BIOSTATISTICAL IMPLICATIONS ♦12507
OF DESIGN, SAMPLING, AND
MEASUREMENT TO HEALTH
SCIENCE DATA ANALYSIS

Gary G. Koch, Dennis B. Gillings, and Maura E. Stokes

Department of Biostatistics, School of Public Health,
University of North Carolina, Chapel Hill, North Carolina 27514

INTRODUCTION

One of the reasons the field of biostatistics is considered difficult is that many advantageous statistical methods are currently available, but the extent and relevance of their application to policy, evaluation, and research questions in the health sciences is often limited by analytical assumptions that are hard to interpret. Two basic issues underly this dilemma: (*a*) the distinction between the study population (that is investigated) and the target population (for which conclusions are formulated), as assumptions are needed to facilitate linkages between them, and (*b*) the role of the measurement process in enhancing such linkages. Further, it is important to consider the ways in which study design sets a framework for interpretation of observed associations. In other words, sampling and measurement processes determine the framework for statistical analysis together with the population for which statistical results are relevant, and study design affects the strength of conclusions regardless of their generalizability.

The basic objective of this chapter is to discuss the relevance of sampling and measurement processes to two related issues: the linkage of analytical results for a study population to further derivations for a target population; and the similarities among related strategies for the analysis of data involving different measurement scales. Primary attention is given to reviewing

163

several areas of statistical literature that are useful in health science applications. More specifically, the following topics are discussed with examples:

1. The implications of coverage, sampling error, and measurement error aspects of research design to the validity of generalizations from a study to a target population. A special case is the difference between how these issues are addressed in randomized vs nonrandomized clinical trials with historical controls (see analyses of Table 2 and Table 4).
2. Randomization statistical methods for testing hypotheses about finite populations in either an observational or a randomized study (see analyses of Tables 1 through 5). The similarity between methods commonly applied to data on different measurement scales (nominal, ordinal, interval) is discussed.
3. Large sample generalized chi-square methods for analyzing categorical data. Both weighted least squares and maximum likelihood methods are presented, with emphasis given to differences in interpretation between additive and multiplicative models (see Tables 1 through 3).
4. Large sample chi-square methods for the analysis of ordinal data. Both nonparametric rank methods and generalized chi-square methods are considered alternative strategies (see Table 4).
5. Large sample methods for testing hypotheses and fitting models to censored survival data in follow-up studies (see Table 5).
6. Large sample methods for testing hypotheses and fitting models to estimates based upon complex sample surveys (see Table 6).

With the intent of integrating the multiple directions of discussion to be undertaken, this chapter groups common statistical methods into general types and emphasizes issues that underly their application to analogous questions. Thus, although the interplay among the multiple objectives of this discussion may cause parts to appear difficult at a first reading, its ultimate intent is to resolve some paradoxes and explain relevant subtleties of biostatistics as practiced today.

RESEARCH DESIGN CONSIDERATIONS

Research design is one of the most important determinants of statistical analysis strategy because it guides the linkage between what is observed and how it can be interpreted. More generally, this linkage has been referred to as *internal validity* (1). Further, the synthesis of research design with assumptions that extend its scope is the basis of *external validity*. Because such assumptions are external to study design, some substantive justification is required to ensure their plausibility. As a consequence, two types of statistical strategies are of interest for most research investigations: 1. *local population analyses* directed at internal validity and 2. *extended population analyses* directed at external validity.

Because strategies 1 and 2 are concerned with different questions, one, and its corresponding methods, cannot be said to be better than the other. However, the differences between them are important because of implications for interpretation. The most relevant consideration is the distinction between the sampling and measurement processes that generate the data and a more general situation that these data are claimed to represent. We will use the term *sampling process* to imply coverage and sampling error and the term *measurement process* to encompass response (or measurement) error, as they relate to the US Bureau of the Census total sample survey error decomposition (see 2–5), and analysis of variance decompositions for experimental data (see 6, 7). *Coverage* is the extent to which all possible types of subjects are either included or are eligible for inclusion in the study; *sampling error* is the extent to which subjects are different with respect to the true or idealized expected values for phenomena under study; and *response error* is the extent to which multiple observations of the same phenomenon for the same subject are different from each other.

Sampling Process Issues

Most research data in the health sciences can be classified according to one of the following three types of sampling processes:

1. Historical data from all subjects in a study population having a natural (i.e. geographic or temporal) or fortuitous definition.
2. Experimental data involving the random allocation of subjects in a study population to different treatments.
3. Sample survey data involving the random selection of subjects from a larger study population.

Another type of sampling process occasionally used is the synthesis of processes 2 and 3, i.e. the random allocation of treatments to subjects from a randomly selected sample. This type of sampling process provides both experimental and survey data.

LOCAL POPULATION ANALYSIS   A similarity among the sampling processes 1 through 3 is their linkage to a corresponding study population for local population analyses. However, the coverages of their respective populations are different because of the extent to which they involve randomization; i.e. historical data with no randomization usually have only isolated coverage of a convenient population; experimental data with random allocation have multifold coverage for the experiences under alternative treatments of a protocol restricted population; and sample survey data with random selection usually have wide coverage of some large scale population.

An important issue for each of processes 1 through 3 is the extent to which nonresponse reduces coverage. Alternatively, assumptions about incomplete data are required in order for the actual coverage of the study population, through an extended population analysis, to be equivalent to the ideal coverage that would have existed if response was 100%. As a result, the topic of incomplete data has received extensive discussion in recent statistical literature. A review of issues and strategies for sample survey data is given in (8), and for experimental data in (9–11).

Finally, as indicated in standard references on sampling [e.g. (12) and (13)] or experimental design (e.g. 14–17), the unit of randomization can be subjects, clusters of subjects, subjects within clusters of subjects, or more sophisticated extensions. Furthermore, randomization may be undertaken restrictively in subsets (called strata or blocks) with equal or unequal probabilities. In survey research, these considerations lead to stratified, multi-stage cluster probability random samples; whereas in experimental design research, they lead to repeated measurements (or split-plot) experiments.

EXTENDED POPULATION ANALYSIS   For many biostatistical applications, the target population of interest is often more extensive than the study population. For extended population analyses, assumptions about sampling errors are required for each of the sampling processes 1 through 3. If the principal analysis objective is detecting associations between outcome measures and demographic, diagnostic, and environmental variables, then one assumption that can be used to link observed data to the target population is that there are no sampling errors among the outcome measure true values (or conceptual expected values) for subjects with the same characteristics. Under this condition, partitioning subjects according to explanatory variables may provide a *homogeneous stratification framework* that allows one to view the variation among subjects with the same characteristics as response error.

If the homogeneous stratification assumption is considered reasonable, then historical data, experimental data, and sample survey data represent equivalent sampling frameworks from an extended population analysis point of view. More specifically, all are equivalent to stratified simple random sampling with replacement (in reference to response error) from the correspondingly structured target population provided that (*a*) the *stratum* to which a subject belongs is identifiable without response error and (*b*) the measurement process for the outcome measure reports the same distribution of values for the same phenomenon, regardless of the stratum to which a subject belongs. Under these conditions, there are no sampling errors within strata; associations between outcome measures and explanatory variables are investigated in terms of across-strata variation relative to within-strata response error. Consequently, the only important aspect of the sampling process for extended population analyses is that its scope be comprehensive and include enough subjects from a sufficient number of strata so that (a) the across-strata variation provides meaningful information about the outcome measure and (b) the within-strata variation provides an adequate basis for assessing the plausibility of the homogeneous stratification assumption. For this reason, large sample size together with representation of all strata are critical requirements for such analysis. The specific selection process (e.g. clustering) is of no technical importance because the data are viewed as equivalent to a stratified simple random sample. Moreover, this framework is equivalent to probability distributional sampling (e.g. binomial, exponential, normal, etc) or stochastic process sampling (e.g. Poisson) discussed in standard references (e.g. 18, 19) if the stratified population structure can be presumed known. As a result, data analysis can be based on general methods with optimal theoretical properties. Finally, the statistical issues associated with incomplete data are also more straightforward because both the observed and missing data may be assumed to come from the same underlying distribution.

In summary, although extended population analyses are of interest for many investigations and are straightforward to apply, they should be viewed with caution because they are based on assumptions external to the data. Any conclusions are tentative until they are supported by similar studies for other locations and time periods or until they are accepted as reproducible in principle.

Measurement Process Issues

The measurement process is concerned with the manner by which data are obtained and the form in which they are expressed. For both of these aspects of data collection, the basic objective is for the data to be relevant, reliable, and valid (see 20). A measurement process is *relevant* if it provides information of substantive interest. It is *reliable* if it yields consistent values for the same phenomena in the sense of minimal response error. More specifically, the general concept of reliability also encompasses the following:

1. Precision—the extent to which multiple observations of the same phenomenon for the same subject by the same observer are similar.
2. Objectivity—the extent to which multiple observations of the same phenomenon for the same subject by different observers are similar.

3. Constancy—the extent to which the phenomenon under study is stable in value within the same subject (i.e. tends not to fluctuate due to intrinsic biological variability, etc).
4. Congruence—the extent to which multiple measures of multiple aspects for the same phenomenon within the same subject are in general agreement.

Finally, a measurement process is considered *valid* if it is relevant, reliable, and yields values that provide a convincing basis for the evaluation of the research questions for which the study of the observed phenomena was undertaken. In this regard, validity can be based on intuitive grounds (*face validity*), substantive theoretical grounds (*construct validity*), agreement among experts (*consensual validity*), association with other measures that are accepted as valid (*correlational validity*), and association with some type of correct decision pertaining to the research objectives of the study (*predictive validity*).

DATA ACQUISITION METHODS   The manner by which data are collected for investigations in the health sciences can be classified according to communication mode and time orientation.

Communication modes   Self-reported questionnaires, telephone interviews, and personal interviews represent the three most commonly used communication modes for obtaining data. Of these the self-reported questionnaire is the least expensive. It also has the advantage of reflecting the subject's personal expression of the information that is sought without the potential bias that may arise in reaction to an interviewer who may be perceived in either a positive or negative light. However, in many situations, the subject may not understand a questionnaire sufficiently to provide accurate information, and so the use of interviews is preferable provided that any bias associated with it is minimal. Finally, many medical diagnostic or evaluation procedures require a personal interview, either in terms of laboratory tests or physician examination, because the patient may have no personal knowledge of the phenomena under study.

Time orientations   Cross-sectional and longitudinal acquisition represent the two types of time orientations for collecting data. Cross-sectional data are collected at a single point of time. Furthermore, many cross-sectional studies are retrospective if they collect additional information about subjects' past history. For this type of study, any association between past history and current status should be viewed cautiously because a cross-section of subjects may be biased to include an excess with past histories that are compatible with current availability. For example, subjects for whom the association does not apply may have died and so this feature is not represented.

Longitudinal studies are prospective because they are concerned with the future experience of subjects. One type of longitudinal study involves the successive evaluation of subjects at regular time intervals with respect to one or more outcome measures and is often termed *repeated measurements study.* Alternatively, follow-up studies that monitor the status of a subject until the occurrence of a defined event are also longitudinal.

DATA EXPRESSION   The form in which data are expressed can be classified according to two basic dimensions. These are measurement scale and structure.

Measurement scales   Nominal, ordinal, interval, and ratio scales are the four main types of measurement frameworks. Nominal scales are the crudest, as they provide only an indication of whether a subject belongs to a particular category. Ordinal scales involve values that can be ranked from poorest to best, and thus give directional information. Interval scales provide numerical measurement on a continuous scale and demand that equal differences between points have the same meaning regardless of location. Although such scales may seem applicable to many situations, caution should be observed. For example, a reduction in weight of 20 pounds from 160 pounds may be considered healthy for a 5'4" male, but it may be dangerous for a 6'6" male. Finally, ratio scales require that equal ratios as well as equal differences of measured values have the same meaning regardless of the locations of those measured values.

The measurement scale is important because it determines the type of information available for statistical analysis. In particular, contingency table (or categorical data) methods are used for nominal data and ordinal data that are expressed in discrete categories; nonparametric rank methods are used for ordinal data for which continuous values are available; and parametric methods based upon assumed sampling processes are used for interval and/or ratio data.

Data structure   The data structure for an investigation can involve either a single outcome measure, and be called *univariate,* or several outcome measures, in which case it is *multivariate.* Further, it can include duplicate determinations by the same, or different observers to explore reliability and response error.

Finally, an investigation can be multifactorial and be concerned with associations between outcome measures and accompanying explanatory variables such as demographic, diagnostic, and environmental factors.

Research Design Examples

HISTORICAL DATA   The term *historical data* is used to describe research designs that do not involve the application of any type of explicit probability randomization process to the subjects under study. Some examples are:

1. Studies of extent of injury for all persons in automobile accidents during a particular time period in some geographic area (see Table 1).
2. A nonrandomized prospective study of the outcome of medical treatment in comparison to the experience of an historical control population who previously received another treatment (see Table 2).
3. A cross-sectional study to explore associations between current health status and aspects of work environment and previous medical history (see Table 3).

For these and other situations with a natural, fortuitous, or specially-selected sample such as case/control studies or health services resource utilization assessments in a community setting, the subjects under study are representative only of themselves. For this reason, a local population analysis identifies associations in this restricted setting. Alternatively, if certain assumptions can be justified, extended population analysis is possible and more comprehensive questions can be addressed.

EXPERIMENTAL DATA   The term *experimental data* is used to describe research designs that involve random allocation of a population of subjects to treatment groups. Such randomization may be applied separately in several clinics of a multicenter study, in which case it is stratified or restricted (see Table 4), or it may be applied to the overall patient population, ignoring the clinic (or assumed to be equivalent to such an allocation process as in Table 5).

An example of an experimental study, which is considered later, is a clinical trial to compare four surgical treatments of duodenal ulcer for eligible patients at 17 participating hospitals. The outcome measures of interest are dumping syndrome severity (an ordinal scaled measure of an undesirable sequela of surgery) and patient follow-up status with respect to death, recurrence, or reoperation during the five years following treatment. Subjects under study represent themselves and allow a local population analysis. In addition, an extended population analysis may be warranted, depending on the validity of necessary assumptions.

Table 1 Driver status with respect to serious injury cross-classified according to vehicle size, vehicle age, and vehicle model year for 1966, 1968–1972 North Carolina multiple vehicle accidents with left side or front impact for sober drivers traveling at moderately high speed

Vehicle size	Vehicle age in years	Model year	Driver status re serious injury		Percentage accidents serious injury		Simplified linear model[a]		Model predicted percentage serious	
			No	Yes	Estimate	SE	Specifi- cation (X)	WLS parameter estimates ± SEs	Estimate	SE
Small	0–2	≤66	119	31	20.7	3.3	100	21.5 ± 1.3	21.5	1.3
Small	0–2	67–69	262	61	18.9	2.2	101	−3.3 ± 0.7	18.5	1.2
Small	3–5	≤66	255	66	20.6	2.3	100	−3.0 ± 1.2	21.5	1.3
Small	3–5	67–69	171	42	19.7	2.7	101		18.5	1.2
Middle	0–2	≤66	143	29	16.9	2.9	110		18.3	0.9
Middle	0–2	67–69	405	67	14.2	1.6	111		15.3	0.8
Middle	3–5	≤66	297	69	18.9	2.0	110		18.3	0.9
Middle	3–5	67–69	223	49	18.0	2.3	111		15.3	0.8
Standard	0–2	≤66	137	31	18.5	3.0	120		15.0	1.1
Standard	0–2	67–69	624	87	12.2	1.2	121		12.0	0.8
Standard	3–5	≤66	470	82	14.9	1.5	120		15.0	1.1
Standard	3–5	67–69	407	50	10.9	1.5	121		12.0	0.8

[a] $Q_W(DF = 9) = 4.53$ is nonsignificant with $P > 0.50$ for goodness of fit.

Table 2 Liver function outcome status for treatment and historical control populations of overdose patients cross-classified according to diagnostic risk status and time to hospital admission

Diagnostic risk status	Time to hospital admission	Group	Liver function outcome status		Percentage		Simplified logistic model[a]		Model predicted percentages severe	
			Severe	Not severe	estimate	severe SE	Specification (X)	ML parameter estimates ±SEs	Estimate	SE
Moderate	Early	Treatment	7	55	11.3	4.0	1000	-2.381 ± 0.356	8.5	2.8
Moderate	Early	Control	4	19	17.4	7.9	1001	1.740 ± 0.432	24.9	7.2
Moderate	Delayed	Treatment	3	14	17.6	9.2	1010	1.122 ± 0.324	22.1	6.4
Moderate	Delayed	Control	3	2	60.0	21.9	1011	1.278 ± 0.436	50.5	10.4
Moderate	Late	Treatment	1	0	100.0	38.5[b]	1020		46.6	15.0
Moderate	Late	Control	2	1	66.7	27.2	1021		75.8	11.8
High	Early	Treatment	6	12	33.3	11.1	1100		34.5	8.8
High	Early	Control	6	2	75.0	15.3	1101		65.4	10.8
High	Delayed	Treatment	3	4	42.9	18.7	1110		61.8	9.2
High	Delayed	Control	3	0	100.0	18.7[b]	1111		85.3	6.2
High	Late	Treatment	5	1	83.3	15.2	1120		83.2	8.4
High	Late	Control	6	0	100.0	10.5[b]	1121		94.7	3.4

[a]Qp(DF = 8) = 5.25 is nonsignificant with $p > 0.50$ for goodness of fit.
[b]Standard error estimate based upon adjustment of 0 frequencies to 0.5 as discussed in (35) and (51).

Table 3 Employee complaint status with respect to byssinosis symptoms, cross-classified according to workplace condition, years of employment, and smoking history for participants in a 1973 pulmonary function survey at a large textile corporation

Workplace condition	Years employment	Smoking re past 5 years	Complaint status re byssinosis symptoms		Byssinosis symptoms prevalences/1000		Simplified linear model for prevalence rates[a]		Model predicted prevalences	
			Yes	No	Estimate	SE	Specification (X)	WLS parameter estimates ± SEs	Estimate	SE
Dusty	<10	Yes	30	203	128.8	21.9	1101	12.0 ± 1.6	140.1	20.1
Dusty	<10	No	7	119	55.6	20.4	1100	33.8 ± 19.0	45.8	18.9
Dusty	≥10	Yes	57	161	261.5	29.8	1111	100.6 ± 27.0	240.7	24.9
Dusty	≥10	No	11	81	119.6	33.8	1110	94.3 ± 25.0	146.4	26.4
Not Dusty	<10	Yes	14	1340	10.3	2.7	1000		12.0	1.6
Not Dusty	<10	No	12	1004	11.8	3.4	1000		12.0	1.6
Not Dusty	≥10	Yes	24	1360	17.3	3.5	1000		12.0	1.6
Not Dusty	≥10	No	10	986	10.0	3.2	1000		12.0	1.6

[a] $Q_W(DF = 4) = 4.68$ is nonsignificant with $p > 0.25$ for goodness of fit.

Table 4 Dumping syndrome severity for duodenal ulcer patients treated with one of four randomly assigned operations at four participating hospitals

Hospital	Operation[a]	Dumping syndrome severity			Standardized uniform average score		Simplified linear model[b]		Model predicted average scores	
		None	Slight	Moderate	Estimate	SE	Specification (X)	WLS parameter estimates ± SEs	Estimate	SE
1	V + D	23	7	2	0.172	0.052	1 0.00	0.200 ± 0.026	0.200	0.026
1	V + A	23	10	5	0.263	0.058	1 0.25	0.172 ± 0.058	0.243	0.017
1	V + H	20	13	5	0.303	0.057	1 0.50		0.287	0.018
1	GR	24	10	6	0.275	0.058	1 0.75		0.330	0.028
2	V + D	18	6	1	0.160	0.055	1 0.00		0.200	0.026
2	V + A	18	6	2	0.192	0.061	1 0.25		0.243	0.017
2	V + H	13	13	2	0.304	0.058	1 0.50		0.287	0.018
2	GR	9	15	2	0.365	0.058	1 0.75		0.330	0.028
3	V + D	8	6	3	0.353	0.091	1 0.00		0.200	0.026
3	V + A	12	4	4	0.300	0.089	1 0.25		0.243	0.017
3	V + H	11	6	2	0.263	0.078	1 0.50		0.287	0.018
3	GR	7	7	4	0.417	0.090	1 0.75		0.330	0.028
4	V + D	12	9	1	0.250	0.062	1 0.00		0.200	0.026
4	V + A	15	3	2	0.175	0.073	1 0.25		0.243	0.017
4	V + H	14	8	3	0.280	0.070	1 0.50		0.287	0.018
4	GR	13	6	4	0.304	0.080	1 0.75		0.330	0.028

[a] For operations, V + D denotes vagotomy and drainage, V + A denotes vagotomy and antrectomy, V + H denotes vagotomy and hemigastrectomy, GR denotes gastric resection.

[b] $Q_W(DF = 14) = 8.94$ is nonsignificant with $P > 0.50$ for goodness of fit.

Table 5 Follow-up outcome status for duodenal ulcer patients treated with one of four randomly assigned operations

Operation[a]	Follow-up status re 6 months, 24 months, 60 months							Life table survival percentages and (SEs) at times in months			Exponential model[b] survival percentages and (SEs) at times in months		
	Death, recurrence, reoperation during time intervals			Lost to follow-up during time intervals			Patient status satisfactory at 60 months						
	0–6	7–24	25–60	0–6	7–24	25–60		6	24	60	6	24	60
V + D	12	16	26	8	13	36	226	96.4 (1.0)	91.4 (1.5)	82.6 (2.2)	96.7 (0.5)	92.5 (0.6)	84.5 (1.2)
V + A	11	16	19	7	7	35	236	96.6 (1.0)	91.6 (1.5)	85.3 (2.0)	96.7 (0.5)	92.5 (0.6)	84.5 (1.2)
V + H	9	5	10	5	17	24	273	97.4 (0.9)	95.8 (1.1)	92.6 (1.5)	97.7 (0.5)	96.0 (0.7)	92.8 (1.4)
GR	9	15	24	8	11	37	242	97.4 (0.9)	92.9 (1.4)	85.0 (2.0)	96.7 (0.5)	92.5 (0.6)	84.5 (1.2)
Combined	41	52	79	28	48	132	977						
Scores to identify quasi-ordering	0.026	0.078	0.175	0.500	0.515	0.535	0.564	$Q_{KW}(DF = 3) = 14.04$ is significant with $p < 0.01$ for comparison of operations with respect to event survival.					
Life table survival difference scores	−0.970	−0.928	−0.858	0.015	0.051	0.107	0.142	$Q_{KW}(DF = 3) = 14.49$ is significant with $P < 0.01$ for comparison of operations with respect to event survival.					

[a] For operations, V + D denotes vagotomy and drainage, V + A denotes vagotomy and antrectomy, V + H denotes vagotomy and hemigastrectomy, GR denotes gastric resection.

[b] $Q_{W}(DF = 9) = 3.04$ is nonsignificant with $P > 0.50$ for goodness of fit.

SAMPLE SURVEY DATA   Probability random selection of subjects from a larger population leads to *sample survey data.* An example is the Health Interview Survey (HIS) of the National Center for Health Statistics, and an outcome of interest is the estimated number of physician visits per person per year (see Table 6). For this situation, local population analyses relate to the population from which the sample was selected and have straightforward interpretation. Extended population analyses are more awkward because, in this situation, sample survey data are equivalent to historical data (because the population from which they were obtained is a natural, fortuitous, or self-selected sample of some larger target population of interest).

STATISTICAL METHODOLOGY CONSIDERATIONS

Statistical methods for the analysis of historical, experimental, and sample survey research designs for which data are obtained for individual subjects (or experimental units) can be classified into three general classes:

1. *Randomization statistical methods* to test hypotheses about finite populations—For these methods, the only assumption required is randomized allocation of subjects either explicitly (experimental data) or implicitly via the hypothesis itself (historical data). In the latter case it would be important to control for other variables that might influence the observed outcomes, as only explicit randomization can be assumed to balance their effects.
2. *Weighted least squares methods* for large sample chi-square tests of hypotheses for linear model descriptions of variation among a set of estimates and the estimation of model parameters—For these methods, the only required assumption is probability random selection, either explicitly (sample survey data) or implicitly via the homogeneous stratification assumption for extended population analyses.
3. *Maximum likelihood methods* for the estimation and testing of parameters in an assumed structural model—Additional technical assumptions are necessary either in the form of underlying probability distributions (e.g. binomial, exponential, and normal) or stochastic processes (e.g. Poisson). Thus, maximum likelihood methods are mostly restricted to extended population analyses (in which the underlying probability model is viewed as the rationale for the homogeneous stratification assumption or vice versa).

In addition, these three approaches to statistical analysis are of interest for applications involving aggregate data in which the unit of study is a geographic area. However, statistical methods for these situations, such as

Table 6 Estimated physician visits per person per year for the 1973 HIS survey of the US population cross-classified according to residence, family income, and education of head of household

Residence	Family income (1,000's)	Education family head (years)	HIS physician visits per person per year		Simplified linear model		Model predicted physician visits per person per year	
			Estimate	SE	Specification (X)	WLS parameter estimates ± SEs	Estimate	SE
SMSA	<5	<12	6.15	0.18	111	4.18 ± 0.11	5.95	0.07
SMSA	<5	12	6.17	0.41	111	0.66 ± 0.11	5.95	0.07
SMSA	<5	>12	6.31	0.49	111	1.12 ± 0.09	5.95	0.07
SMSA	5–15	<12	4.73	0.13	110		4.83	0.07
SMSA	5–15	12	4.98	0.17	110		4.83	0.07
SMSA	5–15	>12	6.08	0.19	111		5.95	0.07
SMSA	≥15	<12	4.82	0.25	110		4.83	0.07
SMSA	≥15	12	4.70	0.18	110		4.83	0.07
SMSA	≥15	>12	5.66	0.16	111		5.95	0.07
Non-SMSA	<5	<12	5.08	0.26	101		5.30	0.11
Non-SMSA	<5	12	5.36	0.44	101		5.30	0.11
Non-SMSA	<5	>12	4.58	0.58	101		5.30	0.11
Non-SMSA	5–15	<12	4.14	0.15	100		4.18	0.11
Non-SMSA	5–15	12	4.32	0.19	100		4.18	0.11
Non-SMSA	5–15	>12	5.06	0.29	101		5.30	0.11
Non-SMSA	≥15	<12	4.42	0.37	100		4.18	0.11
Non-SMSA	≥15	12	4.49	0.33	100		4.18	0.11
Non-SMSA	≥15	>12	4.48	0.31	101		5.30	0.11

simultaneous structural equation models and time series models, and the issue of ecological correlation are outside the scope of this paper. Some references in which they are discussed include (21–24).

A more explicit understanding of methods 1 through 3 can be gained by considering the general data array in Table 7, in which $h = 1,2,\ldots,q$ indexes a set of strata for which the respective sampling and/or measurement processes are independent (via the study design or equivalent assumptions). Such strata correspond to sets of subjects for whom there is interest in comparisons or relationships involving a set of subpopulations indexed by $i = 1,2,\ldots,s$ and a set of outcome measures (or response variables) indexed by $j = 1,2,\ldots,d$. The subjects within the i-th subpopulation of the h-th stratum are indexed by $l = 1,2,\ldots,n_{hi}$. Thus y_{hijl} denotes the observed value for the j-th response variable for the l-th subject in the i-th subpopulation of the h-th stratum. Finally, potentially important aspects of structure for the subpopulations and/or strata are expressed through *intervening variables* indexed by $k = 1,2,\ldots,w$. Examples of intervening variables w_{hik} include indicator (dummy) variables and quantitative scores for cross-classifications that underly the subpopulations or strata.

Some applications in which this general framework is useful are as follows:

1. Automobile accident studies exploring associations between driver injury and motor vehicle model year—Strata correspond to impact site, impact speed, vehicle size, and vehicle age; subpopulations correspond to vehicle model year classifications; and the outcome measure corresponds to extent of injury. Otherwise, the actual value of vehicle weight (or an equivalent index for ranges of it) is an intervening variable (see Table 1).

2. A multicenter randomized clinical trial to compare four surgical operations for duodenal ulcer, undertaken at four hospitals—Strata correspond to hospitals; subpopulations correspond to operations; and the outcome measure is dumping syndrome severity. Otherwise, an index of the proportional amount of stomach removed (0.00, 0.25, 0.50, 0.75) is an intervening variable (see Table 4).

3. A national sample survey of health services utilization—Strata correspond to design factors such as region of the country; subpopulations correspond to domains based on education, income, and urban vs rural area of residence; and the outcome measure is estimated number of physician visits. Otherwise, indexes (or indicators) for education and income are intervening variables (see Table 6).

More generally, the data array in Table 7 encompasses the following research design considerations:

Table 7 General format for data array

Stratum	Subpopulations (groups or domains)	Subjects in subpopulations	Within strata × subpopulation scaling factor	Response variables		
				1	2 $\cdots$	d
1	1	1	$w_{111}\cdots w_{11w}$	y_{1111}	y_{1121}	$\cdots y_{11d1}$
1	1	2	$w_{111}\cdots w_{11w}$	y_{1112}	y_{1122}	$\cdots y_{11d2}$
$\cdots$	$\cdots$	$\cdots$	$\cdots$			
1	1	n_{11}	$w_{111}\cdots w_{11w}$	$y_{111n_{11}}$	$y_{112n_{11}}$	$\cdots y_{11dn_{11}}$
1	2	1	$w_{121}\cdots w_{12w}$	y_{1211}	y_{1221}	$\cdots y_{12d1}$
1	2	2	$w_{121}\cdots w_{12w}$	y_{1212}	y_{1222}	$\cdots y_{12d2}$
$\cdots$	$\cdots$	$\cdots$	$\cdots$			
1	2	n_{12}	$w_{121}\cdots w_{12w}$	$y_{121n_{12}}$	$y_{122n_{12}}$	$\cdots y_{12dn_{12}}$
$\cdots$	$\cdots$	$\cdots$				
$\cdots$	$\cdots$	$\cdots$				
1	s	1	$w_{1s1}\cdots w_{1sw}$	y_{1s11}	y_{1s21}	$\cdots y_{1sd1}$
1	s	2	$w_{1s1}\cdots w_{1sw}$	y_{1s12}	y_{1s22}	$\cdots y_{1sd2}$
$\cdots$	$\cdots$	$\cdots$	$\cdots$			
1	s	n_{1s}	$w_{1s1}\cdots w_{1sw}$	$y_{1s1n_{1s}}$	$y_{1s2n_{1s}}$	$\cdots y_{1sdn_{1s}}$
2	1	1	$w_{211}\cdots w_{21w}$	y_{2111}	y_{2121}	$\cdots y_{21d1}$
2	1	2	$w_{211}\cdots w_{21w}$	y_{2112}	y_{2122}	$\cdots y_{21d2}$
$\cdots$	$\cdots$	$\cdots$	$\cdots$			
2	1	n_{21}	$w_{211}\cdots w_{21w}$	$y_{211n_{21}}$	$y_{212n_{21}}$	$\cdots y_{21dn_{21}}$
$\cdots$	$\cdots$	$\cdots$				
$\cdots$	$\cdots$	$\cdots$				
2	s	1	$w_{2s1}\cdots w_{2sw}$	y_{2s11}	y_{2s21}	$\cdots y_{2sd1}$
2	s	2	$w_{2s1}\cdots w_{2sw}$	y_{2s12}	y_{2s22}	$\cdots y_{2sd2}$
$\cdots$	$\cdots$	$\cdots$	w			
2	s	n_{2s}	$w_{2s1}\cdots w_{2sw}$	$y_{2s1n_{2s}}$	$y_{2s2n_{2s}}$	$\cdots y_{2sdn_{2s}}$
$\cdots$	$\cdots$	$\cdots$				
$\cdots$	$\cdots$	$\cdots$				
$\cdots$	$\cdots$	$\cdots$				
q	1	1	$w_{q11}\cdots w_{q1w}$	y_{q111}	y_{q121}	$\cdots y_{q1d1}$
q	1	2	$w_{q11}\cdots w_{q1w}$	y_{q112}	y_{q122}	$\cdots y_{q1d2}$
$\cdots$	$\cdots$	$\cdots$				
q	1	n_{q1}	$w_{q11}\cdots w_{q1w}$	$y_{q11n_{q1}}$	$y_{q12n_{q1}}$	$\cdots y_{q1dn_{q1}}$
$\cdots$	$\cdots$	$\cdots$				
$\cdots$	$\cdots$	$\cdots$				
q	s	1	$w_{qs1}\cdots w_{qsw}$	y_{qs11}	y_{qs21}	$\cdots y_{qsd1}$
q	s	2	$w_{qs1}\cdots w_{qsw}$	y_{qs12}	y_{qs22}	$\cdots y_{qsd2}$
$\cdots$	$\cdots$	$\cdots$	$\cdots$			
q	s	n_{qs}	$w_{qs1}\cdots w_{qsw}$	$y_{qs1n_{qs}}$	$y_{qs2n_{qs}}$	$\cdots y_{qsdn_{qs}}$

1. The $s \geqslant 2$ subpopulations can be multifactorial, corresponding to two or more evaluation (or comparison) factors. These may be either treatment, demographic, diagnostic, and/or environmental factors. Pertinent aspects of underlying measurement scales are expressed through the $\{w_{hik}\}$.

2. The q strata can be multifactorial, corresponding to the cross-classification of two or more demographic, diagnostic, and environmental factors. Such factors are sometimes called *control variables* to reflect two considerations: (*a*) the need to incorporate them in the analysis of the relationship between subpopulations and outcome measures as a consequence of either stratified randomization in the research design for local population analyses or support of the homogeneous stratification assumption for extended population analyses, and (*b*) their peripheral role as explanatory variables of secondary interest for purposes of interpretation. Otherwise, the special case of $q = 1$ corresponds to a nonstratified population.

3. The special case of $d = 1$ response variable represents a univariate analysis situation. The general case of $d \geqslant 2$ is multivariate. Moreover, the data for each response variable can be presumed to be ordinally scaled, as a nominally scaled measure with r possible outcomes can be expressed in terms of r corresponding binary indicator variables (i.e. dummy variables that are 1 for presence of an attribute and 0 for absence). Thus, y_{hijl} can be analyzed in terms of either their actual values (binary, interval, and ratio scales) or their ranks (ordinal scales).

Randomization Methods for Local Population Analysis

Because the subjects in historical and experimental studies have not been selected by probability random sampling from some larger target population, they are only representative of themselves from a local population analysis point of view. The questions of statistical interest for this framework are concerned with associations between the response variables and the subpopulations. For the special case of $q = 1$ stratum (for which the subscript h is dropped), this type of question can be expressed in terms of the randomization *hypothesis of no association*, H_{OR}, directed at identifying differences between subpopulations regarding level of response. A precise statement for statistical purposes is as follows:

H_{OR}: There is no association between the response variables and the subpopulations in the sense that the observed partition of the data vectors $y_{il} = (y_{ill}, \ldots, y_{idl})'$ into subpopulations can be regarded as equivalent to a successive set of simple random samples of sizes $n_1, n_2, \ldots, n_s$ subjects from the finite population of $\sum_{i=1}^{s} n_i = n$ subjects in their pooled combination.

More generally, for q strata it can be expressed in terms of the randomization *hypothesis of no partial association,* H_{OP}, directed at identifying differences between subpopulations regarding level of response for all strata simultaneously:

H_{OP}: For each of the strata $h = 1, 2, \ldots, q$, there is no relationship between the response variable and the subpopulations in the sense that the observed partition of the data vectors $y_{hil} = (y_{hill}, \ldots, y_{hidl})'$ into subpopulations can be regarded as equivalent to a successive set of stratified simple random samples of sizes $n_{h1}, n_{h2}, \ldots, n_{hs}$, respectively, from their corresponding pooled combinations.

STATISTICAL TEST OF H_{OR} The hypothesis H_{OR} implies that the $(n!/\pi^s_{i=1} n_i!)$ possible allocations of the n subjects' data vectors to the s subpopulations are equally likely. For experimental data with subpopulations corresponding to randomized treatments, this statistical framework is a direct consequence of the structure of their design relative to the equivalent hypothesis of no treatment differences. For historical data, the statistical framework is induced by the inherent nature of the hypothesis itself even though such data have not been obtained by probabilistic methods.

Univariate analysis   For the case of $d = 1$ response variable (for which the subscript j is dropped), one type of test statistic for H_{OR} is the randomization one-way analysis of variance statistic $Q_R = (n-1)S^2_a/S^2_t$, where $S^2_a = \Sigma^s_{i=1} n_i(\bar{y}_i-\bar{y})^2$ is the sum of squares for the variation among the subpopulation observed means $\bar{y}_i = (\Sigma^{n_i}_{l=1} y_{il}/n_i)$ about their H_{OR} common expected value $\bar{y} = (\Sigma^s_{i=1}\Sigma^{n_i}_{l=1} y_{il}/n)$, and $S^2_t/n = \{\Sigma^s_{i=1} \Sigma^{n_i}_{l=1} (y_{il}-\bar{y})^2/n\}$ is the H_{OR} finite population common variance for the $\{y_{il}\}$. If the sample sizes for the respective subpopulations are moderately large (e.g. $n_i \geqslant 20$), then Q_R has an approximate chi-square distribution with degrees of freedom (DF) $= (s-1)$. On the other hand, for small sample situations (e.g. all $n_i \leqslant 5$), the significance of Q_R should be evaluated by exact permutation methods (25). Finally, if the y_{il} are rank transformations of ordinal data, then $Q_R = Q_{KW}$ where Q_{KW} is the Kruskal-Wallis (26) rank analysis of variance statistic; and if the y_{il} are 0 and 1 according to a binary indicator, then $Q_R = (n-1)Q_P/n$ where Q_P is the Pearson chi-square statistic for the $(s \times 2)$ contingency table for the subpopulations vs the binary response.

Another type of test statistic for H_{OR} can be formulated by directing attention at the association between the y_{il} and one or more of the intervening variables w_{ik}. For this purpose, the multiple correlation randomization statistic $Q_{CR} = (n-1)R^2_{y,w}$ where $R_{y,w}$ is the finite population multiple correlation coefficient for the least squares prediction of the y_{il} as a linear function of the intervening variables $w_{il}, \ldots, w_{it}$. If the overall sample size n is moderately large and not overly concentrated in a single subpopulation (i.e. $n \geqslant 50$ and many of the $n_i \geqslant 1$), then Q_{CR} has an approximate chi-square distribution with $DF = t$ (where it is assumed that the w_{ik} are nonredundant in the sense that their corresponding matrix $\mathbf{W}$ for all subjects has full rank $t < s$). Because this aspect of Q_{CR} only involves the n_i in a collective as opposed to an individual sense, its application is of particular interest when s is moderately large but most of the n_i are small. Finally, for the special case of $t = 1$ intervening variable (for which the subscript k is dropped), the statistic Q_{CR} can also be expressed as $Q_{CR} = (F-E)^2/V$ where $F = \Sigma^s_{i=1} \Sigma^{n_i}_{l=1} w_i y_{il}$ is a linear function of the observed values y_{il}, $E = n \, \bar{w} \, \bar{y}$ where $\bar{w} = \Sigma^s_{i=1} n_i w_i/n$ is its H_{OR} expected value, and $V = \{\Sigma^s_{i=1} n_i (w_i - \bar{w})^2\} S^2_t/n^2 (n-1)$ is its H_{OR} variance. Thus, the correlation statistic Q_{CR} can be interpreted as a comparison of the squared difference between the observed and H_{OR} expected values for a linear function of the data to the corresponding H_{OR} variance. In this form, Q_{CR} is identical to the Spearman rank correlation test statistic for the situation in which both the w_{ik} and y_{il} are rank transformations of ordinal data. Furthermore, if both the w_{ik} and y_{il} are binary indicators then $Q_{CR} = (n-1)Q_P/n$ where Q_P is the Pearson chi-square statistic for the 2 $\times$ 2 contingency table for their cross-classification; alternatively, if n_{11} denotes the number of subjects with $w_{ik} = y_{il} = 1$, $n_{1.}$ denotes the number with $w_{ik} = 1$, and $n_{.1}$ denotes the number with $y_{il} = 1$, then $Q_{CR} = (n_{11}-m_{11})^2/V$ where $m_{11} = (n_{1.}n_{.1}/n)$ is the H_{OR} expected value for n_{11} and $V = n_{1.}n_{.1} (n-n_{1.}) (n-n_{.1})/n^2 (n-1)$ is the H_{OR} variance for n_{11}.

Multivariate analysis For the case of d response variables, the multivariate randomization one-way analysis of variance statistic $Q_{MR} = (n-1) \{tr(\mathbf{S}_a \mathbf{S}^{-1}_t)\}$ where $\mathbf{S}_a$ is among subpopulations means sum of products matrix, $(\mathbf{S}_t/n)$ is the presumed nonsingular H_{OR} population covariance matrix for the $\{y_{il}\}$, and tr denotes the trace operation for a matrix (i.e. the sum of diagonal elements). If the sample sizes for the respective subpopulations are sufficiently large (e.g. $n_i \geqslant 20 \sqrt{d}$), then Q_R has an approximate chi-square distribution with $DF = (s-1)d$.

Two special cases of Q_{MR} are of interest. If all the y_{il} are rank transformations of corresponding ordinal response variables, then $Q_{MR} = Q_{MKW}$ where Q_{MKW} is the multivariate Kruskal-Wallis statistic discussed in (27). An application in which this type of statistic is useful is repeated measurement (or split-plot) experiments involving the evaluation of the same subject for the same ordinally scaled, outcome measure under two or more experimental and/or observational conditions (e.g. different sites of the body, different times subsequent to treatment, different stimuli, different observers). This topic is discussed in (17) and (28). Furthermore, if the y_{il} are $d = (r-1)$ binary indicators for any subset of $(r-1)$ of the r possible outcomes of a nominally scaled response variable, then $Q_{MR} = (n-1)Q_P/n$ where Q_P is the Pearson chi-square statistic for the $(s \times r)$ contingency table for the sub-populations vs the r-category response.

STATISTICAL TEST OF H_{OP} The hypothesis H_{OP} implies that the hypothesis H_{OR} holds simultaneously for all strata $h = 1, 2, \ldots, q$. For this reason, statistical tests for it can be undertaken by various types of across strata combinations of the frameworks previously described for tests of H_{OR}. In particular, one family of test statistics for H_{OP} is total randomization partial association statistics $Q_T = \Sigma^q_{h=1} Q_h$ where Q_h is a test statistic for H_{OR} like Q_R, Q_{CR}, Q_{MR} for the h-th stratum. If the sample sizes $\{n_{hi}\}$ are sufficiently large for the corresponding chi-square statistics $\{Q_h\}$ to have approximate chi-square distributions with $\{(DF)_h\}$, then Q_T has an approximate chi-square distribution with $DF = \Sigma^q_{h=1} (DF)_h$.

Alternatively for most situations in which H_{OP} is of interest, a somewhat different approach is more useful. It is based on the across strata sums $G_{ij} = \Sigma^q_{h=1} n_{hi} (\bar{y}_{hij} - \bar{y}_{h.j})$ of the differences between the within stratum observed value sums for the i-th treatment and their H_{OP} expected values. These quantities are then compared to their corresponding H_{OP} covariance matrix in a manner that takes into account the restrictions $\Sigma^s_{i=1} G_{ij} = 0$. More specifically, these considerations lead to the average multivariate randomization partial association statistic $Q_{AMR} = G'V^{-1}_G G$ where G is the vector of G_{ij}'s for all d responses for any subset of $(s-1)$ subpopulations and $V_G = \Sigma^q_{h=1} V_{G,h}$ is the sum of corresponding within stratum covariance matrices. If the overall (across-strata) sample size is moderately large for each subpopulation (e.g. $\Sigma^q_{h=1} n_{hi} \geqslant 30 \sqrt{d}$), then Q_{AMR} has an approximate chi-square distribution with $DF = (s-1)d$. In view of this consideration, Q_{AMR} is more widely applicable than its total partial association counterpart Q_{TMR} because its sample size requirements for an approximate chi-square distribution are potentially much less stringent, i.e. they are based on the across-strata sums $\{\Sigma^q_{h=1} n_{hi}\}$ in contrast to their within-stratum components $\{n_{hi}\}$. Another important advantage of Q_{AMR} is that it is more powerful than Q_{TMR} with respect to alternatives for which the pattern of subpopulation differences is similar within the strata. On the contrary, if such patterns are conflicting (i.e. in opposite directions), then Q_{TMR} is preferable from the point of view of power, but this advantage must be achieved at the cost of its increased sample size requirements.

For situations in which the association between the y_{hijl} and one or more of the intervening variables w_{hik} are of interest, multivariate partial correlation test statistics analogous to Q_{AMR} can be formulated in terms of the across strata sums $F_{jk} = \Sigma^q_{h=1} \Sigma^s_{i=1} w_{hik} n_{hi} (\bar{y}_{hij} - \bar{y}_{h.j})$ of the differences between linear functions of the within-stratum observed values and their H_{OP} expected values. More specifically, for the special case of $d = 1$ response variable (for which the subscript j is dropped) and $t = 1$ intervening variable (for which the subscript k is dropped), this framework leads to the partial correlation randomization test statistic $Q_{PCR} = F^2/V$ where $V = \Sigma^q_{h=1} V_h$ is the sum of the H_{OP} variance V_h for the within stratum linear functions $F_{hi} = \Sigma^q_{h=1} \Sigma^s_{i=1} w_{hi} n_{hi} (\bar{y}_{hi} - \bar{y}_h)$. If the overall (across strata) sample size is moderately large and not overly concentrated in a single subpopulation (i.e. $\Sigma^q_{h=1} \Sigma^s_{i=1} n_{hi} \geqslant 50$ and many of the $n_{hi} \geqslant 1$ for each h), then Q_{PCR} has an approximate chi-square distribution with DF $= 1$. Thus, Q_{PCR} represents a relatively powerful test statistic for testing H_{OP} against alternatives involving similar within stratum monotonic association between the response variable and the intervening variables because the pertinent information for its evaluation is concentrated in a single degree of freedom. On the contrary, Q_{PCR} is not recommended for situations involving nonmonotone associations or conflicting directions for within stratum monotone associations.

Finally, two special cases of Q_{PCR} are of particular interest. If the y_{hil} and w_{hi} are within stratum rank transformations of ordinal data, then Q_{PCR} is a partial rank correlation test statistic. Furthermore, if both the y_{hil} and the w_{hi} are binary indicators, then $Q_{PCR} = Q_{CMH}$ where Q_{CMH} is the Mantel-Haenszel (29) refinement of a strategy suggested by Cochran (30) for combining information in a set of q 2 $\times$ 2 contingency tables. In this regard its more well-known expression is $Q_{CMH} = \Sigma^q_{h=1} (n_{h11} - m_{h11})^2/\Sigma^q_{h=1} V_h$ where n_{h11}, m_{h11}, and V_h have the same definitions for the h-th stratum as previously cited in reference to the binary case of Q_{CR} for a single stratum.

SUMMARY COMMENT   As indicated in the previous discussion, randomization test statistics can be formulated for many different types of situations involving univariate or multivariate data structures, nominal, ordinal, interval, or ratio measurement scales, and with or without the information in the factor scalings. For all of these situations, the probability model implied by the hypotheses is used to construct expected values and covariance matrices for specific linear functions of the data that are directed at the comparison or associations of interest. These quantities are then combined together to form test statistics with approximate chi-square distributions. Thus, all of the methods described here as well as other related ones can be viewed as being based on the same general principles. Further discussion of these types of methods is given in (31), (32), and (33).

Weighted Least Squares Methods for Fitting Variational Models

For data like that displayed in Table 7, there is often interest in testing linear hypotheses concerning the variation among the elements of a $(u \times 1)$ vector F of estimates that pertain to one or more aspects of the association between the outcome measures and the factors underlying the subpopulations and strata. If the sample sizes n_{hi} are sufficiently large for such estimates to have an approximate normal distribution with the $(u \times 1)$ vector μ of large sample expected values (or population values), then such hypotheses can be expressed in the general form

$$H_{OW}: W\mu = 0_w$$

where W is a $(w \times u)$ matrix of *contrast constraints* (i.e. the elements in its rows add to 0) with known coefficients and full rank w and 0_w is a $(w \times 1)$ vector of 0's. Furthermore, if V_F denotes any large sample (consistent) estimate of the covariance structure for F, then the Wald (34) statistic $Q_W = F'W' \{WV_FW'\}^{-1}WF$ can be used to test H_{OW} via its approximate chi-square distribution with DF $= w$ under the conditions stated here.

The hypothesis H_{OW} can be interpreted as a goodness of fit test for describing μ in terms of the variational model $\mu = X\beta$ where X is a $(u \times t)$ *model specification (or design) matrix* of known coefficients with full rank $t = (u - w)$, which is orthogonal to W in the sense that $WX = 0_{wt}$ is a $(w \times t)$ matrix of 0s, and β is a $(t \times 1)$ vector of unknown parameters. In other words, $\mu = X\beta$ implies $W\mu = WX\beta = 0_w$ and vice versa. This linkage of W and X is often expressed by calling W the *constraint formulation* of the model and calling X the *freedom equation* or model specification formulation. Moreover, it also provides the rationale for calling X a variational model which characterizes μ in a manner compatible with the hypothesis H_{OW}. For this reason, it is of descriptive interest regardless of whether such variation can be interpreted in terms of any structural model pertaining to some underlying probability distribution or stochastic framework for the data.

If goodness of fit for a model X is considered adequate, then the weighted least squares method described by Grizzle et al (35) can be used to obtain the estimate $b = (X'V_F^{-1} X)^{-1}X'V_F^{-1}F$ for the parameter vector β and the estimate $V_b = (X'V_F^{-1}X)^{-1}$ for its covariance matrix. Moreover, for large samples, b is equivalent to any optimal estimate for β and has an approximate multivariate normal distribution. As a result, Wald statistics can also be used to test linear hypotheses

$$H_{OC,W}: C\beta = 0_c$$

concerning its parameters, where C is a $(c \times t)$ matrix with known coefficients and full rank c. These test statistics, $Q_{W,C} = b'C'\{CV_bC'\}^{-1}Cb$, have approximate chi-square distributions with $DF = c$ under $H_{OC,W}$. Furthermore, they are identically equal to the amount by which the goodness of fit statistic Q_W would increase in order to be a simultaneous test of H_{OW} and $H_{OC,W}$—in the sense that $H_{OC,W}$ implies $\beta = Z\gamma$, where Z is a $[t \times (t - c)]$ matrix of full rank $(t - c)$ and γ is a $[(t - c) \times 1]$ parameter vector; and so in combination with H_{OW} implies $\mu = XZ\gamma$ which is equivalent to $W_C\mu = 0_{(w+c)}$ where W_C is a $[(w+c) \times u]$ matrix orthogonal to XZ. As a result, Q_W and $Q_W(C)$ represent additive components for the goodness of fit statistic for the simplified model $\mu = X_C\gamma$ (where $X_C = XZ$) implied by $H_{OC,W}$. Additional components can be included in this chi-square partition by further specifications of hierarchical sequences of models X_C (or constraints W_C). For purposes of completeness, the identity model $X_0 = I_u$, where I_u is the $(u \times u)$ diagonal matrix of 1's, can be viewed as the initial model in such sequences because it involves no constraints; also its parameter vector $\beta_0 = \mu$, which implies that the corresponding estimates $b_0 = F$, and that C matrix tests pertaining to β_0 are identical to W matrix tests pertaining to μ. Thus, both the testing of hypotheses W and the fitting of variational models X can be undertaken in terms of the same conceptual framework.

Finally, some examples of the types of functions F in which the application of weighted least methods have been useful include the following:

1. The analysis of proportions for the distribution of a nominal response variable, linear functions of proportions for an average score of an ordinal response variable, and logarithmic functions of proportions for relative aspects of nominal and ordinal data [see Tables 1, 3, 4 and (35)].
2. The analysis of correlated marginal proportions for repeated measurement experiments involving the evaluation of the same subject for the same nominal or ordinal response variable under two or more conditions (see 36).
3. The analysis of life table based survival rates [see Table 5 and (37)].
4. The analysis of summary indexes like measures of agreement between two or more observers (see 38 or 39).
5. The analysis of ratio estimates based on complex probability sample surveys [see Table 6 and (5)].

For all of these situations, the assumptions that are required for the use of Wald statistics and weighted least squares methods for fitting variational models X are directly linked to the research design. They are:

1. Probability random selection either explicitly via the research design (sample survey data) or implicitly via the stratified simple random sam-

pling assumption for extended population analysis (historical and experimental data).

2. Sufficiently large sample size for $\mathbf{F}$ to have an approximate multivariate normal distribution.
3. Sufficiently large sample size and available information to obtain a consistent estimate $\mathbf{V_F}$ for the covariance matrix of $\mathbf{F}$.

Thus, the application of weighted least squares methods is advantageous when the above minimal assumptions are satisfied and the status of other assumptions concerning some underlying probability distribution or stochastic process framework for the data is either unknown and/or introduces superfluous complexity into the analysis of $\mathbf{F}$. Otherwise, the principal limitation of the scope of weighted least squares methods is their requirement of very large sample sizes (e.g. $\Sigma^q_{h=1} \Sigma^s_{i=1} n_{hi} \geqslant 1000$).

Maximum Likelihood Methods for Structural Models

When the objectives of a research investigation are concerned with the association between outcome measures and factors underlying the subpopulations and strata, their analysis can be based upon either a variational or structural point of view. With the variational approach, estimates that describe the phenomena of interest are formed initially and then provide the statistical framework for addressing study questions. Alternatively, with the structural approach, an underlying probability distribution (e.g. binomial, exponential, normal) or stochastic process (e.g. Poisson) is assumed a priori on the basis of substantive arguments to characterize the statistical behavior of a data array and, as before, provide the framework for addressing study questions.

Although these two points of view appear distinct, they overlap in many applications because estimates from a variational approach may be identical to those from a structural approach. In other cases, estimates may be motivated by a structural rationale even though a specific structural framework is not assumed (e.g. estimates of survival subsequent to treatment for some disease may be viewed as varying among subjects in accordance with an exponential function, even though there is no biological basis for the assumption that its corresponding population distribution is exponential).

If the variational approach has no underlying technical framework, then weighted least squares methods as described in the previous section must be used, as the only information such methods require is a set of descriptive estimates and corresponding estimated covariance matrices. However, the price that is paid for this generality is large sample size requirements to ensure approximate normality. For this reason, when moderate sample sizes (e.g. $100 \leqslant \Sigma^q_{h=1} \Sigma^s_{i=1} n_{hi} \leqslant 1000$) are under study, the depth of application may be limited. Thus, if refined analysis of such moderate sample sizes is necessary, then it must be based upon a structural approach that has a plausible underlying probability distribution or stochastic process framework.

One structural method that is extensively used is maximum likelihood as discussed in (40–43). With this method, maximization of the assumed probability function or "likelihood" for the data (e.g. product normal, product binomial, product Poisson) with respect to the model structure is used to obtain parameter estimates. Moreover, differences between maximized logarithms of such probability functions for hierarchically related models (e.g. $\mu = XZ\gamma$ nested in $\mu = X\beta$) are used to obtain approximate chi-square tests for corresponding model simplification hypotheses (e.g. $C\beta = 0$).

Although maximum likelihood methods are straightforward in concept, they should be applied with caution to small and moderate sample size situations because the extent of their optimal statistical properties is linked to large samples also. However, for them, large sample considerations pertain to the estimates that are obtained through the way in which the maximum likelihood method uses the information in the model in combination with the research design sampling considerations. Thus, their use is advantageous when the sample size is sufficiently large for the model structure to imply that the maximum likelihood estimates of its parameters have an approximate multivariate normal distribution.

Finally, the overlap of the variational and structural approaches also carries over to an analogous overlap between weighted least squares methods and maximum likelihood methods. If estimates to which weighted least squares are applied are also maximum likelihood estimates from some preliminary structural model, and if the sample size is sufficiently large that estimates have an approximate multivariate normal distribution, then the parameter estimates for simplified models from either weighted least squares or maximum likelihood methods are equivalent, having the same large sample expected values and covariance matrix. Further, the estimates from these two methods are typically optimal under these conditions, in which case they are called BAN (Best Asymptotically Normal) estimates in the sense of Neyman (44). Some examples in which this asymptotic equivalence is specifically recognized include the following:

1. Multiple linear regression models for independent univariate normally distributed data with common variance. In this case both maximum likelihood methods and weighted least squares methods lead to the same estimates of the regression coefficients as ordinary unweighted least squares.
2. Log-linear models for the analysis of multi-way contingency tables based upon large sample cross-classifications of categorical data from a product multinomial distribution. An important aspect of this situation is

that stratified simple random sampling from a very large population is a research design based sufficient assumption for the product multinomial distribution. Thus, the use of maximum likelihood methods for these situations can be based upon either a variational or structural point of view.

3. Log-linear models for the analysis of large values of Poisson counts (i.e. values ≥ 10).
4. Survival models for the time to occurrence of vital events for the analysis of large groups of homogeneous subjects.

For further discussion of the application of maximum likelihood methods to these types of situations as well as more generally, see (33, 42, 43, 45).

UNIVARIATE NORMAL MULTIPLE LINEAR REGRESSION MODEL
The observed data $\{y_{hil}\}$ for $d = 1$ response variable (for which the subscript j is dropped) are assumed to have been obtained independently from normal distributions with common within subpopulation expected values $\{\mu_{hil} = \mu_{hi}\}$ and common (overall) variance σ^2. Also, the vector μ of the $\{\mu_{hil} = \mu_{hi}\}$ is assumed to be characterized by the linear regression model $\mu = X\beta$ where X is a known design matrix with full rank t and β is an unknown parameter vector. The log-likelihood for this situation has the form

$$\log_e L = - \frac{n}{2} \log(2\pi) - \frac{n}{2} \log(\sigma^2) - \frac{1}{2\sigma^2} (y - X\beta)' (y - X\beta)$$

where y is the vector of $\{y_{hil}\}$ and $n = \Sigma_{h=1}^q \Sigma_{i=1}^s n_{hi}$ is the overall sample size. The maximum likelihood estimate $\hat{\beta}$ for β is obtained by differentiating $\log_e L$ with respect to β and solving the resulting linear equations. Thus, it can be readily verified that $\hat{\beta} = (X'X)^{-1}X'y$, which is also the unweighted least squares estimate. The covariance matrix for $\hat{\beta}$ is $V_\beta = (X'X)^{-1}\sigma^2$. Because the error mean square

$$s_e^2 = (y-X\hat{\beta})' (y- X\hat{\beta})/(n-t)$$

is an unbiased estimate for σ^2 such that $(n - t) s_e^2/\sigma^2$ has the chi-square distribution with $DF = (n - t)$, any hypothesis of the type $H_0 : C\beta = 0$ where C is a matrix with full rank c can be tested in terms of the quadratic ratio statistic

$$QR = (n-t)\hat{\beta}'C'\{C(X'X)^{-1} C'\}^{-1}C\hat{\beta}/cs_e^2$$

which has the F-distribution with $DF = [c, (n - t)]$ under H_0.

MULTINOMIAL MULTIPLE LOGISTIC REGRESSION   The observed data $\{y_{hijl}\}$ are assumed to have been obtained independently from multinomial distributions with common within subpopulation probability vectors $\pi_{hi} = (\pi_{hi1}, \ldots, \pi_{hir})'$, where $\{\pi_{hij}\}$ denotes the expected value of the binary indicator variables $\{y_{hijl}\}$ corresponding to the $\{j\text{-th}\}$ outcome of an $r = (d+1)$ category nominal or ordinal response variable. Thus, if $n_{hij} = \Sigma^{n_{hi}}_{l=1} y_{hijl}$ denotes the number of subjects observed with the j-th response outcome for the i-th subpopulation of the h-th stratum and if $\mathbf{n}_{hi} = (n_{hi1}, \ldots, n_{hir})'$ denotes their composite frequency vector [with n_{hir} being obtained via the subtraction $n_{hir} = (n_{hi} - \Sigma^d_{j=1} n_{hij})$], then the likelihood function for the data has the general form

$$L = \Pi^q_{h=1} \Pi^s_{i=1} n_{hi}! \; \Pi^r_{j=1} (\pi_{hij}{}^{n_{hij}} / n_{hij}!),$$

where the $\{\pi_{hij}\}$ satisfy the natural constraints $\{\Sigma^r_{j=1} \pi_{hij} = 1\}$.

If the $\{\pi_{hij}\}$ are compatible with the model constraints $\mathbf{W}\log_e \pi = 0$ where $\pi = (\pi'_{11}, \ldots, \pi'_{qs})'$, $\log_e$ transforms a vector to the vector of natural logarithms, and $\mathbf{W}$ is a full rank matrix of contrasts that are linearly independent of the rows of the matrix $\mathbf{U}$ corresponding to the natural constraints, it then follows that the $\{\pi_{hij}\}$ may be represented by the multiple logistic model

$$\pi_{hi} = \exp(\mathbf{X}_{hi}\beta)/\{\mathbf{1}'_r \exp(\mathbf{X}_{hi}\beta)\}$$

where $\exp$ transforms a vector to the vector of exponential functions and $\mathbf{1}_r$ is an $(r \times 1)$ vector of 1's. In this framework, the $\{\mathbf{X}_{hi}\}$ are $(r \times t)$ submatrices of the full $(qrs \times t)$ design matrix $\mathbf{X} = (\mathbf{X}'_{11}, \ldots, \mathbf{X}'_{qs})'$ such that $\mathbf{W}\mathbf{X} = 0$ (which is implied by the model's corresponding log-linear constraints) and $\mathbf{U}\mathbf{X} = 0$ (which is implied by the natural constraints). Finally, the denominators of the π_{hi} are standardizing constants with respect to the natural constraints $\mathbf{1}'_r \pi_{hi} = 1$.

The maximum likelihood estimate $\hat{\beta}$ for β is obtained by substituting the model expression for the $\{\pi_{hi}\}$ into the expression for $\log_e L$, and then differentiating with respect to β. This process leads to the nonlinear equations $\mathbf{X}'\mathbf{n} = \mathbf{X}'\mathbf{m}$ where $\mathbf{n} = (\mathbf{n}'_{11}, \ldots, n'_{qs})'$ is the composite vector of observed frequencies and $\mathbf{m}$ is the composite vector of predicted frequencies $\mathbf{m}_{hi} = n_{hi} \hat{\pi}_{hi}$ for which $\hat{\pi}_{hi}$ is obtained by substituting $\hat{\beta}$ into the model expression for π_{hi}. In most applications, these equations do not have an explicit solution. For this reason, iterative numerical methods are usually required. Here, two specific types of alogrithms have been found useful. If h, i, and j correspond to a multi-way cross-classification of factors and responses and $\mathbf{X}$ corresponds to a hierarchical model of main effects and interactions (such that for any included interaction term all related interactions of the same or lower order are also included), then the iterative proportional fitting algorithm described in (43) can be used to determine $\mathbf{m}$ first and then $\hat{\beta}$ by subsequent transformation. The principal advantage of this approach is that it can be applied efficiently to multi-way cross-classifications involving contingency tables with a very large number of cells (e.g. $qrs \geqslant 200$). Its primary disadvantage is its limitation in scope to hierarchical models and the further requirement that such models be specifiable in terms of marginal tables (which are linked to their distinct sets of highest order interactions) with all cells being non-null. Alternatively, for situations in which the number of cells is not very large (i.e. $qrs < 200$), the Newton-Raphson method (or equivalently iterative weighted least squares), described in (42), can be used directly to solve for β. The advantage of this approach is that its scope includes any full rank model X that is of interest. On the contrary, its principal limitation is its prohibitively large cost when qrs is large (e.g. $qrs \geqslant 200$) or t is large (e.g. $t \geqslant 40$).

Finally, regardless of the manner in which $\hat{\beta}$ is computed, its estimated covariance matrix can be expressed in the form

$$V_{\beta} = \{\Sigma^q_{h=1} \Sigma^s_{i=1} \, n_{hi} \, X'_{hi}[D_{\pi_{hi}} - \pi_{hi} \, \pi'_{hi}]X_{hi}\}^{-1}$$

where $D_{\pi_{hi}}$ is a diagonal matrix with π_{hi} down the main diagonal. Thus, statistical tests of hypotheses $H_0 : C\beta = 0$ can be either undertaken by Wald statistics for $C\hat{\beta}$ relative to its covariance matrix $CV_{\beta}C'$ or by log-likelihood reduction statistics for the difference between the maximized log-likelihood with respect to $\hat{\beta}$ for X vs the maximized log-likelihood with respect to $\hat{\gamma}$ for the model XZ implied by H_0 (through its equivalent specification as $\beta = Z\gamma$ where Z is orthogonal to C), which multipled by (-2) yields an approximate chi-square statistic with $DF = $ Rank (C). For further discussion of alternative test statistics for H_0, see (32).

POISSON MULTIPLE LOG-LINEAR REGRESSION   The observed data $\{y_{hijl}\}$ are assumed to represent total counts for independent Poisson streams corresponding to d types of rare events (e.g. different accident types) which are under study in the subpopulations of the respective strata. The expected values $\{\mu_{hijl}\}$ of the $\{y_{hijl}\}$ are assumed to be the products of known exposure measures $\{N_{hijl}\}$ and common within subpopulation event rate parameters $\{\lambda_{hij}\}$. In other words, $\mu_{hijl} = N_{hijl} \, \lambda_{hij}$. Thus, the likelihood function for the data has the general form

$$L = \Pi^q_{h=1} \, \Pi^s_{i=1} \, \Pi^d_{j=1} \, \Pi^{n_{hi}}_{l=1} \, \{[\exp(-N_{hijl} \, \lambda_{hij})] \, (N_{hijl}\lambda_{hij}) \, ^{y_{hijl}}/y_{hijl}!$$

If the $\{\lambda_{hij}\}$ are compatible with the log-linear model constraints $W[\log_e\lambda] = 0$ where $\lambda = (\lambda_{111}, \lambda_{112}, \ldots, \lambda_{qsr})'$, $\log_e$ transforms a vector to the vector of natural logarithms, and W is a full rank matrix of known coefficients, it then follows that the $\{\lambda_{hij}\}$ may be represented by the multiplicative model $\lambda = \exp(X\beta)$ where $\exp$ transforms a vector to the vector of exponential functions. In this framework X is the $(qrs \times t)$ full rank design matrix that is implied by the models' constraints through the orthogonality condition $\mathbf{WX} = \mathbf{0}$.

The maximum likelihood estimate $\hat{\beta}$ for β is obtained by substituting the model representation for the $\{\lambda_{hij}\}$ into the expression for $\log_e L$, and then differentiating with respect to β. This process leads to the nonlinear equations $\mathbf{X'y} = \mathbf{X'm}$ where $\mathbf{y} = (y_{1111}, \ldots, y_{11d1}, y_{1121}, \ldots y_{qsdn_{qs}})$ is the composite vector of observed counts and $\mathbf{m}$ is the corresponding composite vector of expected counts $m_{hijl} = N_{hijl} \hat{\lambda}_{hij}$ where the $\{\hat{\lambda}_{hij}\}$ are obtained via $\hat{\lambda} = \exp(\mathbf{X}\hat{\beta})$. In most applications, these equations do not have an explicit solution. For this reason, iterative numerical methods like those described previously for multiple logistic regression are usually required.

The covariance matrix for the maximum likelihood estimates $\hat{\beta}$ has the form $V_\beta = \{\mathbf{X'D}_\mu\mathbf{X}\}^{-1}$ where $\mathbf{D}_\mu$ is a diagonal matrix with the quantities $\{\mu_{hijl}\}$ down the main diagonal. Thus, statistical tests of hypotheses $H_0: \mathbf{C}\beta = \mathbf{0}$ can be undertaken by Wald statistics for $\mathbf{C}\hat{\beta}$ relative to its estimated covariance matrix $\mathbf{C}V_\beta \mathbf{C'}$ or by log-likelihood reduction statistics for the difference between the maximized log-likelihoods for the model $\mathbf{X}$ and the model $\mathbf{XZ}$ where $\mathbf{Z}$ is orthogonal to $\mathbf{C}$ [multiplied by (–2) to yield an approximate chi-square statistic with DF = Rank (C)].

Finally, because the conditional distribution of the $\{y_{hijl}\}$, given that the sums $\{y_{hi.l} = \Sigma^d_{j=1} y_{hijl}\}$ over event types j are fixed, is an independent set of multinomial distributions with subtotal frequency parameters $\{y_{hi.l}\}$ and within subpopulation probability parameters

$$\pi_{hijl} = \{\mu_{hijl}/ \Sigma^d_{j=1} \mu_{hijl}\} = \{N_{hijl} \lambda_{hij}/\Sigma^d_{j=1} N_{hijl} \lambda_{hij}\},$$

it follows that models for the $\{\lambda_{hij}\}$ imply models for the $\{\pi_{hijl}\}$. Furthermore, if the exposure measures can be presumed to be independent of event type in the sense that $N_{hijl} = N_{hi*l}$, then

$$\pi_{hijl} = \pi_{hij} = \{\lambda_{hij}/ \Sigma^d_{j=1} \lambda_{hij}\} = \{\exp(\mathbf{x'}_{hij}\beta)/\Sigma^d_{j=1} \exp(\mathbf{x'}_{hij}\beta)\}$$

where $\mathbf{x'}_{hij}$ is the (hij)-th row of $\mathbf{X}$; and this respresentation of $\{\pi_{hij}\}$ can be verified to be the multiple logistic regression model. Thus, log-linear models for the $\{\lambda_{hij}\}$ imply multiple logistic models for the conditional probabilities $\{\pi_{hij}\}$ given fixed sums over j, under the condition of equal exposure with respect to j. However, because the exposure measure that actually applies to the $\{y_{hijl}\}$ is the product of both the true exposure and the reporting rate, the assumption of equal exposure should be viewed cautiously because such an assumption simultaneously requires equal true exposure and equal reporting rates.

Alternatively, if the principal objective of analysis is subpopulation comparisons, and if the true exposures $\{\nu_{hil}\}$ are the same for all event types, and if reporting rates $\{\phi_{hjl}\}$ are the same for all subpopulations so that the N_{hijl}

satisfy the multiplicative model $N_{hijl} = \nu_{hil}\phi_{hjl}$, then cross-product subpopulation ratios of event type ratios (i.e. odds ratios) are compatible with the representation

$$\frac{\pi_{hijl}\ \pi_{hi'j'l}}{\pi_{hi'jl}\ \pi_{hij'l}} = \frac{N_{hijl}\ \lambda_{hij}\ N_{hi'j'l}\ \lambda_{hi'j'}}{N_{hi'jl}\ \lambda_{hi'j}\ N_{hij'l}\ \lambda_{hij'}}$$

$$= \frac{\nu_{hil}\ \phi_{hjl}\ \lambda_{hij}\ \nu_{hi'l}\ \phi_{hj'l}\ \lambda_{hi'j'}}{\nu_{hi'l}\ \phi_{hjl}\ \lambda_{hi'j}\ \nu_{hil}\ \phi_{hj'l}\ \lambda_{hij'}}$$

$$= (\lambda_{hij}\ \lambda_{hi'j'}/\lambda_{hi'j}\ \lambda_{hij'})$$

$$= \exp\{(\mathbf{x}_{hij} - \mathbf{x}_{hi'j} - \mathbf{x}_{hij'} + \mathbf{x}_{hi'j'})'\ \beta\}.$$

Thus, odds ratios with respect to the $\{\pi_{hijl}\}$ are equal to odds ratios with respect to the $\{\lambda_{hij}\}$ under the condition that exposure measures satisfy a multiplicative model with respect to true exposure and reporting rate.

In summary, if the exposure measures are actually known, then the Poisson log-linear model framework can be used to deal directly with the λ_{hij}. However, if they are not known, then multinominal logistic regression methods can be used to deal with either ratios $\{\lambda_{hij}/\lambda_{hij'}\}$ under the equal exposure assumption $N_{hijl} = N_{hi*l}$ for event types j, or with cross-product ratios $\{\lambda_{hij}\ \lambda_{hi'j'}/\lambda_{hi'j}\ \lambda_{hij'}\}$ under the multiplicative model exposure assumption $N_{hijl} = \nu_{hil}\ \phi_{hjl}$. Otherwise, it should always be recognized that multiple logistic models may be of interest in their own right regardless of any linkage to underlying Poisson stochastic processes.

SURVIVAL PROPORTIONAL HAZARDS REGRESSION MODEL   The observed data $\{y_{hil}\}$ for $d = 1$ response variable, for which the subscript j is dropped, are assumed to have been independently obtained from common within subpopulation time to event distributions belonging to some family such as exponential, Weibull, extreme value, etc. If $P_{hi}(y)$ denotes the cumulative probability distribution function for the i-th subpopulation of the h-th stratum, then the proportional hazards regression model for the data has the general form

$$\Lambda_{hi}(y) = \{\exp(\mathbf{x'}_{hi}\beta)\}\Lambda(y)$$

where $\Lambda_{hi}(y) = \{(dP_{hi}/dy)/1 - P_{hi}(y)\}$ is the hazard function for the distribution $P_{hi}(y)$, $\mathbf{x'}_{hi}$ is the (hi)-th row of the model specification matrix $\mathbf{X}$ of known constants and β is the unknown parameter vector, and $\Lambda(y)$ is the basic hazard function for the family to which the $P_{hi}(y)$ belong. From this framework, likelihood functions can be constructed in a manner that takes into account the available information for both observed failures for whom the y_{hil} are known and the censored information for subjects for whom failure is known to be subsequent to the time of last observation y^*_{hik} From such expressions, maximum likelihood estimates can be obtained by iterative numerical methods. Similarly, hypotheses can be tested in terms of differences between maximized log-likelihoods. For more detailed information concerning these types of models and their application see (45).

HISTORICAL DATA EXAMPLES

This section is concerned with statistical analyses for three types of investigations involving historical data collected during specific time periods from populations in a particular geographic area. Because the subjects are not obtained by probability random sampling methods from a larger target population, they are representative only of themselves and constitute a local population. Two statistical strategies are of interest for these situations. One is directed at the local population itself, the other at a more extensive target population from which the subjects are presumed to have been selected by stratified simple random sampling. Both of these involve similar methods, but the interpretation of results is fundamentally different because the limited conclusions about the local population require minimal assumptions, whereas broader conclusions pertaining to the target population may have questionable validity because of controversy over the assumptions.

Example 1: Highway Safety—A Total Population of Events

This example is based on research undertaken at the University of North Carolina by Stewart (46) in order to study the relationship between the severity of driver injury in automobile accidents and crash configuration, road conditions, automobile type, and driver demographic status. The data in Table 1 give frequencies of whether the driver experienced severe injury (e.g. a bleeding wound, fracture) or a fatal injury cross-classified according to vehicle size (small, middle, large), vehicle age (0 to 2 years, 3 to 5 years), and vehicle model year (1966 or before, 1967 to 1969). Data were not available for 1967 because of a system backlog at that time. The (local) population is all 1966, 1968 to 1972 police-reported North Carolina multiple vehicle accidents with left side or front impact for sober drivers traveling at a moderately high speed.

A principal purpose of this investigation was a comparison of the likelihood of serious injury for accident involved drivers for 1966 model or before automobiles and 1967 to 1969 automobiles with respect to the "second collision" between driver and vehicle interior subsequent to the "first collision" between the vehicle and some other vehicle or object. This comparison would help evaluate safety improvement standards regarding lap and shoulder belt restraint systems, energy absorbing steering columns, and protected dash board that were introduced by the 1966 Highway Safety Act. Because the likelihood of serious injury is related to many factors concerning the accident, the analysis of its association with model year must be undertaken for a homogeneous population of accidents in order to allow cause and effect interpretations. The definition of the population under study according to crash configuration, driver status, vehicle size, and vehicle age is considered adequate for homogeneity (see 46 for further discussion).

LOCAL POPULATION ANALYSIS   For the study population of 1966, 1968 to 1972 North Carolina accidents, all of the frequencies in Table 1 are fixed constants that describe historical events as opposed to realizations of random variables for a broader population. However, there is still interest in questions of whether the observed distribution of injury severity is random across the subpopulations defined by vehicle weight X vehicle age X model year cross-classification. More specifically, such questions can be expressed in terms of either randomization hypotheses of *no multiple (or joint) association:*

H_{OR}: Injury severity is distributed in accordance with random partition with respect to vehicle weight X vehicle age X model year cross-classification, i.e. the 12 subpopulations can be regarded as an exhaustive set of 12 simple random samples (without replacement) from the fixed population of all accidents in Table 1;

or hypotheses of *no partial association* for one (or more) components of the cross-classification after stratification adjustment for the others:

H_{OP}: For each vehicle weight X vehicle age stratum, injury severity is distributed in accordance with random partition with respect to model year, i.e. the two model year subpopulations can be regarded as a set of two stratified simple random samples (without replacement) from the fixed population corresponding to the vehicle weight X vehicle age cross-classification.

Statistical test of H_{OR}   The hypothesis H_{OR} implies that the frequencies for the 12 X 2 situation in Table 1 have a multiple hypergeometric distribution with fixed margins for injury severity (for the pooled subpopulations) and for each cell of the vehicle size X vehicle age X model year cross-classification. Thus, test statistics for H_{OR} can be expressed in terms of multivariate comparisons of differences between observed frequencies and H_{OR} expected frequencies to corresponding estimates of H_{OR} variance and/or covariance structure. As discussed in (32) or (47), these considerations lead to the well-known Pearson chi-square statistic Q_P. However, the rationale for using Q_P for local population analysis of historical data has been emphasized as opposed to its use for the analysis of simple random samples from larger target populations. For the data in Table 1, $Q_P = 33.50$ with DF = 11 is significant with $p < 0.01$. Because this result contradicts the acceptance of H_{OR}, the variation in the percentages of accidents involving severe injury for the vehicle size X vehicle age X model year cross-classification is more extensive than typically would have been expected. It is concluded that injury severity is different across the twelve vehicle size X vehicle age X model year subpopulations.

Statistical test of H_{OP}   The hypothesis H_{OP} implies that the frequencies in Table 1 corresponding to each vehicle size X vehicle age stratum have independent hypergeometric distributions with corresponding fixed historical marginal distributions for injury severity and model year. From this framework, several types of test statistics for H_{OP} can be formulated. One of these is the sum of the within stratum Pearson chi-square statistics for model year vs injury severity. For the data in Table 1, this *total partial association statistic* $Q_{TP} = 8.93$ with DF = 6 (1 DF for each 2 X 2 table and 6 tables in aggregate) is nonsignificant with $0.15 < p < 0.20$. Thus, this result demonstrates one of the principal limitations of Q_{TP}, which is relatively weak power directed at a broad alternative.

For many investigations, the questions of interest are linked to narrow alternatives that are concerned with whether within-stratum associations (e.g. smaller percentages of severe injuries in 1967 to 1969 automobiles than in 1966 or before automobiles) are sufficiently consistent to contradict H_{OP}. This does not require that all associations be similar in strength or direction, but rather that those in one direction are sufficiently strong to cause the combined association to be statistically significant. A test statistic that is directed at such narrow alternatives can be formulated in terms of the general strategy originally described by Cochran (30) and Mantel-Haenszel (29) and further elaborated in (31) and (32). It is based upon the comparison of the sum of the across strata differences between the within stratum observed frequencies and H_{OP} expected frequencies to the corresponding sum of within strata estimates of H_{OP} variance and/or covariance structure, and, accordingly, has an approximate chi-square distribution with DF = 1 for sufficiently large samples (e.g. all frequencies in the model year vs injury severity marginal table exceed 10). For the data in Table 1, the across strata sum of the observed numbers of drivers with serious injury was $n(66,yes) = 308$; the across strata sum of H_{OP} expected values was $m(66,yes) = 282.2$; and the across strata sum of H_{OP} variances was $v(66,yes) = 120.62$. Thus, the average partial association (or Cochran/Mantel-Haenszel) statistic $Q_{CMH} = (25.8)^2/(120.62) = 5.52$ is significant with $0.01 < p < 0.05$. Because this result represents a statistical contradiction to H_{OP} with respect to a narrow alternative of a priori interest, it implies that there is a partial association between injury severity and model year after stratification adjustment. Also, this partial association can be interpreted as indicating that the 9.1% difference between the observed and expected numbers of drivers with serious injury relative to expected is greater than what would have been anticipated if the data within the respective strata had been a random partition of the corresponding subpopulations.

Although Q_{CMH} is advantageous with respect to the detection of similar patterns of association across the strata, it has relatively poor power for situations in which the within stratum relationships are heterogeneous and have conflicting directions. If these alternatives are also of interest, then broader statistical methods like Q_{TP} must be used at the cost of either reduced power against consistent within stratum relationships, or increased sample size. In summary, the rationale underlying the use of Q_{CMH} to test H_{OP} is an illustration of what is more generally known as the *broad hypothesis vs narrow alternative argument,* with H_{OP} being the broad hypothesis and consistent within stratum relationships being the narrow alternative. As was the case with this example and many other applications, it is one of the most effective strategies for dealing with many questions of statistical interest within the scope of the available data.

Conclusion   There is a statistically significant association between injury severity and the vehicle size X vehicle age X model year cross-classification for 1966, 1968 to 1972 North Carolina multiple accidents under consideration. Furthermore, there is a significant partial association between injury severity and model year after stratification adjustment for vehicle size X vehicle age. Finally, because the data in Table 1 pertain to a reasonably homogeneous partition of a total population of events, these associations are a statistical indication that safety improvements in 1967 to 1969 automobiles were one of the causes for reduced likelihood of injury. This conclusion applies only to the local population described in Table 1. Also, because the data in Table 1 constitute a population rather than a sample, viewing the data as random is a consequence of the probability structure induced by H_{OR} and H_{OP}. Note that once these hypotheses are rejected, so is their corresponding implied probability structure. Thus, other types of analysis such as the estimation of parameters and standard errors for underlying statistical models and the construction of confidence intervals cannot be undertaken in this framework, as these methods require assumptions that link the local population under study to some more extensive target population. Because such assumptions are considered plausible for the data in Table 1, their extended population analysis is discussed in the next section.

EXTENDED POPULATION ANALYSIS Because injury severity is influenced by the accident environment rather than fortuitous factors associated with geography and date, there is a reasonable basis for assuming the data in Table 1 are a stratified simple random sample from the vehicle size X vehicle age X model year cross-classification for a target population. Unfortunately, this target population cannot be specified through deductive logic because it is based on judgment and is subject to controversy. It may be any of the following:

1. All accidents of the same type described in Table 1 for any location in the United States during 1966, or 1968 to 1972.
2. All accidents of the same type described in Table 1 for North Carolina for an unspecified time period relative to the model year and vehicle age constraints.
3. All accidents of the same type described in Table 1 for any location in the United States during an unspecified time period relative to the model year and vehicle age constraints.
4. A purely hypothetical population of accidents of the same type described in Table 1.

The statistical analysis is similar for any of these target populations even though the interpretations of results are fundamentally different in scope and, correspondingly, susceptibility to criticism. A subtle but important issue is that the data are assumed to be a stratified simple random sample rather than an unrestricted simple random sample. As a result, the basis of generalization from the sampled local population to the target population is the extent to which their within stratum distributions of injury severity can be viewed as similar. Further, no assumptions about the similarity of among strata distributions of accident environments are needed, as attention is directed at the relationship of injury severity to the strata rather than prediction of the joint injury severity X strata cross-classification. In other words, as long as the estimates of percentage severe injury for a stratum like standard size, 3 to 5 years old 1967 to 1969 automobiles are applicable to a defined target population, then comparisons among strata estimates are similarly meaningful, regardless of whether such accident types are more or less prevalent in the target population than in North Carolina during 1966, 1968 to 1972.

The assumption of stratified simple random sampling implies that frequencies in Table 1 have independent binomial distributions. To test hypothesis

H^*_{OR}: Injury severity has the same binomial distribution for all vehicle size X vehicle age X model year strata the same Pearson chi-square statistic Q_P for local population analysis can be used because H^*_{OR} implies H_{OR} for the conditional hypergeometric distribution of the frequencies in Table 1 under H^*_{OR}, given that the distribution for the pooled strata is fixed. Similarly, the local population test statistics for H_{OP} can be used when testing

H^*_{OP}: For each vehicle size by vehicle age stratum, injury severity has the same binomial distribution for the vehicle model year subpopulations.

Thus, although the extended population and local population analysis frameworks are different, common methods are applicable. However, the principal objective of extended population analysis is to explain the variation among the binomial distributions for the respective strata in terms of a regression model and to test hypotheses about model parameters. An appropriate method is weighted least squares asymptotic regression.

Weighted least squares analysis for a linear model Differences between estimated percentages of severe injury for strata can be investigated by testing linear hypotheses among them relative to corresponding estimates of variance based upon the assumed stratified simple random sampling framework. If sample sizes are sufficiently large (e.g. so that all frequencies in Table 1 exceed 5), then Wald (34) statistics have an approximate chi-square distribution with degrees of freedom equal to the dimension of the hypothesis. More formally, let μ denote the (12 X 1) vector of population values (or large sample expected values) for the (12 X 1) vector F of estimated percentages of severe injury. Then linear hypotheses concerning differences among the elements of μ can be expressed in the general form

H_{OW}: $W \mu = O_w$

where W is a (w X 12) matrix of contrast constraints (i.e. the elements in its rows add to 0) with known coefficients and full rank w and O_w is a (w X 1) vector of 0's. If V_F denotes a large sample (consistent) estimate of the variance/covariance structure for F, then the Wald chi-square statistic for H_{OW} is the matrix product (quadratic form)

$$Q_W(DF = w) = F'W'\{W \ V_F W'\}^{-1}WF.$$

In applications, both statistical significance (where $p < 0.05$) and nonsignificance ($p > 0.10$) for Q_W are interpretable. Statistical significance indicates that differences specified by W may be important. On the other hand, nonsignificance implies that variation in μ can be explained using a lower dimensional (t X 1) parameter vector β where $t = (12 - w)$. This would require using the linear model $\mu = X \beta$ where X is a (12 X t) *design* matrix of known coefficients with full rank t and X is orthogonal to W, meaning that $\mathbf{W}\,\mathbf{X} = \mathbf{O}_{w,t}$, where $\mathbf{O}_{w,t}$ is a ($w \times t$) matrix of 0's. In other words, $\mu = \mathbf{X}\,\beta$ implies $\mathbf{W}\,\mu = \mathbf{O}_w$ and vice-versa. Thus, if Q_W is not significant, the linear model using $\mathbf{X}$ adequately represents differences in μ. The linkage of $\mathbf{W}$ and $\mathbf{X}$ is often expressed by calling $\mathbf{W}$ the *constraint formulation* of the variational model and calling $\mathbf{X}$ the *freedom equation* or *model specification* formulation.

For the data in Table 1, the following preliminary hypotheses were tested with Wald chi-square statistics:

1. Equal differences between model years across all vehicle size by vehicle age strata (i.e. no vehicle size $\times$ model year interaction, no vehicle age $\times$ model year interaction, and no vehicle size $\times$ vehicle age $\times$ model year interaction; or equivalently model year effects and size $\times$ age effects are additive). For this hypothesis, we can use

$$
\mathbf{W}_1 =
\begin{bmatrix}
\text{Small} & \text{Small} & \text{Small} & \text{Small} & \text{Mid.} & \text{Mid.} & \text{Mid.} & \text{Mid.} & \text{Stand.} & \text{Stand.} & \text{Stand.} & \text{Stand.} \\
0\text{--}2 & 0\text{--}2 & 3\text{--}5 & 3\text{--}5 & 0\text{--}2 & 0\text{--}2 & 3\text{--}5 & 3\text{--}5 & 0\text{--}2 & 0\text{--}2 & 3\text{--}5 & 3\text{--}5 \\
{\leqslant}66 & 67\text{--}69 & {\leqslant}66 & 67\text{--}69 & {\leqslant}66 & 67\text{--}69 & {\leqslant}66 & 67\text{--}69 & {\leqslant}66 & 67\text{--}69 & {\leqslant}66 & 67\text{--}69 \\
1 & -1 & -1 & 1 & 0 & 0 & 0 & 0 & 0 & 0 & 0 & 0 \\
1 & -1 & 0 & 0 & -1 & 1 & 0 & 0 & 0 & 0 & 0 & 0 \\
1 & -1 & 0 & 0 & 0 & 0 & -1 & 1 & 0 & 0 & 0 & 0 \\
1 & -1 & 0 & 0 & 0 & 0 & 0 & 0 & -1 & 1 & 0 & 0 \\
1 & -1 & 0 & 0 & 0 & 0 & 0 & 0 & 0 & 0 & -1 & 1
\end{bmatrix}
$$

and $Q_W(\text{DF} = 5) = 2.14$ is nonsignificant with $p > 0.50$.

2. No differences between 0 to 2 years vehicle age and 3 to 5 years vehicle age subpopulations for each vehicle size $\times$ model year stratum (i.e. no vehicle age effects in any sense). For this hypothesis,

$$
\mathbf{W}_2 =
\begin{bmatrix}
1 & 0 & -1 & 0 & 0 & 0 & 0 & 0 & 0 & 0 & 0 & 0 \\
0 & 1 & 0 & -1 & 0 & 0 & 0 & 0 & 0 & 0 & 0 & 0 \\
0 & 0 & 0 & 0 & 1 & 0 & -1 & 0 & 0 & 0 & 0 & 0 \\
0 & 0 & 0 & 0 & 0 & 1 & 0 & -1 & 0 & 0 & 0 & 0 \\
0 & 0 & 0 & 0 & 0 & 0 & 0 & 0 & 1 & 0 & -1 & 0 \\
0 & 0 & 0 & 0 & 0 & 0 & 0 & 0 & 0 & 1 & 0 & -1
\end{bmatrix}
$$

and $Q_W(\text{DF} = 6) = 3.81$ is nonsignificant with $p > 0.50$.

3. Equal differences between small vs middle and middle vs large vehicle sizes for each vehicle age $\times$ model year stratum (i.e. homogeneity of increment effects for increasing vehicle sizes; or equivalently, vehicle size effects are linear). For this hypothesis,

$$
\mathbf{W}_3 =
\begin{bmatrix}
1 & 0 & 0 & 0 & -2 & 0 & 0 & 0 & 1 & 0 & 0 & 0 \\
0 & 1 & 0 & 0 & 0 & -2 & 0 & 0 & 0 & 1 & 0 & 0 \\
0 & 0 & 1 & 0 & 0 & 0 & -2 & 0 & 0 & 0 & 1 & 0 \\
0 & 0 & 0 & 1 & 0 & 0 & 0 & -2 & 0 & 0 & 0 & 1
\end{bmatrix}
$$

and $Q_W(\text{DF} = 4) = 2.14$ is nonsignificant with $p > 0.50$.

4. The hypotheses 1, 2, and 3 simultaneously (i.e. no vehicle age effects and additive model year and linear vehicle size effects). For this hypothesis, W_4 is a (9 X 12) matrix that can be formed by combining W_1, W_2, and W_3 and then deleting redundant rows; and $Q_W(DF = 9) = 4.53$ is nonsignificant with $p > 0.50$.

The hypothesis 4 leads to the simplified linear model indicated in Table 1, which is shown with parameter estimates and their standard errors. These parameters can be interpreted as (a) a reference cell parameter corresponding to the percentage severe injury for small size 0 to 2-year-old, 1966 or before automobiles, (b) a linear decrement effect for increasing vehicle size, (c) a decrement effect for 1967 to 1969 model year automobiles. Predicted values and their estimated standard errors from this model are given in the last two columns of Table 1 for percentages of severe injury for each stratum. These quantities represent smoothed estimates that reflect conclusions from hypotheses 1 to 4. Also, standard errors for these predicted values are smaller than those for the original estimated percentages of severe injury because they are based on a common framework for all strata with extraneous sources of variation removed.

In summary, the relationship between percentage of severe injury and the vehicle size X vehicle age X model year cross-classification can be represented by additive model year effects and linear vehicle size effects. The estimated percentage of severe injury is highest at 21.5% for small size, 0 to 2-year-old, 1966 or before automobiles; it is significantly ($p < 0.05$) less for 1967 to 1969 automobiles than 1966 or before automobiles by 3.0% for all vehicle size X vehicle age strata; and it is progressively less ($p < 0.01$) for increasing vehicle sizes by 3.3% and 6.5% for all vehicle age X model year strata.

Weighted least squares analysis for multiplicative models   The additive model in Table 1 is useful for interpreting effects of vehicle size and model year in terms of changes in percentage of severe injury. Although these quantities have a simple definition, they may not be effective for evaluation purposes because they do not state explicitly relative differences. One way of dealing with this question is to use the ratios of 3% relative to the predicted values for percentages of severe injury for 1966 or before automobiles; i.e. $(3.0/21.5) = (0.14)$ for small vehicles, $(3.0/18.3) = (0.16)$ for middle size vehicles, and $(3.0/15.0) = (0.20)$ for large size vehicles. Thus, the 3.0% absolute difference corresponds to fractional reductions ranging from 0.14 to 0.20. These are substantial relative differences.

Hypothesis testing and model formulation can be directed at either absolute measures or relative measures but not both at the same time. Linear models provide a simplified structure for the interpretation of absolute differences. Relative differences among subpopulations can be investigated from either of two points of view:

1. Exponential models for multiplicative relationships among the percentages of severe injury.
2. Logistic models for multiplicative relationships among the ratios of percentages for severe vs not severe injury (i.e. the odds of severe injury vs not severe injury).

Wald statistics can be used to test hypotheses H_{OW} for the exponential model 1 by revising the definition of F to the (12 X 1) vector of logarithms of the percentages of severe injury and μ to the corresponding (12 X 1) vector of natural logarithms of population values. Also, weighted least squares methods can be used to fit models X to μ via F on this logarithmic scale; as a result, the exponential transformations (i.e. reverse of taking natural logarithms) of the parameter estimates b represent relative measures for subpopulation comparisons of ratios of percentages of severe injury. Similarly, these same methods can be applied to the logistic model 2 except that F becomes the (12 X 1) vector of logarithms of ratios of percentages severe vs not severe injury (i.e. logits or log odds), and μ becomes the (12 X 1) vector of natural logarithms of similar ratios of population values. Then exponential transformation of parameter estimates b represent relative measures of the odds of severe vs not severe injury. So linear methods can be used to investigate nonlinear relationships such as 1 and 2 if they can be transformed to a linear framework.

For the data in Table 1, the same simplified structure X that was formulated for the linear model analysis is also satisfactory for the exponential and logistic model. The goodness of fit statistic for the exponential model is $Q_W(DF = 9) = 5.99$, $p > 0.50$, and the estimated fractional reduction in percentage of severe injury for 1967 to 1969 model years relative to 1966 or before is 0.16 ± 0.06. Alternatively, the goodness of fit statistic for the logistic model is $Q_W(DF = 9) = 5.65$, $p > 0.50$, and the estimated fractional reduction in the odds for severe vs not severe injury for 1967 to 1969 model years relative to 1966 or before is 0.19 ± 0.07. Thus, for this example, linear, exponential, and logistic models are equally effective for investigating the variation among the percentages of severe injury. They lead to the same simplified structure X and provide relative measures for model year comparisons that have similar interpretations. In this case, the choice among them is a matter of personal taste and computational convenience. On the other hand, for some applications, one of these models may be preferable because of more parsimonious structure or easier interpretation. Note that logistic models do have the technical advantage of always yielding predicted values for percentages in the 0 to 100 range, whereas linear and exponential models may give predicted values outside this range. Usually for large samples, this issue is not of practical importance because models with impossible predicted values tend to be contradicted by significantly large goodness of fit statistics, but such issues are different for small samples (i.e. many cell frequencies less than 5). Even though Wald statistics may often provide reasonable results for small samples, their technical validity requires large samples and so another method is required. One method in extensive use is maximum likelihood as discussed in (40–43). With this method, parameter values that maximize the multinomial probability function for the observed data provide the parameter estimates, and differences between maximized logarithms of probability functions for hierarchically related models are used to obtain approximate chi-square test statistics for hypotheses. One cautionary statement is in order. Maximum likelihood methods also require large samples for statistical properties of the procedure to be optimal. However, the large sample considerations relate to model structure, not individual cell frequencies, so sample size should be sufficiently large for the parameter estimates to have an approximate multivariate normal distribution.

Maximum likelihood often involves the solution of nonlinear equations using iterative calculations. For logistic models and their generalizations discussed in (42, 43) the algorithms are easily computerized. However, for linear, exponential, and other types of models that may give predicted values outside the 0 to 100 range, the calculations may be unacceptably difficult or expensive. Computational convenience is one of the principal reasons that logistic models are used extensively for maximum likelihood applications to small sample situations. A specific illustration is given later in Table 2.

Conclusions The relationship between injury severity and the vehicle weight X vehicle age X model year cross-classification in Table 1 is explained adequately by a linear, or an exponential, or a logistic model with the same structure **X.** For each of these frameworks, both the model year and the equal increment vehicle weight parameter are statistically significant ($p < 0.05$). However, their interpretations are different because the linear model involves additive effects, whereas the exponential and logistic models use multiplicative effects.

Further, these conclusions appear valid for a more extensive target population, notably other parts of the United States and other time periods. However, additional support for the latter conclusion through other similarly oriented studies would seem necessary.

OTHER EXTENDED POPULATION ANALYSES   Sometimes there is interest in the use of data like those in Table 1 for predicting the joint injury severity X strata cross-classification for some target population. Stronger assumptions are required because both within-strata accident severity and across-strata distributions of accident environment are involved. If the across-strata distribution for the target population is known from other sources, then, in combination with the within-strata percentages, it yields estimates for the joint injury severity X strata distribution. This two-stage procedure, which is similar to raking / synthetic estimation reviewed in (48, 49), is also applicable when the across-strata distribution for the target population is known only partially in terms of marginal distributions, provided that higher order relationships are negligible (see 50 for related discussions of indirect standardization).

Another framework of interest is where the joint injury severity X strata frequencies in Table 1 can be assumed to have independent Poisson distributions with population (expected) values that are the product of unknown rate parameters and partially or completely known exposure (denominator) values. Because this multiplicative structural model is a general formulation of the case of equal exposure values, which implies the logistic model for the within stratum distribution of injury severity, its rate parameters can be analogously interpreted as relative measures of association for components of the joint injury severity X strata cross-classification. Finally, although maximum likelihood or weighted least squares methods can be used for estimation and hypothesis testing for this Poisson regression model, provided sample size is adequate, results should be viewed with even more caution than those from the stratified simple random sampling analyses because stronger assumptions are involved.

Example 2: A Nonrandomized Clinical Study with a Historical Control

The data in Table 2 are from a study comparing the prospective experience of a population of patients receiving an antidote for a suicidal-intent overdose of a medical product with a historical control population of patients treated by general support. The outcome measure is whether a laboratory test for liver function was severe. A critical issue is the validity of an evaluation based on a comparison of liver function status for patients receiving the antidote relative to expected status under supportive treatment so that uncontrolled aspects of the overdose experience are taken into account. The statistical strategy is to compare treatment and control populations within risk status strata. These strata may be viewed as matched sets within which patients are presumed to have similar risk and hence similar expected outcome if there is no difference between treatment and control. On the contrary, the extent to which the treatment patients consistently have more favorable outcomes than controls supports treatment efficacy. Risk status is controlled through a diagnostic risk status index (moderate, high) for certain blood assays and a time to hospital admission index (early, delayed, late).

LOCAL POPULATION ANALYSIS   Because patients were neither selected by probability random sampling nor assigned to treatment by random allocation, they are representative only of themselves and all frequencies in Table 2 are fixed. However, as in Table 1, hypotheses like H_{OR} and H_{OP} can still be investigated via an induced randomization structure. The hypothesis of primary interest is of type H_{OP} and concerns the partial association of liver function status and treatment population after stratification adjustment for risk.

Statistical test of H_{OP}   The Cochran/Mantel-Haenszel statistic (Q_{CMH}) is used to test H_{OP} because this test is powerful for detecting consistent differences in favor of one treatment. For the data in Table 2, $Q_{CMH} = 8.01$ is significant with $p < 0.01$, using the chi-square $DF = 1$ approximation to its distribution. However, because the numbers of patients in the strata are fairly small, the exact method described in (52) and (53) is also used to test H_{OP}. With this procedure, the exact one-tailed p-value is $p_e = 0.0051$ confirming that there is a partial association between liver function status and treatment vs control. This partial association can be described as a 20.4% relative difference between the 25 observed patients with severe liver function status in the treatment population and the 31.4 expected patients if treatment and control were a random partition of a common population.

Conclusion   There is a statistically significant association between liver function status and treatment vs historical control components of the local population. This association can be interpreted as a statistical indication that the antidote is more effective than supportive treatment provided that the following assumptions are plausible:

1. There is no selection bias with respect to study inclusion for the patients in each population.
2. Data collection procedures for liver function status and stratification indexes for the patients in each population are equivalent, i.e. the same values are reported for the same phenomena.
3. Diagnostic risk status and time to hospital admission provide a homogeneous stratification framework for each population, i.e. the patients within each stratum of each population have similar risk regarding liver function status.

Because the validity of these assumptions is difficult to assess, the interpretation of a nonrandomized clinical study with a historical control is inherently controversial and ultimately depends upon the reproducibility of findings in other patient populations. Additional discussion of the statistical problems of analyzing studies with historical controls is given in (54), (55), (56), and (57).

EXTENDED POPULATION ANALYSIS   The data in Table 2 may be assumed to be a stratified simple random sample from a target population analogous to that described in Example 1. The rationale for this is that for patients within each stratum of treatment and control, liver function status has no relationship with patient characteristics such as age, sex, and previous medical history, or with the time and place of occurrence.

Because many of the frequencies for this example are small, maximum likelihood methods are used to fit logistic models to the data, which leads to the simplified structure X shown in Table 2 together with corresponding parameter estimates and their estimated standard errors. These parameters can be interpreted as follows with respect to the natural logarithm of the ratio of the percentage severe vs not severe for liver function outcome status:

1. A reference cell parameter for patients in the treatment population with moderate diagnostic risk status and early hospital admission.
2. An increment effect for high diagnostic risk status.
3. An equal (linear) increment effect for increasing time to hospital admission.
4. An increment effect for the control population.

Predicted values from this model and their estimated standard errors are given in the last two columns of Table 2. The differences between treatment and historical control populations vary considerably across strata, ranging from 11.5% for patients with high diagnostic risk and late hospital admission to 30.9% for patients with high diagnostic risk status and early treatment. Returning to the multiplicative framework, the odds for severe vs not severe liver function status are 3.6 times greater in the historical control population than the treatment population for all strata. Thus, the logistic model permits the difference between treatment and control to be expressed in terms of a single relative parameter even though the absolute difference between them varies substantially among the strata. In contrast to the previous example, data in Table 2 illustrate a situation in which the interpretations of absolute and relative differences are not the same.

Example 3: A Cross-Sectional Prevalence Study

This example is based on a 1973 survey of the respiratory health of 6631 employees at 14 plants of a large cotton textile manufacturing corporation.

One of the objectives of this study, which is described in (58) and (59), was the investigation of the relationship between the reported prevalence of employee complaints for symptoms associated with the respiratory ailment byssinosis and the occupational environment. The data in Table 3 represent frequencies for employee complaint status cross-classified according to workplace for entire employment period (dusty, not dusty), duration of employment period (< 10 years, ≥ 10 years), and smoking status during the past five years (yes, no) for a local population of 5419 employees for whom such information was available. Because these data refer only to a subset of employees of a single corporation at a particular time point, careful consideration must be given to the objectives of their statistical analysis.

1. Conclusions should be directed toward the existing respiratory health status of current employees as it relates to their need for health services programs as opposed to the historical developments leading to that status.
2. The cross-classification of workplace, duration of employment, and smoking status represents a set of strata for which the variation in existing respiratory health status may indicate different levels of need for health services as opposed to a framework for evaluating the risk factors for its historical development.

Stringent assumptions, external to the data, would be required if this cross-sectional study were to be taken as equivalent to a longitudinal study. For the present example, these assumptions may include occupational migration having no relationship with complaint status, symptoms remaining present once they occur for employees whose entire employment involves the same work environment, and the relationship of complaint status with length of employment being the same regardless of the initial date of employment (i.e. no cohort effects).

LOCAL POPULATION ANALYSIS As in the previous examples, there was no selection of employees by probability sampling—they represent only themselves. All frequencies in Table 3 are considered fixed, but hypotheses like H_{OR} and H_{OP} can still be investigated through the randomization structures induced. For H_{OR}, the Pearson chi-square statistic $Q_p = 550.4$ with DF = 7 is significant with $p < 0.01$, indicating that the variation among prevalences of byssinosis symptoms for the workplace $\times$ employment duration $\times$ smoking status strata is more extensive than expected under a random partition of a common population. The Cochran/Mantel-Haenszel chi-square statistics with DF = 1 are as follows for the three specifications of H_{OP}:

1. $Q = 392.2$ for workplace after stratification adjustment for employment duration and smoking status.
2. $Q = 10.4$ for smoking status after stratification adjustment for workplace and employment duration.
3. $Q = 13.6$ for employment duration after stratification adjustment for workplace and smoking status.

Thus, there is significant variation with $p < 0.01$ for each dimension of the cross-classified strata after adjustment for the other two.

EXTENDED POPULATION ANALYSIS   The more complete analysis reported in (59), shows that race, sex, and somewhat more refined definitions of workplace and employment duration sources of variation were all compatible with the hypothesis H_{OP} of no partial association after strata adjustment. If the assumption that this same general structure also applies to some more extensive target population is reasonable, then the analysis of the data from a corresponding stratified simple random sampling point of view becomes useful.

Because the frequencies in Table 3 are sufficiently large to suggest that the prevalences for byssinosis symptoms have approximately normal distributions, Wald statistics are used to test hypotheses concerning them. On the linear scale, this approach leads to the detection of significant interactions with $p < 0.01$ for workplace $\times$ smoking and workplace $\times$ employment duration. Furthermore, these interactions can be interpreted as corresponding to the dissimilarity of significance ($p < 0.01$) for the smoking status and employment duration sources of variation in the dusty workplace, but nonsignificance ($p > 0.25$) for the not dusty workplace. These conclusions are incorporated in the simplified variational model X for this example, which is shown in Table 3 together with its estimated parameters and their standard errors. These parameters can be interpreted as follows: 1. A reference cell parameter for employees in the not dusty workplace with $\geqslant 10$ years employment and nonsmoking status during the 5 years prior to the survey. 2. An increment effect for the dusty workplace. 3. An increment effect for $\geqslant 10$ year employment for employees in the dusty workplace. 4. An increment effect for smoking for employees in the dusty workplace. Predicted values from this model and their estimated standard errors are given in the last two columns of Table 3. Examination of these quantities further clarifies the workplace $\times$ smoking and workplace $\times$ employment duration interactions by indicating no variation at all with respect to employment duration and smoking status in the not dusty workplace and an additive relationship in the dusty workplace. Finally, an analysis of these data can be undertaken with a logistic model, but then the workplace $\times$

smoking and workplace X employment interactions are less apparent ($0.05 < p < 0.10$) than with the additive model. Thus, the additive model is considered to provide a more useful analytical framework for this example.

A RANDOMIZED CLINICAL TRIAL EXAMPLE

Let us consider an example of a true experiment in which associations can be interpreted more strongly as indicative of cause and effect. In particular, the data are from a clinical trial to compare four surgical operations for treatment of duodenal ulcer. Suitably eligible patients at 17 participating hospitals were randomly assigned on an equal probability basis to one of the following treatments: (*a*) vagotomy and drainage, (*b*) vagotomy and antrectomy (removal of approximately 25% of the distal stomach), (*c*) vagotomy and hemigastrectomy (removal of approximately 50% of the stomach), (*d*) gastric resection (removal of approximately 75% of the stomach). Although extensive information about patients was available, attention here is restricted to the severity of the *dumping syndrome,* an undesirable sequela of surgery for duodenal ulcer, and follow-up status with respect to death, recurrence, or reoperation at 6 months, 24 months, and 60 months. Other aspects of this study are discussed in (60).

Example 4: Analysis of Ordinal Data for Dumping Syndrome Severity

Because dumping syndrome severity was expressed as none, slight, or moderate, its relationship to treatment for four of the participating hospitals is investigated in terms of the contingency table shown in Table 4. As for the historical data examples, two types of analysis strategies are of interest. One is directed at the local population of patients who participated in the study, and the other at some more extensive population who may be treated with one of the four operations at any hospital in the future.

LOCAL POPULATION ANALYSIS   The research design for this investigation involved randomization, so data for each treatment within each hospital provide an estimate for the distribution of dumping syndrome severity that would be expected if it had been administered to all patients. If there is no relationship between dumping syndrome severity and operation, then the four target populations corresponding to the four treatment groups would be identical as regards dumping syndrome severity, and the randomized structure of the research design would imply that the data satisfied the hypothesis of no partial association, H_{OP}.

H_{OP}: For each hospital, dumping syndrome severity is distributed at random with respect to the four treatments. Data for the respective treatments can be regarded as a stratified set of simple random samples from the fixed populations corresponding to the hospitals.

Thus, H_{OP} can be interpreted as a hypothesis of no treatment differences.

Statistical test of H_{OP}   Although many test statistics for H_{OP} are available, those exploring relationships that involve the ordering of dumping syndrome severity and operation are of most interest. Another important issue is that the across hospital combination of within hospital relationships provides an overall indication of whether such relationships are sufficiently consistent to contradict H_{OP}. Thus, the analysis strategy can be based upon the broad hypothesis vs narrow alternative argument where H_{OP} represents the broad hypothesis and similar increasing relationships between dumping syndrome severity and amount of stomach removed represents the narrow alternative.

With these comments in mind, the partial correlation extension of the Cochran/Mantel-Haenszel statistic discussed in (31) and (32) is used to test H_{OP} with respect to two scales:

1. Within hospital standardized rank (or ridit) scores for both dumping syndrome severity and operation with ties taken into account via midranks; more specifically the score a_{hj} assigned to the j-th dumping syndrome category for the n_h patients at the h-th hospital has the form $a_{hj} = (n_{hjf} + \frac{1}{2}n_{hj} + \frac{1}{2})/n_h$ where n_{hj} is the number of patients with the j-th outcomes and $n_{hjf} = \Sigma^{(j-1)}_{k=1} n_{hk}$ is the number of patients with a more favorable response; the score w_{hi} assigned to the i-th treatment has a similar definition.
2. Standardized uniform scores, i.e. 0 for none, 0.5 for slight, and 1.0 for moderate dumping syndrome severity and 0.00, 0.25, 0.50, and 0.75 for operation.

For each of these scores, a partial correlation randomization test statistic can be constructed in the general form $Q_{PCR} = (F-E)^2/V$ where $F = \Sigma_h \Sigma_i \Sigma_j w_{hi} a_{hj} n_{hij}$ is sum of the products of the frequencies in Table 4 and their corresponding dumping syndrome and treatment scores, E is the H_{OP} expected value for F, and V is the H_{OP} variance for F. If the overall sample size is moderately large (e.g. $\Sigma n_h \geqslant 50$ and many of the $n_{hij} \geqslant 1$), then Q_{PCR} has an approximate chi-square distribution with DF = 1. For the data in Table 4, $Q_{PCR} = 6.92$ with $p < 0.01$ for standardized rank scores, and $Q_{PCR} = 6.34$ with $0.05 > p > 0.01$ for standardized uniform scores. Thus, both of these results suggest differences among the operations whereby the dumping syndrome severity increases with the increasing amount of stomach removed. The principal advantage of the rank scores is that they provide a straightforward framework for comparison, requiring no assumptions about the structure of the ordinal scales for dumping syndrome severity and amount of stomach removed. A disadvantage is that their results may be difficult to interpret in terms of the original measurement scale. Alternatively, uniform scores provide a useful descriptive framework for summarizing the relationship between amount of stomach removed and the average of the proportion of patients for whom the dumping syndrome severity was at least slight and the proportion for whom it was at least moderate. It should be remembered that uniform scores are sometimes controversial because they appear to require equal spacing for ordinal categories like none, slight, moderate. However, this issue applies only when the mean score is being interpreted as a generalized estimate for the proportion moderate and for which "slight" is viewed as half-way between "none" and "moderate." Thus, uniform scores always provide a reasonable basis for investigation, but may not be the most appropriate when a more meaningful framework is available [e.g. natural scales indicative of costs or levels of impaired activity or derived scales from certain types of statistical models such as those discussed in (61), (62), and (63)].

Discussion   A randomized study permits a comparison of treatments that is more convincing than the nonrandomized study vs historical control situation, which assumes comparability of two populations under the assumption of a homogeneous stratification structure. Of course, the validity of the comparisons is dependent on data collection procedures for dumping syndrome severity being equivalent for the four operations. For example, if patients with more stomach removed were monitored more closely than those with less surgery, then their apparently more severe dumping syndrome status may be a consequence of reporting bias. For this reason, objective data obtained by methods that are unrelated (or blinded) to any information concerning a patient's treatment status are as essential to the validity of randomized studies as they are to other types of studies.

In summary, the randomized structure of the research design for this example permits statistical comparisons that do not require any other technical assumptions. However, the relevance of this comparison depends on the coverage of the patient population under study and the quality of the dumping syndrome data. Thus, a randomized study is not necessarily more informative than a nonrandomized study unless its coverage is as broad and its data are valid and are as reliable. More simply, although randomization can be a very important component of the validity of a well-designed clinical study, it is neither a necessary nor sufficient component.

EXTENDED POPULATION ANALYSIS   As before, the data in Table 4 are assumed to be a stratified simple random sample from some target population.

The standardized uniform scale provides a quantitative description of the ordinal categories for dumping syndrome severity. Average scores of the form $(0.5\ P_S + P_M)$ where P_S is the proportion of patients with slight dumping syndrome severity and P_M is proportion with moderate severity are used to investigate the variation among the hospital X treatment strata. An advantage of these mean scores as a basis of analysis is that their incorporation of the information in both P_S and P_M supports the plausibility of approximate normal distributions for their statistical behavior even though many of the frequencies in Table 4 are small. Thus, Wald statistics can be used to test hypotheses and weighted least squares methods used to fit variational models. This leads to the simplified model X shown in Table 4 together with corresponding parameter estimates and estimated standard errors. These parameters can be interpreted as follows:

1. A reference cell parameter for patients at any hospital who were administered vagotomy and drainage.
2. An equal (linear) increment for increasing amounts of stomach removed for the respective operations.

For further information concerning the analysis which led to the model X as well as the methods which were used to fit it, see (64, 65).

Predicted values from this model and their estimated standard errors are given in the last two columns of Table 4. Examination of these quantities indicates that for each operation, there is no variation among the hospitals with respect to the standardized uniform scaling of dumping syndrome severity. This conclusion is an important feature of the extended population analysis because it supports the assumption that the experience of patients at the four hospitals in Table 4 is representative of some larger population of patients. In other words, if there is variation among the hospitals, then their self-selected (by willingness and/or ability to participate) nature may limit the extent to which results may be generalized. More importantly, if there is hospital X operation interaction, then a similar statement applies to the comparison of operations. Alternatively, however, if such sources of variation can be statistically eliminated through the partition of each hospital's patients into strata according to, say, demographic, medical history, and medical environment characteristics, then generalization to other target populations may be realistic.

Discussion   Patient inclusion criteria for a randomized study are critical for generalization to more extensive target populations. In this regard, if the scope of a randomized study is too narrow in terms of patient eligibility or patient consent to participate, its results may not be as convincing as those from a nonrandomized study vs historical control situation with considerably broader coverage and a suitably homogeneous stratification structure. Clinical studies involving randomized treatment allocation should be conducted in a carefully controlled manner with strict adherence to the research design protocol and maintenance of data quality and include participating hospitals (or clinics) that encompass broad coverage of patients. Such a well-designed randomized study is often considered to be the most appropriate scientific framework for the comparison of alternative medical treatments in an objective manner and is subject to only minimal criticism.

SURVIVAL DATA EXAMPLE

For many clinical studies, the principal objective is to compare two or more treatments with respect to the length of time until occurrence of some well-defined event, such as death from chronic disease, recurrence of infectious disease, failure of dental restorative procedure, and emergence of psychological or developmental traits. Data are obtained by follow-up of subjects who, ultimately, are classified into one of three categories:

1. The vital event did not occur as of the end of the maximal follow-up period for the study (e.g. 5 years). These subjects are called *overall survivors*.
2. The vital event did not occur as of the time of last follow-up, but subsequent observation of the subject was impossible because of some competing event, unavailability due to change of address or disinterest (i.e. follow-up losses), or the closing date for data collection for the study. These subjects are called *withdrawals*.
3. The vital event occurred during the follow-up period either in an exact sense (e.g. date of death) or in terms of the interval between the last time of follow-up prior to its detection and the first time of follow-up afterward (e.g. events based upon diagnostic evaluations of subjects at periodic visits). These subjects may be called *occurrences*, although more specific labels, such as deaths, recurrences, and failures, are more common.

Example 5: Survival Analysis of Randomized Trial for Duodenal Ulcer

For the duodenal ulcer study of example 4, a composite vital event of interest was operation failure as defined by the occurrence of death, ulcer recurrence, or the need for reoperation during a 5-year follow-up period with intermediate evaluation visits at 6 months and 24 months. The resulting data for all participating hospitals combined (under the assumption of no variation among them) are given in Table 5.

If there were no withdrawals (i.e. follow-up losses) for this study, then the length of the follow-up period would be the same for all subjects. As a result, the statistical issues for the analysis of the time to event data in Table 5 would be the same as those for the ordinal data in Table 4. Then rank methods could be used for local population analysis and weighted least squares or maximum likelihood methods could be undertaken for extended population analysis. However, when withdrawals are present, some information is censored, i.e. withdrawals are neither overall survivors nor occurrences. A major source of difficulty is that the ranking of withdrawals relative to survivors and occurrences and to themselves is not entirely clear. For example, a withdrawn patient at 2 years has better survival than an occurrence patient at 6 months, but uncertain status relative to an occurrence at 5 years. Thus, the appropriate use of withdrawal information is an important statistical issue which must be addressed. A critical assumption that is implicit in all of the subsequent discussion is that withdrawal is unrelated to occurrence of the event under study. This means that the unobserved experience of withdrawn subjects is equivalent to the observed experience of subjects who did not withdraw. As indicated in (45), even though this assumption is often taken for granted, it should be viewed cautiously because it may be unrealistic and make interpretation of findings difficult and even ambiguous. Finally, the population coverage and data quality considerations discussed for Table 4 apply equally strongly to the analysis of Table 5. Further discussion of the importance of such issues with respect to the design and analysis of longitudinal follow-up studies is given in (57) and (66).

LOCAL POPULATION ANALYSIS   The randomization structure of the research design is used as the framework to test the hypothesis,

H_{OR}: Patient follow-up status regarding death, recurrence, or reoperation is distributed at random with respect to the four treatments and so data are equivalent to a set of simple random samples from the fixed population corresponding to their pooled combination.

As previously indicated, the within-treatment variation among hospitals is assumed negligible so that the stratified within-hospital randomization can be viewed as equivalent to an unrestricted randomization for the pooled hospitals. Consequently, H_{OR} can be interpreted as an hypothesis of no treatment differences. More generally, if there were variation among the hospitals, then the hypothesis of no treatment differences would need to be formulated in a manner analogous to H_{OP} for Table 4.

Statistical test of H_{OR} Because the principal alternatives of interest for H_{OR} are longer survival for at least one treatment vs the others, the basic analytic strategy in the formulation of test statistics for it is to develop and use effectively a quasi-ordering of observed categories for follow-up status. A true ordering is ambitious due to the dilemma of how to treat the withdrawals. One way of identifying a quasi-ordering is to assign scores to the categories in a manner similar to that described in (67) and then to compare their averages for the respective treatment groups via randomization one-way analysis of variance, i.e. generalized Kruskal-Wallis (26) statistics Q_{KW}. More specifically, the score assigned with this approach to the j-th follow-up status category ($j = 1, \ldots, 7$ for Table 5) has the form $a_j = (N + N_{je} - N_{jL} + 1)/2N$, where N_{je} is the number of patients in the combined population of N patients for whom the vital event was experienced in a time interval that preceded the time interval corresponding to the j-th category (regardless of whether j applies to the vital event or lost-to-follow-up), and N_{jL} is the number for whom the vital event occurred after the interval corresponding to the j-th category or after the end of the 60 month follow-up period for those j that apply to the vital event, and $N_{jL} = 0$ for those j that apply to lost-to-follow-up. The +1 is a technical correction of no practical importance. These scores, which identify a quasi-ordering of categories $j = 1, \ldots, 7$, are shown in Table 5. To illustrate the calculation for category $j = 2$, $N = 41 + 52 + 79 + 28 + 48 + 132 + 977 = 1357$, $N_{je} = 41$, and $N_{jL} = 79 + 132 + 977 = 1188$. This gives $a_j = (1357 + 41 - 1188 + 1)/2714 = 0.078$. The generalized Kruskal-Wallis statistic is obtained from them by forming $Q_{KW} = (N-1)S_a^2/S_t^2$ where S_a^2 denotes the among-treatments sum of squares and S_t^2 denotes the total sum of squares for the one-way analysis of variance of these scores. This one-way analysis of variance is carried out for $N = 1357$, and each patient receives a score according to the category to which that patient belongs. So all patients in category $j = 2$ receive a score of 0.078. If the overall sample size is moderately large (e.g. at least 20 patients per treatment of whom at least 10 have experienced the vital event), then Q_{KW} has an approximate chi-square distribution with DF = (number of treatments − 1). For the data in Table 5, $Q_{KW} = 14.04$ with DF = 3 is significant with $p < 0.01$. Thus, the variation of patient follow-up status among operations is greater than would have been expected if the experiences of the patients were a random partition of a common population.

Although the scores a_j are simple to apply, they have been criticized for not making as much use of the information of the follow-up status categories to develop a quasi-ordering as is feasible, and for this reason are unnecessarily conservative (in the sense of correspondingly less statistical power for tests of H_{OR} against certain related alternatives). On the other hand, any quasi-ordering has an arbitrary ring even though an underlying justification may be formulated. Additional discussion of this issue and other aspects of the use of scores for statistical tests of H_{OR} is given in (66), (68), (69), and (70).

Another type of framework that can be used to test H_{OR} involves comparison of the difference between the sum of the observed survival experience and the sum of the expected survival experience to a corresponding estimate of H_{OR} covariance structure in a manner similar to the life table method described by Mantel (71). The observed survival experience for the i-th treatment group during the k-th time interval is the sum f_{ik} of the number of its subjects for whom the vital event is known to have occurred after the k-th interval (if at all) plus half the number of subjects for whom withdrawal occurred during the k-th interval (i.e. withdrawals are regarded as occurring uniformly during the interval so that hypothetical complementary pairs of subjects whose summed survival for that interval equals its length are considered equivalent to a single subject who was observed to survive its entire length). The expected survival experience for the i-th treatment group has the form $m_{ik} = (f_{*k} g_{ik} / g_{*k})$ where g_{ik} is the difference between the number of subjects in the i-th group for whom the vital event was known not to have occurred prior to the k-th interval (i.e. for whom there was exposure to risk during the interval) and half the number of subjects for whom withdrawal occurred during the k-th interval; and $f_{*k} = \Sigma_i f_{ik}$ and $g_{*k} = \Sigma_i g_{ik}$ are the combined population counterparts of the $\{f_{ik}\}$ and $\{g_{ik}\}$. The resulting sum $G_i = \Sigma_k (f_{ik} - m_{ik})$ of the difference between the total observed survival experience and the total expected survival experience for the respective time intervals may be also expressed in the form $G_i = \Sigma_j c_j n_{ij}$ where n_{ij} is the number of subjects in the i-th treatment group with the j-th follow-up status, and the c_j are the life table survival difference scores implied by the identity of the two definitions of the G_i. These scores, which are shown in Table 5, may also be used to obtain a generalized Kruskal-Wallis statistic via one-way analysis of variance computations. For the data in Table 5, the resulting $Q_{KW} = 14.49$ with DF = 3 is significant with $p < 0.01$. Thus, the conclusion is the same as for the previous analysis. Other discussion of some of the statistical properties of the test statistic Q_{KW} based on life table survival difference scores, which is sometimes called the log rank statistic or the generalized Savage statistic, is given in (45), (70), and (72). Furthermore, for an extended population analysis setting in which the time to event data have continuous survivorship functions that are in a multiplicative power relationship to one another, it has been shown to be an optimal procedure according to theoretical criteria. For this reason, Peto et al (66), as well as many other statisticians, recommend it as the best procedure to test H_{OR} for most longitudinal randomized studies.

So far in example 5 the ordering of operations has not played any role, as it did for the dumping syndrome data in Table 5, for the reason that no substantive basis existed for anticipating a monotone relationship between the time to event follow-up data and the amount of stomach removed. In fact, a nonmonotone relationship for which the most favorable outcomes occurred for an intermediate operation was anticipated as being as likely as any other type of treatment difference. Finally, if there had been important covariables such as age and patient's medical history which, potentially, had a strong relationship with follow-up status, then refinements of the statistics Q_{KW} that account for the covariables could have been used. Two relevant strategies are randomization rank analysis of covariance as described by Quade (73) and analogous counterparts of the extended population analysis versions of the regression methods for survival data described by (74–76).

EXTENDED POPULATION ANALYSIS   In the same way as example 4, the data in Table 5 are assumed to be a stratified simple random sample from some target population. Because no underlying stochastic process is known to characterize these follow-up data, life table procedures are used to summarize the experience of each treatment group in terms of estimated survival percentages at 6, 24, and 60 months. With this approach, described in (77, 78), effective use of the incomplete information for withdrawals is achieved through the actuarial determination of the estimated survival percentage for the i-th treatment group at the end of the k-th time interval as the product function $F_{ik} = 100 \, \Pi^k_{k'=1} \, (f_{ik'}/g_{ik'})$ where $f_{ik'}$ and $g_{ik'}$ are estimated survival experience and exposure to risk for the i-th treatment group for the k'-th interval as defined previously in reference to the log-rank test statistic. Because the frequencies of occurrence for the vital events are moderately large for the respective time intervals (i.e. the corresponding $n_{ij} \geqslant 5$), the F_{ik} have an approximate normal distribution for which the covariance structure can be estimated by matrix methods given in (79). Thus, Wald statistics test hypotheses concerning estimated survival percentages shown in Table 5, and weighted least squares can be used to fit variational models that describe them. Model predicted values for estimated survival percentages are shown in the last 3 columns of Table 5, which are based upon a linear model with the following parameters fitted to the natural logarithms of estimated survival percentages:

1. A reference cell parameter corresponding to the logarithm of the common predicted value for the percentage of patients who are alive without recurrence or need for reoperation shortly after treatment regardless of operation.

2. A linear decrement parameter over time at 6, 24 and 60 months representing the logarithm of the monthly proportional decrease in nonoccurrence percentages for all operations except vagotomy and hemigastrectomy (V + H).
3. A linear decrement parameter over time at 6, 24, and 60 months for vagotomy and hemigastrectomy.

Examination of these predicted values indicates that vagotomy and hemigastrectomy is the most effective treatment.

Additional discussion of the use of Wald statistics and weighted least squares methods to analyze time to event data is given in (37) and (79). More generally, for many types of follow-up studies, either exact time to failure information is available or there is interest in accounting for relevant covariables. In these cases, data cannot be summarized as in Table 5 with samples that are sufficiently large for the type of analysis described here. However, if an underlying stochastic process like the proportional hazards model discussed in (45) and (74–76) is considered appropriate, maximum likelihood methods can be used to estimate parameters and predict survival percentages at different levels of covariables. These latter quantities have an interpretation analogous to the Kaplan-Meier (80) extension of the life table survival estimation procedure in which times of occurrence are distinct and known exactly. These methods have been recommended in (66) and elsewhere as flexible and useful for investigating multivariate relationships.

A COMPLEX SAMPLE SURVEY EXAMPLE

Example 6: Analysis of Health Interview Survey Data

This example is based upon data from the 1973 Health Interview Survey (HIS) of the United States conducted by the National Center for Health Statistics (81). A multi-stage probability sampling plan was implemented to provide a continuous nationwide sample of the civilian, noninstitutionalized United States population during 1973. Furthermore, the survey was designed so that weekly samples were additive across time.

One response variable of interest for HIS is number of physician visits. For each household member, visit experiences were reported for the two weeks prior to the interview in order to reduce recall errors. Information was combined across the entire sample to produce estimates for an average number of physician visits per person per year.

Often, for surveys like HIS there is interest in comparisons among multiway cross-classified domains (i.e. subpopulations that do not correspond to strata used in the survey design). Because domain estimates are from a complex probability sample, their analysis should be based upon an appropriately estimated covariance structure. To illustrate how weighted least squares asymptotic regression methods can be used for this purpose, Freeman et al (82, 83) considered the domain estimates for physician visits given in Table 6 for the cross-classification of education of head of household (< 12 years, 12 years, > 12 years), income of household (< 5000, 5000–14999, ≥ 15,000) and location of household (SMSA, Non-SMSA, where SMSA means Standard Metropolitan Statistical Area). The estimated covariance matrix for these estimates was obtained by balanced repeated replication (BRR) as described in (84) and (85). To conserve space, only the estimated standard errors (i.e. the square roots of diagonal elements) are shown in Table 6; otherwise, the correlation structure for the complete matrix is given in (86).

Patterns of variation among domain estimates in Table 6 can be explored using linear regression models. As a preliminary, hypotheses about constraints W were tested with Wald statistics and led to the following results:

1. There were some differences among domain estimates; Qw (DF = 17) = 216.85 is significant with $p < 0.01$.
2. There were similar differences between residence subdomains across all income X education domains (i.e. no residence X income interaction, no residence X education interaction, and no residence X income X education interaction; equivalently, residence effects and education X income joint effects are additive); Q_W (DF = 8) = 7.90 is nonsignificant with $p > 0.25$.
3. There were no differences among the subdomains with < 12 years or 12 years of education and $5000 to $14999 or > $15000 income for each residence, and no differences among subdomains with either < $5000 income or > 12 years of education for each residence, together with hypothesis 2 simultaneously; Q_W (DF = 15) = 17.56 is nonsignificant with $p > 0.25$.

Hypothesis 3 leads to the simplified linear model in Table 6. Weighted least squares estimates of parameters and their standard errors are also listed. These parameters can be interpreted as: 1. a reference cell parameter corresponding to domains with non-SMSA residence, ≥ $5000 income, and ≤ 12 years of education, 2. an increment for SMSA residence, and 3. an increment for either < $5000 income or > 12 years of education. Predicted values and estimated standard errors from this model are given in Table 6. As indicated previously, these smoothed estimates incorporate the conclusions from hypotheses 2 and 3, and they have smaller estimated standard errors than the original domain estimates. Thus, for both the SMSA and non-SMSA residence, there are two levels of physician visits according to income X education, with the higher level corresponding to < $5000 income or $>$ 12 years of education and the lower level corresponding to $\geqslant$ \$5000 income and $\leqslant$ 12 years of education; otherwise, for all income X education domains, there were on average 0.66 more physician visits for persons with SMSA residence than those without. Finally, other applications of weighted least squares methods to complex sample survey data are given in (5), (87), and (88).

In summary, this analysis is straightforward in concept because data were obtained directly from the 1973 United States target population by probability sampling methods. In this sense, its conclusions are general to the entire United States. However, if a different population is of interest, assumptions that link it to the sample must be formulated and justified. Then the analysis of sample surveys would be on the same basis as the analysis of historical data and attention would need to focus on the unweighted information. The analysis strategy would be similar to examples in Tables 1 to 3. Unfortunately, the interpretation of results is not definitive because they are based on an extended population analysis for an historical data framework rather than probability sampling.

SUMMARY AND DISCUSSION

A common theme in this chapter is the extent to which general statements can be substantiated, based on a particular data set subjected to rigorous statistical analysis. Magical remedies that will attain the elusive goal of clear cut generalization are not prescribed. Instead, the scope of generalization that may be possible is given attention and illustrated extensively. Of course, as with most fundamental truths, the bottom line is intuitively obvious: namely, the more generality demanded, the more assumptions required and the less defensible the conclusions; but intuition alone is not sufficient to eliminate the need for a thorough and formal discussion of the matter. The major burden is justifying assumptions rather than securing a larger computer or more software. Little coverage that will help the practitioner has been given to justifying assumptions because emphasis has been on statistical rather than substantive issues. However, the authors are crucially aware of overall priorities and do not intend to imply that statisticians should put on blinkers and merely race around the track under the jockey's whip.

Recognizing the statistical intricacies related to generalization is an important first step, but tangible progress comes only when the statistical analyst understands clearly the startling similarities within what, apparently, is a divergent set of analytical tools. A type of "generalized analysis of variance" can be used in most cases to explore questions of interest. This catch-all phrase would cover all the Q (quadratic form, or χ^2) and QR (quadratic ratio, or F) statistics developed in the more theoretical sections of the paper. The statistical procedures for categorical vs ordinal vs interval data have been developed separately, the analogies between them are not always well understood, and so there is confusion. However, there really is unity underneath it all, which this paper has tried to summarize.

The third major point is the importance of focusing on the question of interest and, in so doing, sharpening the subsequent statistical analysis. Such focus is achieved through identifying narrow alternatives to the broad hypothesis that is under exploration. The statistical test that has power to detect the narrow alternative should be the procedure of choice.

Other issues that have received attention in the chapter may be said to be subsidiary to these three key points. But several secondary issues deserve highlighting. In particular, the distinction between structural and variational models is an important one that is not well-known. The notion of a variational model provides a statistical rationale for the legitimacy of analyzing a historical data set that is not a legitimate sample of any real population but merely an available data set accumulation. Further, the variational approach may be convenient on computational grounds, or the structural may be preferable because of underlying substantive arguments.

A further aspect of this choice of approach is the selection of an additive vs a multiplicative (log linear) model. Here, there is no mathematical decision to make, but one that should be based on subject matter arguments. Additive models have an intuitive appeal and are easy to interpret; the analysis can be carried out in the same units as the measurements were taken. In the absence of a theory specifying a different form, or other considerations, linear models are preferred. In many cases, similar conclusions would be reached regardless of which type of model was chosen (see example 1) and in this case there is no reason to complicate the analysis and interpretation. However, when a multiplicative structure is natural because of the question of interest, log-linear models represent the proper strategy.

On a different note, the homogeneous stratification assumption has been presented with more pomp than is deserved, but the notion is important. In simple language it corresponds to the assumption that all the relevant variables have been measured. Then generalization to a target population that extends the study design can be argued and defended. But, does the analyst know the relevant variables? One can, and should, proceed according to the best knowledge available. That is, after all, how progress has been made throughout history—the opportunity to generalize further should not be refuted solely on the grounds of current limitations. The interplay of methodology and balanced judgment is vitally important in these situations and must be underscored continually.

One final comment is needed to restore some balance that is not present in the chapter. Design should be the essence of a statistician's role in health science endeavors. Unfortunately, study design often gets inadequate professional attention, partly because statisticians tend to operate in a therapeutic mold rather than a preventive one. The well designed study does eliminate many of the problems that would otherwise challenge the ingenuity of the data gymnast. Such gymnastics are needed and play an important role but should not represent the sole priorities of statisticians or even the most important ones. The classroom wisdom of early involvement and careful design should be the two major commandments of statistical practice. Then many of our current controversies regarding interpretation would be resolved because they would have been prevented in advance.

ACKNOWLEDGMENTS

This research was supported in part by the US Bureau of Health Manpower, HRA, through grant number 5–DO4–AH–01649–01, and the US Bureau of the Census through Joint Statistical Agreement JSA 79–16. The authors would like to thank Robert Lehnen and J. Richard Stewart for helpful comments with respect to the preparation of the manuscript. They also would like to express their appreciation to JoAnn DeGraffenreidt, Julie MacMillan, and Bea Parker for their conscientious typing of the manuscript.

Literature Cited

1. Campbell, D. T., Stanley, J. C. 1963. Experimental and quasi-experimental designs for research on teaching. In *Handbook of Research on Teaching,* ed. N. L. Gage, 171–246. Chicago: Rand McNally
2. Hansen, M. H., Hurwitz, W. N., Madow, W. G. 1953. *Sample Survey Methods and Theory.* Vols. I, II. New York: Wiley
3. Hansen, M. H., Hurwitz, W. N., Bershad, M. A. 1961. Measurement errors in censuses and surveys. *Bull. Int. Stat. Inst.* 38(II):359–74
4. Koch, G. G. 1973. An alternative approach to multivariate response error models for sample survey data with applications to estimators involving subclass means. *J. Am. Stat. Assoc.* 68: 906–13
5. Koch, G. G., Freeman, D. H. Jr., Freeman, J. L. 1975. Strategies in the multivariate analysis of data from complex surveys. *Int. Stat. Rev.* 43(1):59–78
6. Wilk, M. B., Kempthorne, O. 1955. Fixed, mixed, and random models in the analysis of variance. *J. Am. Stat. Assoc.* 50:1144–67

7. Koch, G. G., Tolley, H. D. 1975. A generalized modified $-\chi^2$ analysis of categorical data from a complex dilution experiment. *Biometrics* 31(1):59–92
8. Madow, W., Rizvi, H. 1979. On incomplete data: A review. *Proc. ASA Surv. Res. Methods Sect.* In press
9. Rubin, D. G. 1974. Characterizing the estimation of parameters in incomplete data problems. *J. Am. Stat. Assoc.* 69:467–74
10. Hartley, H. O., Hocking, R. R. 1971. The analysis of incomplete data. *Biometrics* 27:783–823
11. Stanish, W. M., Gillings, D. B., Koch, G. G. 1978. An application of multivariate ratio methods for the analysis of a longitudinal clinical trial with missing data. *Biometrics* 34:305–17
12. Cochran, W. G. 1963. *Sampling Techniques.* New York: Wiley. 2nd ed.
13. Kish, L. 1965. *Survey Sampling.* New York: Wiley
14. Federer, W. T. 1955. *Experimental Design.* New York: Macmillan
15. Scheffe, H. 1959. *The Analysis of Variance.* New York: Wiley
16. Winer, B. J. 1971. *Statistical Principles*

in Experimental Design. New York: McGraw-Hill. 2nd ed.

17. Koch, G. G., Amara, I. A., Stokes, M. E., Gillings, D. 1980. Some views on parametric and non-parametric analysis for repeated measurements. *Int. Stat. Rev.* In press

18. Hogg, R. V., Craig, A. T. 1970. *Introduction to Mathematical Statistics.* London: Macmillan. 3rd ed.

19. Cramer, H. 1945. *Mathematical Methods of Statistics.* Princeton: Princeton Univ. Press

20. Suchman, E. A. 1967. *Evaluative Research: Principles and Practice in Public Service & Social Action Programs,* pp. 115–31. New York: Russell Sage Foundation

21. Box, G. E. P., Jenkins, G. M. 1970. *Time Series Analysis.* San Francisco: Holden-Day

22. Theil, H. 1971. *Principles of Econometrics.* New York: Wiley

23. Langbein, L. I., Lichtman, A. J. 1978. *Ecological Inference.* Sage Univ. Pap. Ser. Quant. Appl. Soc. Sci. Beverly Hills & London: Sage Publ.

24. Goldberger, A. S. 1964. *Econometric Theory.* New York: Wiley

25. Lehmann, E. L. 1959. *Testing Statistical Hypotheses.* New York: Wiley

26. Kruskal, W. H., Wallis, W. A. 1953. Use of ranks in one criterion variance analysis. *J. Am. Stat. Assoc.* 46:583–621

27. Puri, M. L., Sen, P. K. 1971. *Nonparametric Methods in Multivariate Analysis.* New York: Wiley

28. Koch, G. G. 1969. Some aspects of the statistical analysis of 'split plot' experiments in completely randomized layouts. *J. Am. Stat. Assoc.* 64:485–505

29. Mantel, N., Haenszel, W. 1959. Statistical aspects of the analysis of data from retrospective studies of disease. *J. Natl. Cancer Inst.* 22:719–48

30. Cochran, W. G. 1954. Some methods for strengthening the common χ^2 test. *Biometrics* 10:417–51

31. Mantel, N. 1963. Chi-square test with one degree of freedom: Extensions of the Mantel-Haenszel procedure. *J. Am. Stat. Assoc.* 58:690–700

32. Landis, J. R., Heyman, E. R., Koch, G. G. 1978. Average partial association in three-way contingency tables: A review and discussion of alternative tests. *Int. Stat. Rev.* 46:237–54

33. Koch, G. G., Bhapkar, V. P. 1980. Chi-square tests. In *Encyclopedia of Statistical Sciences,* ed. N. L. Johnson, S. Kotz. New York: Wiley. In press

34. Wald, A. 1943. Tests of statistical hypotheses concerning several parameters when the number of observations is large. *Trans. Am. Math. Soc.* 54:426–82

35. Grizzle, J. E., Starmer, C. F., Koch, G. G. 1969. Analysis of categorical data by linear models. *Biometrics* 25:489–503

36. Koch, G. G., Landis, J. R., Freeman, J. L., Freeman, D. H., Lehnen, R. G. 1977. A general methodology for the analysis of experiments with repeated measurement of categorical data. *Biometrics* 33:133–58

37. Johnson, W. D., Koch, G. G. 1978. Linear models analysis of competing risks for grouped survival times. *Int. Stat. Rev.* 46:21–51

38. Landis, J. R., Koch, G. G. 1977. The measurement of observer agreement for categorical data. *Biometrics* 33:159–75

39. Landis, J. R., Koch, G. G. 1977. An application of hierarchical kappa-type statistics in the assessment of majority agreement among multiple observers. *Biometrics* 33:363–74

40. Walker, S. H., Duncan, D. B. 1967. Estimation of the probability of an event as a function of several independent variables. *Biometrika* 54:167–79

41. Cox, D. R. 1970. *The Analysis of Binary Data.* London: Methuen

42. Nelder, J. A., Wedderburn, R. W. M. 1972. Generalized linear models. *J. R. Stat. Soc. A* 135(3):370–84

43. Bishop, Y. M. M., Fienberg, S. E., Holland, P. W. 1975. *Discrete Multivariate Analysis.* Cambridge: MIT Press

44. Neyman, J. 1949. Contributions to the theory of the χ^2 test. *Proc. 1st Berkeley Symp. Math. Stat. Probab.,* pp. 239–72

45. Breslow, N. E. 1975. Analysis of survival data under the proportional hazards model. *Int. Stat. Rev.* 43(1):45–58

46. Stewart, J. R. 1975. An analysis of automobile accidents to determine which variables are most strongly associated with driver injury: Relationships between driver injury and vehicle model year. *Univ. North Carolina Hwy Safety Res. Cent. Tech. Rep.*

47. Birch, M. W. 1965. The detection of partial association. II. The general case. *J. R. Stat. Soc. B* 27:111–24

48. Freeman, D. H. Jr., Koch, G. G. 1976. An asymptotic covariance structure for testing hypotheses on raked contingency tables from complex sample surveys. *Proc. ASA Soc. Stat. Sect.* 1976, pp. 330–35

49. Purcell, N. J., Kish, L. 1979. Estimation for small domains. *Biometrics* 35:365–84

50. Breslow, N. E., Day, N. E. 1975. Indirect standardization and multiplicative models for rates, with reference to the age adjustment of cancer incidence and relative frequency data. *J. Chronic Dis.* 28:289–303

51. Berkson, J. 1955. Maximum likelihood and minimum χ^2 estimates of the logistic function. *J. Am. Stat. Assoc.* 50: 130–62

52. Gart, J. J. 1971. The comparison of proportions: A review of significance tests, confidence intervals and adjustments for stratification. *Rev. Int. Stat. Inst.* 39:148–61

53. Thomas, D. G. 1975. Exact and asymptotic methods for the combination of 2X2 tables. *Comp. Biomed. Res.* 8: 423–46

54. Byar, D. P., Simon, R. M., Friedewald, W. T., Schlesselman, J. J., DeMets, D. L., Ellenberg, J. H., Gail, M. H., Ware, J. H. 1976. Randomized clinical trials. *N. Engl. J. Med.* 295:74–80

55. Chalmers, T. C., Block, J. B., Lee, S. 1970. Controlled studies in clinical cancer research. *N. Engl. J. Med.* 287(2): 75–78

56. Gehan, E. A. 1978. Comparative clinical trials with historical controls: a statistician's view. *Biomedicine* 28:13–19

57. Peto, R., Pike, M. C., Armitage, P., Breslow, N. E., Cox, D. R., Howard, S. V., Mantel, N., McPherson, K., Peto, J., Smith, P. G. 1976. Design and analysis of randomized clinical trials requiring prolonged observation of each patient. I. Introduction and design. *Brit. J. Cancer* 34:585–612

58. Martin, C. F., Higgins, J. E. 1976. Byssinosis and other respiratory ailments: A survey of 6631 cotton textile employees. *J. Occup. Med.* 18:455–62

59. Higgins, J. E., Koch, G. G. 1977. Variable selection and generalized chi-square analysis of categorical data applied to a large cross-sectional occupational health survey. *Int. Stat. Rev.* 45:51–62

60. Johnson, W. D., Grizzle, J. E., Postlethwait, R. W. 1970. Veterans Administration cooperative study of surgery for duodenal ulcer. I. Description and evaluation of method of randomization. *Arch. Surg.* 101:391–95

61. Gurland, J., Lee, I., Dahm, P. A. 1960. Polychotomous quantal response in biological assay. *Biometrics* 9:382–98

62. Bock, R. D., Jones, L. V. 1968. *The Measurement and Prediction of Judgment and Choice.* San Francisco: Holden-Day

63. Andrich, D. 1979. A model for contingency tables having an ordered response classification. *Biometrics* 35:403–15

64. Koch, G. G. 1977. The interface between statistical methodology and statistical practice. *Proc. ASA Soc. Stat. Sect.,* 1977, pp. 205–14

65. Koch, G. G., Grizzle, J. E., Semenya, K., Sen, P. K. 1978. Statistical methods for evaluation of mastitis treatment data. *J. Dairy Sci.* 61(6):830–47

66. Peto, R., Pike, M. C., Armitage, P., Breslow, N. E., Cox, D. R., Howard, S. V., Mantel, N., McPherson, K., Petro, J., Smith, P. G. 1977. Design and analysis of randomized clinical trials requiring prolonged observation of each patient. II. Analysis and examples. *Brit. J. Cancer* 35:1–39

67. Gehan, E. A. 1965. A generalized Wilcoxon test for comparing arbitrarily singly censored samples. *Biometrika* 52:203–23

68. Breslow, N. E. 1970. A generalized Kruskal-Wallis test for comparing K samples subject to unequal patterns of censorship. *Biometrika* 57:579–94

69. Brown, B. W. Jr., Hollander, M., Korwar, R. M. 1974. Nonparametric tests of independence for censored data with applications to heart transplant studies. In *Reliability and Biometry, Statistical Analysis of Lifelength,* ed. F. Proschan, R. J. Serfling, pp. 327–54. Philadelphia: SIAM

70. Peto, R., Peto, J. 1972. Asymptotically efficient rank invariant test procedures. *J. R. Stat. Soc. A* 135:185–206

71. Mantel, N. 1966. Evaluation of survival data and two new rank order statistics arising in its consideration. *Cancer Chemother. Rep.* 50:163–70

72. Peto, R., Pike, M. C. 1973. Conservatism of the approximation $\Sigma(O-E)^2/E$ in the logrank test for survival data or tumor incidence data. *Biometrics* 29: 579–83

73. Quade, D. 1967. Rank analysis of covariance. *J. Am. Stat. Assoc.* 62: 1187–200

74. Breslow, N. E. 1974. Covariance analysis of censored survival data. *Biometrics* 30:89–100

75. Cox, D. R. 1972. Regression models and life tables (with discussion). *J. R. Stat. Soc. B* 34:187–220

76. Kalbfleish, J. D., Prentice, R. L. 1973. Marginal likelihoods based on Cox's regression and life model. *Biometrika* 60:267–78

77. Berkson, J., Gage, R. P. 1952. Survival curve for cancer patients following

treatment. *J. Am. Stat. Assoc.* 47: 501–15

78. Cutler, S. J., Ederer, F. 1958. Maximum utilization of the life table method in analyzing survival. *J. Chronic Dis.* 8:699–712

79. Koch, G. G., Johnson, W. D., Tolley, H. D. 1972. A linear models approach to the analysis of survival and extent of disease in multidimensional contingency tables. *J. Am. Stat. Assoc.* 67: 783–96

80. Kaplan, E. L., Meier, P. 1958. Nonparametric estimation from incomplete observations. *J. Am. Stat. Assoc.* 53: 457–81

81. National Center for Health Statistics 1974. Current estimates from the Health Interview Survey 1973. *Vital and Health Statistics.* Ser. 10. No. 95. DHEW Pub. No. (HRA) 75-1522. Rockville, MD: Public Health Service

82. Freeman, D. H. Jr., Freeman, J. L., Brock, D. B., Koch, G. G. 1976. Strategies in the multivariate analysis of data from complex surveys. II. An application to the United States Health Interview Survey. *Int. Stat. Rev.* 44(3): 317–30

83. Freeman, D. H. Jr., Freeman, J. L., Koch, G. G., Brock, D. B. 1976. An analysis of physician visit data from a complex sample survey. *Am. J. Public Health* 66(10):979–83

84. McCarthy, P. J. 1969. Pseudoreplication: Half-samples. *Rev. Int. Stat. Inst.* 37(3):239–64

85. Kish, L., Frankel. M. R. 1970. Balanced repeated replications for standard errors. *J. Am. Stat. Assoc.* 65:1071–94

86. Freeman, D. H. Jr., Brock, D. B. 1977. The role of covariance matrix estimation in the analysis of complex sample survey data. In *Survey Sampling and Measurement,* ed. K. N. Namboodiri, pp. 121–40. New York: Academic

87. Freeman, D. H. Jr. 1977. Modeling prevalence rates based on complex sample survey data. *J. Chronic Dis.* 30: 769–79

88. Makuc, D., Gillings, D. B. 1978. An analysis of complex surveys at two points in time to evaluate health status. Proc. ASA Soc. Stat. Sect., San Diego, 1978, pp. 710–15

Ann. Rev. Public Health 1980. 1:227–53

LONG-TERM CARE: Can Our ❖12508
Society Meet the Needs of Its Elderly?

Robert L. Kane and Rosalie A. Kane

The Rand Corporation, Santa Monica, California 90406

INTRODUCTION

This chapter addresses our society's response to the need to provide long-term care (LTC) to the elderly. Such an analysis reveals a great deal about social values in the United States. For this purpose, we define long-term care as physical care over a prolonged period for those incapable of sustaining themselves without this care. We have further restricted our attention to the elderly, thus shifting the focus of analysis away from the more than 400,000 chronically ill and disabled children and young adults in this country (1). In drawing these boundaries, we do not imply that the elderly are the only group needing attention, but that the aged represent a group at particularly high risk of needing LTC.

The Target Population

Because population projections suggest that an increasing proportion of future societies will be elderly, growing attention has been focused on the role of the nursing home. This chapter traces the growth of nursing homes, examines their characteristics, and explores some of the developments that have been suggested to replace the institution as an important component in the care of the elderly.

Although many factors contribute to the rapid growth of nursing homes in this country, the single greatest factor is the aging of our population. Some modest gains in lifespan in the face of a decreasing birth rate have resulted in a rise in the proportion of the population that is 65 years and older from 4% at the turn of the century to almost 11% today. Demographers predict that this proportion will reach 20% by the year 2030. Within the over 65 cohort, the growth spurt has been even more accelerated for

0163-7525/80/0510-0227$01.00

those considered old-old (over 75) (2). This subset is more prone to debilitating illness, less likely to have the necessary social and economic resources to sustain independent living and, therefore, most likely to need nursing home care. About one person in four over age 65 will spend some time in a nursing home (3), and an individual's chances of being admitted to a nursing home increase with age. Currently, about 1.5% of those 65 to 74 years old are living in nursing homes, whereas 10% of those over 75 are nursing home residents.

Is LTC a Medical or Social Program?

Discussions about the role of the nursing home in American society inevitably lead to debates about whether LTC is (or should be) a medical or social program. Current policy reflects use of a medical approach to meet a social need. The breakdown of funding sources for elderly nursing home patients is indicative of the unnatural fit between a social problem and a medical solution. Medicare, the medical insurance program for senior citizens, covers only short, posthospital stays keyed to episodes of illness. Medicare funding covers about 3% of the total money expended on nursing homes in the United States. In contrast, Medicaid, a means-tested medical welfare program, accounts for almost 50% of total nursing home expenditures. Long-term patients are eventually funded by Medicaid when Medicare benefits or private resources are exhausted. Physician care for those over 65 continues to be covered by Medicare, but nursing home care (consisting largely of social services such as housing, homemaking, personal care, and recreation) is construed as a "medical" benefit of the welfare system. Vital social services are thus provided through dollars earmarked as medical.

The general exclusion of the bulk of nonphysician LTC services from Medicare coverage suggests that they are not viewed as strictly within the medical domain. Rather, when an individual's social resources are no longer adequate, medical need has been used as an indicator of eligibility for public assistance (Medicaid). In keeping with this focus, concerns are frequently voiced about the dangers of destroying family responsibility through excessively generous public programs. No evidence is available to suggest that this is the case and several studies suggest that families continue to provide care until demands are excessive (4).

The current proposals advocating a broader array of LTC services to provide alternatives to the nursing home have roots in a long history of ambivalence about the most appropriate means to deliver social welfare services. Thomas (5) describes a periodic swing from indoor (i.e. institutional) to outdoor (i.e. community-based) relief. The relatively recent move to empty the state mental hospitals by transferring patients to the aegis of community mental health centers may be viewed as a part of this movement

(6). Ironically, in that instance, the nursing home was conveniently viewed as a community resource, but it is viewed as an institution when the discussion turns to such programs as home care and day care.

THE NURSING HOME

Historical Development

The nursing home is essentially a post-Depression phenomenon. Although it is possible to trace its ancestry to the almshouses of the Elizabethan Poor Law, for all practical purposes it is a by-product of the Social Security Act and has continued to be shaped by subsequent reforms of that act. The provision of pension funds allowed the purchase of services; the later provision of vendor payments stimulated the growth of the nursing home industry and the accompanying rules and regulations dictated the form of the nursing home.

Dunlop (7) has described the growth of nursing homes over the decade from 1963 to 1973, with the initiative of the Medicare and Medicaid programs as approximate midpoints. He notes that the greatest rate of expansion occurred prior to the implementation of these laws. From 1963 through 1966, the number of nursing home beds per 100 elderly (65 years and over) increased at an annual rate of 8.7%. From 1967 through 1970, the rate was 3.6%; and for 1971 through 1973 it was 6.1%.

This growth in numbers of nursing home beds over the decade represented an overall increase of 117%—from 510,180 to 1,107,358. Thus, by 1974 there were more nursing home beds than acute general hospital beds in this country, and a larger proportion of the former were occupied.

The expansion of the nursing home industry is reflected in the outlay for this type of care. Not only did the dollar volume of such care increase more rapidly than the bed numbers, but the major source of those dollars shifted from the private to the public purse. Figure 1 traces the shift in national nursing home expenditures from 1960 through 1976. Two trends are important to note. First, public expenditures exceeded private expenditures for several years just after the passage of Medicare and Medicaid and have again consistently done so since 1974. Second, with the passage of these laws, the majority of public dollars spent on nursing home care is federal.

As noted earlier, the growth spurt in nursing homes antedated Medicare and Medicaid. Earlier amendments to the Social Security Act provided for vendor payments for nursing home care for portions of the population eligible for welfare and in some states for those deemed medically indigent or unable to bear the medical costs of illness. However, the Medicaid and Medicare programs, particularly the former, have played a major role in shaping the nursing home as we know it today. Through a series of regula-

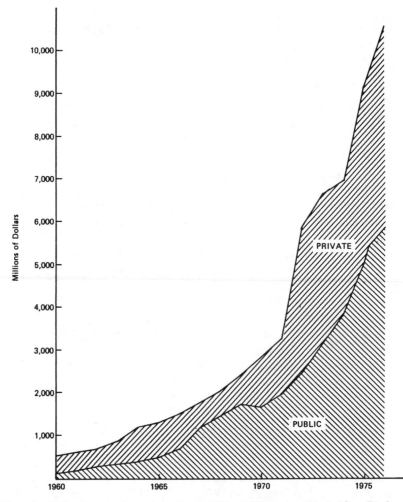

Figure 1   National nursing home expenditures, 1960 to 1976. Source: Adapted from Dunlop
(7) Table 2–3, p. 11.

tions, these programs gradually transformed the model nursing home from
a small family-run, home-based operation of a few beds into a more professionally staffed institution of about 75 to 100 beds designed to meet a variety
of life safety regulations.

A more recent development is the growth of small and large nursing
home chains, as well as the advent of franchised nursing home management
services. This latter phenomenon has, in turn, accelerated development of
a new career line for nursing home managers. Patterns of nursing home

ownership and management are elusive to pin down statistically, not only because shifts are occurring, but also because the information itself is difficult to obtain (8).

Description of the Nursing Home

Although they cover only about half of the patients in nursing homes at any one time, Medicare and Medicaid exert a profound influence through the standards their regulations mandate. To some observers, their effect has been to move the nursing homes toward increasingly resembling miniature hospitals. Many of the current problems related to defining the role of the nursing home in the LTC continuum can be traced to its ambivalent position as a second-class hospital that performs both a medical and a social function.

Table 1 presents some comparative data on the several types of nursing homes. Several points can be emphasized:

1. Nursing homes are generally small operations; the average size is around 75 beds.

Table 1 Selected data on nursing homes by Medicare and Medicaid certification status[a]

		Certification status			
		Both Medicaid and Medicare[b]	Medicaid only		
	Total		SNHs[c]	ICFs[d]	Not certified
All homes (%)	100.0	26.5	26.5	22.4	23.1
Average bed size	75.0	105.0	92.0	57.0	45.0
Percentage Proprietary	76.0	78.0	72.0	79.0	73.0
Average total FTE employees					
per 100 beds	66.3	72.3	68.7	57.5	58.5
Nursing staff	41.4	46.1	42.9	35.8	33.6
RN	4.9	6.5	5.2	2.4	3.7
LPN	5.8	6.4	6.5	4.9	4.2
AID	30.7	33.2	31.2	28.5	25.7
Average occupancy rate (%)	88.2	85.6	89.2	89.2	89.0
Average total monthly charge ($)	479.0	592.0	484.0	376.0	329.0
Median length of stay (yrs)	1.5	1.1	1.7	1.9	2.1

[a] Source: US National Center for Health Statistics, Ser. 13, No. 22, 28, 32 [see ref. (10) for publishing information].

[b] Extended care facilities. This term was used to define facilities "for patients who require skilled nursing and rehabilitation services on a daily basis to help them achieve their optimal level of functioning." Of these homes, 8% were certified by Medicare only.

[c] Skilled nursing homes. This was the Medicaid equivalent of the ECF. SNH and ECF were subsequently merged into a single category, skilled nursing facility (SNF), when Medicare and Medicaid regulations were combined. Of these homes, 35% were certified as both SNFs and ICFs.

[d] Intermediate care facilities, defined as a facility that provides health-related care and services to those who do not need SNF care, an admittedly imprecise definition.

2. Nursing homes are primarily operated under proprietary auspices; about 75% of the homes and 70% of the beds are operated for profit.
3. Nursing homes are not heavily staffed. In all, there is about two thirds of a full-time equivalent person per bed. About two thirds of the staff are nursing personnel.
4. Nursing homes are generally full; over 70% have waiting lists.

These data are based on a national sample. Statistics vary considerably according to geographical location. For example, the breakdown of total nursing home beds per 1000 people age 65 and older ranges from a high of 105 in Minnesota and Wisconsin to a low of under 30 in West Virginia and Florida. Instructively, the occupancy rate is uniformly high, whatever the availability of beds.

The nursing home and the general hospital differ markedly. The latter tends to be larger (in the range of 160 beds), with more personnel (about 250 per 100 beds), and has more advanced technological equipment. Only about 15% of general hospitals are proprietary. Hospital staff are highly professionalized with a hierarchy including physicians and individuals with advanced education in many fields in contrast to nursing homes, which generally are staffed by nursing assistants with some RN supervision. Length of hospital stay is expressed in terms of days rather than months or years. The spectrum of problems treated is shifted toward the more acute. The costs of a single hospital day approach the average monthly nursing home charge. Given these differences, one might be wary about imposing a set of hospital-derived values onto the nursing home.

Although some data on nursing homes are available from national surveys, primarily those conducted by the National Center for Health Statistics (NCHS), much remains unknown. For example, although there is consensus that the nursing home industry has moved increasingly toward chain operations, no precise figures are available as to what proportion of homes or beds are operated by such chains. The best estimate puts the figure at about 35% of beds (9).

Residents

The residents of nursing homes are most easily categorized by their age. Three quarters of the residents are over age 75. About 70% of the residents are female and 75% are 75 and over. From the perspective of the general population, about 5 people per 1000 are in nursing homes, but the proportion rises sharply with age over 65. The data in Table 2 demonstrate, however, that the nursing home residents do not reflect the general US population over age 65. Nursing home residents are more likely to be female, over age 75, white, widowed, or never married.

Table 2 Number and percentage of nursing home residents 65 years and over, August 1973–April 1974, compared with the noninstitutionalized population of the United States 65 years and over in March 1974 by selected characteristics[a]

Characteristic	Nursing home residents 65 years and over	Noninstitutionalized US population 65 years and over
	Number	
Total 65 years and over	961,500	20,602,000
	Percentage	
Total	100.0	100.0
Sex		
Male	27.6	41.4
Female	72.4	58.6
Race/ethnicity		
White	94.8	91.0
All other races	5.2	9.0
Marital status		
Married	12.2	54.3
Widowed	69.4	36.7
Divorced or separated	3.4	3.5
Never married	15.0	5.6
Age		
65–74 years old	17.0	63.5
76 years and over	83.0	36.5

[a] Source: US National Center for Health Statistics Series 13, No. 27.

About 40% of patients enter the nursing home directly from their residences. Another 35% come from general hospitals. The rest come primarily from other institutions like mental hospitals or long-term care specialty hospitals (8%), other nursing homes (14%), or boarding homes (2%).

The nursing home is the repository of the chronically ill. Patients frequently suffer from multiple conditions. Mental illness remains the most prevalent diagnosis. Among the elderly it is called senility (a term lacking in precision and lending itself to judgmental inclusions). Among the young, mental illness and mental retardation are the most common diagnoses. The other major problems affecting one of every three residents are those associated with age: heart disease and arthritis. The prevalence of chronic impairments is accompanied by functional limitations. According to the 1973–1974 national nursing home survey conducted by NCHS, 32% of nursing home patients could not hear a telephone conversation; 46% could not read ordinary newsprint; 28% had lost bowel and bladder control; 51%

had problems with mobility; 31% were either chair-bound or bedridden (10). More than one of these functional limitations commonly occurred in a single individual.

PAYING FOR NURSING HOME CARE

The costs of nursing homes are related to the amount of nursing care and other services given. These costs have increased more than the rate of medical inflation. Using constant 1964 dollars, costs rose almost 40% between 1964 and 1969 and another 15% in the subsequent five-year period.

Although the individual monthly costs of nursing home care are much less than hospital care, the long lengths of stay and the large numbers of residents make the overall costs of nursing homes expensive. Not only are the dollars involved substantial, but the care they purchase is questionable. The investigations into the financing and management of nursing homes in New York State, which were spurred by accusations of fraud and abuse, revealed a distressing state of affairs.

Payment for nursing home care under Medicaid was originally calculated as a fixed per diem cost that varied according to the level and intensity of nursing care, i.e. a patient classified as needing skilled nursing care was paid for at a higher rate than one deemed in need of only intermediate care. However, such a system was viewed as lacking incentives for better quality of care and a more variable approach was inaugurated. As in other areas of nursing home care, the hospital model was adopted. The 1972 amendments to the Social Security Act required that, by July of 1976, states reimburse nursing homes on the basis of reasonable costs. Although this date has long passed, no guidelines have been released defining what is a "cost" and what is "reasonable."

The crux of the issue in defining "reasonable costs" is the degree to which homes should be permitted to make a profit. Because the nursing home industry is primarily proprietary, incentives for investment and services are an important prerequisite for improving the level of care. The difficulty is in calculating the proper base for profits; a controversial issue is whether this should include capital equity as well as current costs (11).

Some costs incurred by nursing homes are fixed and others vary with the intensity of service and occupancy. At the simplest level, these include the general costs of room, board and maintenance, nursing care, other therapies, and medical care. Each may be expected to yield a different rate of return for investors.

A few innovative reimbursement proposals have been put forward to create climates conducive to nursing care. Ruchlin et al (12) proposed a prospective incentive reimbursement scheme in which facilities would be grouped into homogeneous peer categories and paid a mean per diem rate based on four factors: (*a*) dollar ceiling for the peer group, (*b*) occupancy rate, (*c*) health status of patients, and (*d*) facility evaluation. Reimbursement above a fixed range (based on the group mean) would be made only upon documentation that those additional funds were required for quality-related services. Operating surplus for fully compliant homes would be partially distributed to the owners and employees and partially used to purchase capital expansion rights.

Another proposal for achieving quality care at the appropriate level is to hold nursing homes responsible for the provision of minimum custodial care only and to permit residents to purchase all other services on the open market (13). Such a system would, according to its advocates, end placement at an inappropriate level and would have the added psychological benefit of permitting the resident to control his medical care and to make more of his own decisions. The nursing home would become a more home-like environment under these conditions. As a theoretical model this is attractive, but there are many potential problems that would need to be addressed in pilot tests of the plan. How is custodial care to be defined beyond hotel services? If it includes necessary bedside nursing, would a multilevel system again become necessary, or would the patient also purchase intensive nursing services on the open market? Will the services even be available on the open market? And, perhaps most crucial, what safeguards should be developed to protect those residents who do not have the capacity to exercise their purchasing power and who do not have family as guardians? A rather complex administrative system with guardianship mechanisms would surely be necessary.

Kane has proposed a model whereby nursing homes would be paid in proportion to the degree that their patients achieved good outcomes (14). Each patient's outcome would be compared against an individualized prognosis generated from data collected by independent reviewers. Payment would be based on average costs for that class of patient multiplied by a prognostic adjustment factor (PAF). When a patient did better than expected, the PAF would be greater than one; when the outcome was worse than expected, the PAF would be less than one. Such a system is compatible with both prospective and retrospective reimbursement procedures. Its major virtue is its focus on the results of care, thereby minimizing the need for rules and regulations.

QUALITY OF NURSING HOME CARE

Medical Care

Nursing homes are not the favorite haunts of physicians. In one study, only 14% of the active physicians in a metropolitan area participated in nursing home care (15). Closer scrutiny of the care that is provided offers little solace (16). A review of the medical records of nursing home patients in a metropolitan area revealed a substantial number of charts with no evidence of a new observation or a physical examination for six months or more (17).

The doctors' indifference to nursing home care is hardly surprising. Few medical schools offer training in geriatrics (18), and the medical model of seeking definitive treatment is unlikely to find satisfactory application among the pool of patients with multiple chronic problems.

Other disciplines may be more appropriate as primary care givers to nursing home patients. The growth of the nurse practitioner movement offers an attractive alternative to sole reliance on physicians. The philosophy of the nursing profession places more emphasis on caring rather than curing and its traditions encourage nurses to work more comfortably with nursing home staffs to upgrade their skills. The geriatric nurse practitioners would thus appear to provide one solution to the problem of improving the medical care provided to nursing home patients (19).

One demonstration project using a team of geriatric nurse practitioner and social worker provided cause for enthusiasm. The care rendered by the team (supported by physician and clinical pharmacist consultants) was not only better care, by all accounts, but was also cost effective. The savings in other care costs were greater than the entire costs of fielding the team (20).

More recently the utility of the geriatric nurse practitioner, working under telephone supervision of the physician, was again demonstrated. Patients cared for under such a system did as well as or better than a group of control patients (21).

Approaches to Quality of Care Assessment

As we have already noted, the entrance of organized federal programs into LTC has been accompanied by a long series of regulations designed to improve the quality of such institutions. Concern about quality, as reflected in these regulations, has focused on three major areas: (a) the physical features of the plant, (b) the appropriateness of utilization and charges, and (c) the quality of the care itself.

The first concern, the physical structure of the facility, is usually addressed in terms of life safety codes. Scandals about nursing home fires led to a series of increasingly stringent requirements about sprinkler systems, fire doors, corridor widths, fire escapes, and similar concerns. As the cost of upgrading or replacing facilities that had been converted from private homes grew larger, more and more smaller operations closed down to be replaced by purpose-built facilities that resembled hospitals more than homes.

Various statistics have been cited about the extent of inappropriate nursing home use. The Congressional Budget Office (22) has summarized these accounts of inappropriate placement and found a wide range of figures, from 8 to 76% of patients inappropriately placed. Most of these reports depend on the implicit judgments of professionals (usually nurses) as to whether the patient could be equally or better cared for at a less intensive level of care (i.e. intermediate instead of skilled) or by some other means altogether (e.g. home care, day care, or sheltered housing).

Two elements characterize most exploration of the appropriateness of nursing home utilization. First, the majority of discussions are based on implicit judgments without explicit criteria. Second, they presuppose the availability of the alternative forms of care. A convincing set of data suggesting that a majority of nursing home patients could, in fact, do well in some alternative care source currently available has not yet been produced.

Most efforts to review the quality of nursing home care have focused on the structural aspects of such care. The number and type of staff, the condition of the medical records, or the diversity of available services have often been used as proxies for quality of care. As might be expected, for both proprietary and nonprofit facilities, the presence of positive structural attributes is strongly related to the availability of funds as reflected in high daily rates and a lower proportion of welfare clients (23–25). No differences can be shown between the proprietary and nonprofit institutions.

Processes and Outcomes of Care

Fewer models are available to measure quality in the direct processes of nursing home care. One popular approach has been to adopt the medical care evaluation study approach and perform retrospective audits of the management of given problems (26, 27). Other attempts to measure the process of care have relied on a series of checklists of items that should have been performed at certain points in the care process. Deficiency rates are calculated and compared across facilities or across time (28, 29). Both of these approaches have been handicapped by the lack of clearly identifiable standards for care based on knowledge of the link between process and outcome. Reliance on "norms of practice" for development of process criteria would lead to very low standards indeed.

A recent review of the effects of ten Professional Standards Review Organizations (PSROs) to evaluate the quality of nursing home care illustrates the diversity of approaches that might be used (30). Although the emphasis of the PSROs was on measuring the process of care, several different tacks were taken.

One area that appears particularly promising is the attention to the use of drugs among those in nursing homes. Not only do nursing home patients receive a large number of drugs (an average of six) (31), but they are particularly vulnerable to overprescription of psychoactive drugs. A review of drug regimens for nursing home patients thus uncovers multiple deficiencies (32).

In only rare instances has anyone tried to look at changes in patients over time to make any observations that might describe the outcomes of nursing home care. Particularly in an area like nursing home care, in which the relationship between what is done for and what happens to patients is so poorly delineated, outcome assessments are critical.

Gottesman & Bourestom used measures of patient behavior, activities of daily living (ADL), and mental status as outcome measures (33). As with process measures, the occurrence of positive traits was associated with the proportion of private patients and other indicators of more affluent patients. Linn and her colleagues were able to show a relationship between the functional status of patients and such structural measures as RN nursing hours per patient and monthly charges (34). Chekryn & Roos could not demonstrate a relationship between changes in levels of ADL, mental status, life satisfaction, and process of care measures (28). Using a set of utilization review data as a basis for secondary analysis, Kane and his colleagues could show very little change in patient status over time along a number of different dimensions (35).

Quality of Care versus Quality of Life

We have already noted the recurrent confusion surrounding the nursing home's place in society. It is at once the stepchild of the hospital and cousin of the almshouse. This mixed heritage is seen in the difficulties that surround the measurement of quality in long-term care. To the extent that they have been made explicit, such concepts seem to extrapolate from earlier work in medical care. Both the form and the substance harken back to hospital-based procedures. Yet, as we have already noted, the nursing home is quite a different environment, with very different conditions and perhaps different goals. It is more appropriate to talk about quality of life than only about quality of care and, in so doing, to recognize that many of the features of concern may relate to the negative effects of institutionalization.

Although we may be willing to subordinate certain personal needs to avail ourselves of anticipated benefits in the acute care hospital for a finite brief period, it is far less tolerable to accept such sacrifices of personal independence over a longer period, especially when no compensatory benefits are expected. Thus, the fuller definition of health with its emphasis on social and mental status is particularly appropriate to discussions about the quality of life in the nursing home.

Measuring Quality of Life

We have already seen that quality of care is difficult to achieve and to measure; quality of life is an even more elusive commodity, dependent as it is on individual preferences and limited as it may be by individual health, regardless of residence in a nursing home. Insofar as it has been possible to relate particular nursing home settings to the quality of the residents' lives, it seems that positive ratings may also be independent of highly competent technical care. In some ways, in fact, medical technology may produce a well-ordered, hospital-style environment that is more unattractive for a long-term resident.

Few persons perceive nursing home admission as a positive event. Dread and despair are the reactions among the prospective client population. Because of the negative connotations of a nursing home, difficulties arise in determining the facility's own part in providing a high quality of life for residents.

More is known about what is wrong with life in a nursing home than how a program may go about remedying the situation. Books by nursing home residents (36, 37) or by participant observers in long-term care institutions (38) cite the loss of personal freedoms inherent in the role and the extreme difficulty residents may encounter in completing simple actions such as making a telephone call. The former identity of the nursing home residents tends to become subsumed under the classification "patient."

Brody cataloged what she called the "iatrogenic diseases of institutional life" as follows:

Dependency; depersonalization; low self-esteem, lack of occupation or fruitful use of time; geographic and social distance from family and friends and cultural milieu; inflexibility of routines and menus; loneliness; lack of privacy, identity, own clothing, possessions, and furniture; lack of freedom; desexualization and infantalization; crowded conditions; and negative, disrespectful or belittling staff attitudes (39).

It is with such criteria that quality of life can be measured. Some of the items, such as inflexibility of routines and menus, lack of privacy, and negative staff attitudes may be directly attributable to institutional life whereas others such as loneliness, geographic distance from family and friends may also characterize the lives of many elderly persons outside the nursing homes. Little systematic information exists to compare quality of life inside and outside nursing homes and there are no before-after studies to show in what ways the quality of particular patients' lives deteriorates upon admission to a nursing home.

The nursing home has sometimes been called a decision-free environment for its residents. This quality has taken on an extremely ominous note because of our current understanding of the phenomenon that has been called "learned helplessness" (40). According to this theory, when an individual perceives that his actions no longer elicit responses, a syndrome develops characterized by (a) depression, (b) cessation of efforts to influence events, and (c) inability to distinguish when one's actions have actually elicited a response. Learned helplessness has been documented in nursing home residents and a number of field studies (41–43) have shown that startling changes may take place in both affective state and levels of activity when small changes are made that increase actual or perceived control among nursing home residents.

Because individual control is an important dimension affecting the quality of a nursing home resident's life, information is needed about the preferences of particular groups of elderly persons and about which patients fare best under what kinds of conditions. Insufficient data are available, partly because controlled clinical trials of nursing home conditions raise ethical questions and partly because, in many areas, beds are limited and few choices of placement are possible. Given the lack of patient choice, it is impossible to study nursing home preferences by observing movement of patients from facilities with which they are dissatisfied to other facilities. There is some evidence to suggest, however, that the widely known negative effects of relocation of nursing home patients does not occur when the patient himself has requested transfer and is prepared for the move (44).

Fragmentary findings exist to suggest conditions that may be desirable in nursing homes from a quality of life standpoint. Jorgensen & Kane found that patients were most willing to accept nursing home placement if some continuation of their previous lifestyle were possible (45). Silverstone & Wynter discovered that a change to heterosexual living space improved adjustment to nursing home and social behavior in male residents (46). Abdo et al found that the factors most associated with negative adjustment to nursing homes in a group of 20 women were lack of privacy, lack of independence, and distance from families and friends (47). Schoenfield & Hooper made a comparison of institutionalized elderly, finding an association between future commitments (measured by number of planned appointments in the week ahead) and successful aging (48); those in nursing homes tended to have fewer future commitments. Jones hypothesized that crowded conditions caused interpersonal conflict and that friendships tended to be formed, not with people in the same room, but with people several doors away (49). Some of these findings are consistent with the impressions that emerged from nursing homes abroad that homogeneous populations regarding ethnicity and culture, single rooms, separation of the mentally alert from the disorganized, and opportunity to pursue former interests are associated with a quality nursing home environment (50). Studies such as those cited above, however, are not very useful for forming guidelines to assess the quality of life because they are isolated pieces of work that have not generally been repeated and do not form a coherent knowledge base.

MEDICAL VERSUS SOCIAL MODEL

We have not resolved the question of eminent domain. The issue of predominance between the medical and social models for long-term care is not merely a battle for bureaucratic supremacy between two factions of government; it is a fundamental clash of beliefs in the style of life to be pursued and the appropriate manner of its pursuit. This conflict of credos involves questions of both ends and means—the goals and expectations generated by different perspectives and the paths deemed most approachable to reach them. Under the growing pressure of enforced fiscal austerity, a choice is increasingly necessary, and providers and consumers cannot tolerate the ambiguity resulting from assigning equal weight to both approaches.

The social model is attractive because it emphasizes that health care, albeit crucial, is just one of many services needed to raise the quality of life of the aged. Especially with an elderly population, the often dwindling benefits of heroic medical measures must be balanced against the heavy social and psychological costs. Morbidity and disability are conditions of life for the majority of aged people. A medical model allows the conditions to define a range of life circumstances. The very permanence and intractability of these problems argue for societal provisions to protect the elderly from a permanent patient role for decades before their death.

This question of medical versus social model is not merely an issue for academic speculation. It is a primary discussion point for social policy. The current transition in responsibility for enforcing federal regulations around quality of care from Medicare fiscal intermediaries and state officials to PSROs illustrates vividly the dilemma raised by the lack of resolution of the social-medical jurisdictional boundaries.

To the extent that admission to nursing homes is based on the concept of medical necessity, a substantial number of admissions are not necessary. Certainly individuals with equivalent degrees of incapacity are functioning in the community or with lesser amounts of supportive services. (It is estimated that, for every individual in a nursing home, there are at least two equally impaired persons living in the community.)

We have already noted that the nursing home resident has a rather distinct set of social and demographic characteristics. Typically, she is without social resources. The extent of her dependency on the nursing home is the product of her afflictions applied to a weakened host. The familiar public health model with its eternal triangle of host, agent, and environment applies here. From a public health perspective, the separation of social and medical models is an artificial distinction. But in the context of contemporary social policy, the medical route is the means by which social benefits can be extended to a subgroup of the elderly. For this reason, discussions of national health insurance have tended to avoid any mention of long-term care.

ALTERNATIVE FORMS OF LONG-TERM CARE

In the United States we share a common problem with those nations (predominantely in western Europe) in which LTC systems are better developed than ours (50). Our mutual social policy concern is the rising cost of such care. Interest in seeking alternatives to institutional care for the elderly is worldwide.

The enthusiasm for seeking alternatives has created a good deal of confusion (51). The term "alternative" is an imprecise rallying cry; those who gather under its banner imbue the term with different shades of meaning depending on their own goals and reasons for dissatisfaction with the status quo. Some proponents are seeking a source of care to substitute for the institution so that a patient destined to become one of the 5% of institutional residents might be diverted elsewhere. Others have focused on the current population of nursing home residents, deriving estimates of how many might be cared for under alternative auspices. A third group champions a preventive approach, arguing that an investment in various forms of care for the elderly can prevent institutionalization in the future; here there is lack of clarity between the goal of prevention and that of postponement of admission to an institution. Depending on one's definition of the concept "alternative," one may view the nursing home as an organization that should be phased out as soon as possible or as one that should be strengthened as a rehabilitation center facilitating return to the community.

The problem, then, is one of identifying appropriate populations at risk, the strategies that might improve their conditions (or at least minimize the rate of deterioration), and the costs of such approaches. Crucial to this process is measurement of the health and social status of the various elderly populations at risk; without this ability, it is impossible to specify the advantages or disadvantages of various alternatives in terms of their anticipated effects on the service recipients. Definition of anticipated benefits must also differentiate between long-run and short-run benefits—some alternatives may need to be put into place years before their expected benefit in terms of preventing institutional placement, e.g. preretirement counseling. It is always methodologically difficult to demonstrate the effectiveness of the preventive dollar or to make confident decisions about preventive expenditures given future uncertainties.

Costs of Alternatives

In assessing the costs of various alternative strategies, we must apply epidemiological techniques to insure that we are comparing equivalent groups and assessing the relative benefits of alternative approaches. If, for example, alternatives to nursing home care are most useful for those who have a home in the community and if it were found that nursing homes most often serve those who do not at the time of admission have a home in the community, discussions of the comparative effectiveness of the two modalities would be severely compromised. Similarly, any cost effectiveness analysis must consider the full range of the costs of the alternative, including the costs of services provided by family and friends as well as the basic cost of living (52). For these reasons, inappropriate comparisons are often made between institutional care and its alternatives (22).

One major concern about developing additional LTC resources is that they will become supplements rather than replacements. A set of alternatives designed to reduce the proportion of individuals requiring institutionalization would be targeted toward the group in greatest need, but would also have great appeal for those currently functioning with minimal or no support. Providers would be especially attracted to this latter group because they are likely to make fewer demands and to show better results. The provision of increased services could thus lead directly to increased dependency. The likelihood of such an event will depend heavily on our ability to establish appropriate eligibility requirements for such programs. These entrance-monitoring techniques will, in turn, depend heavily on the philosophic orientation of the program, i.e. whether they are viewed as preventive alternatives, substitutive alternatives, or institutionalization alternatives. The degree of utilization of these new programs will depend upon the social and economic incentives that are developed for and within them.

Provision of additional noninstitutional services cannot be expected to have impact on the total amount of nursing home services rendered unless such programs are carefully tailored to meet the needs of an equivalent target group; as stated above, each alternative program will necessarily serve clientele with legitimate needs but without immediate likelihood of entering a nursing home.

Deinstitutionalization

The recent implementation of a deinstitutionalization program in state mental hospitals illustrates the potential problems in efforts to substitute one service delivery system for another. The policy of returning chronic mental hospital patients to the community began in the 1960s and was accompanied by a program of community mental health center development; the latter was expected to meet the direct care needs of the former mental hospital patient. In fact, deinstitutionalization did not lead to better care for the majority of those involved (53, 54) and the newly established mental health centers ultimately emphasized a different clientele for their services. The "deinstitutionalized," who were placed in nursing homes, boarding homes, and single room occupancy hotels, did not find the "community" a hospitable or receptive environment. Although the follow-up information (much of which is sketchy because many state hospitals kept no records of their deinstitutionalized patients) shows that the former state hospital patients were generally almost bereft of services; the new policy direction did not result in less money being spent on mental health services as a whole. A promising reform of the 1960s thus created a problem for the 1970s.

The experience of the mental hospitals in implementing deinstitutionalization makes one cautious of plunging into similar initiatives for current nursing home patients (some of whom are these same former state hospital patients). Several studies have suggested that patients currently placed in nursing homes could be cared for under other auspices (22, 55); however, this is not equivalent to saying that, once in the nursing home, patients may be returned to the community. The ability to leave an institution and return to the community depends on the quality of the institution and its ability to prevent "institutionalization," as well as the availability of appropriate support systems. We have already indicated that avenues of return to the community are often cut off at the time of nursing home admission.

Targeting the Alternatives

Any policy to reduce or change patterns of nursing home care must be based on recognition of the heterogeneous population now found there. For example, the following groups should be considered: the terminally ill patient; the patient needing short-term convalescent care (e.g. for a fracture); the patient who could benefit from intensive rehabilitation procedures; the patient requiring intensive, skilled nursing care; the mentally ill patient; the developmentally disabled; the patient with social needs for shelter and homemaking services who may or may not have additional physical problems; the partially disoriented; or the completely disoriented who may be ambulatory and require supervision. Extremely disparate patients may presently be housed in the same facility, thus making less likely the provision of specialized services to any subgroup. If such patients were to be relocated in the community, clusters of alternative services would be needed to meet the particular needs of the subgroup. Conceivably, too, some subgroups might be better cared for in a modified institutional setting tailored to meet their particular needs.

Table 3 illustrates how the needs of the various target groups currently in the nursing home might be met by different kinds of programs as alternatives. Neither the list of target problems nor the proposed solutions are definitive or exhaustive. Rather the table is provided to illustrate an approach to the problem and to demonstrate the range of services that could

Table 3 Relationship between target groups and possible alternatives

Target group now in nursing home	Community alternatives		Institutional back-up requirement
	Intermediate	Long-range	
Terminally ill	Home health Home hospice Homemaking Counseling	Narcotic law reform	Possibly a hospice
Those who might benefit from rehabilitation	Home health Day hospital		Rehabilitation hospital
Those requiring skilled nursing care	Home health Day hospital Meals-on-wheels Homemaking	Personal care attendant policy	Possibility of acute hospital care when needed
Those who are mentally ill	Halfway house Day hospital Sheltered workshops Day care	Bereavement counseling Identification of high risk groups	Possible need for acute hospital care
Those with social needs and minimal health problems— the frail very old	Sheltered housing Day care Social programming Senior centers Primary health care	Preretirement counseling Reeducation Changed income transfer progs. Employment progs.	Old-age home
The completely disoriented— ambulatory, but needing constant supervision	Foster care		Possibility better services can be provided through institutions

be considered part of the alternative package including home health, sheltered housing, hospice, and foster care. Depending on the target group to be served, alternative clusters of services can be readily conceptualized. The list of target groups is not composed of mutually exclusive categories and some individuals may fit several descriptions.

The far right column refers to the kind of institutional support system that might be needed to maintain the particular group in the community. For example, effective skilled nursing provided at home requires availability of acute hospital beds when needed. In some instances, the ideal institutional alternative may be the plan of choice. Intensive rehabilitation services might be managed on a day-hospital basis (although transportation can create a major obstacle) but some portion of that care might best be provided on an in-patient basis. Similarly, although there are some promising trials of foster care plans for the elderly, perhaps the quality of life of the very disoriented person could best be protected in planned sheltered institutional communities for that group.

This discussion necessarily takes on a hypothetical tone because most of the alternatives mentioned have such limited availability in the United States. In particular, sheltered housing (independent dwelling units with some housekeeping and/or meal services and with an emergency call button system) is popular in Europe, but in its early development stage here. We do not have the range of institutional back-up services in place, either. For instance, old age residential homes, as opposed to nursing homes, are available only on a very limited basis in this country, usually under sectarian auspices.

Research on Alternatives

Several research programs have provided fragmentary evidence about alternatives. In one of the elegant trials conducted to date, Katz and his colleagues conducted a controlled trial of continuous, coordinated home nursing care (56). Comparing an experimental group who received this more intensive service with a control group receiving traditional services, these investigators identified several distinct patterns. The less disabled and the less severely ill showed greater physical and psychological benefits from the care (that is, they deteriorated less rapidly than did the controls). At the other extreme, the most disabled and the most severely ill among the experimental group received more professional services than did the corresponding group of control patients. These findings highlight the need for careful targeting of populations and careful delineation of expectations.

In a quasi-experimental study, Mitchell compared cohorts of Veterans Administration (VA) patients receiving nursing home care and home care (57). She found that the patients with the best prognoses tended to do best on home care. In general, those patients who received home care had fewer limitations in their functional status index, and the functional status index at the outset of the experiment was the best predictor of future functional status. Weissert similarly noted that adult day care is most appropriate for that subset of nursing home patients who should not have been admitted there in the first place or who no longer require services (58).

The US General Accounting Office, with the collaboration of Duke University, is currently addressing the technical problems in making comparisons of program effects (59). Using a standardized instrument to measure various categories of impairment, 118 service agencies in Cleveland have been testing a procedure for disaggregating the actual components of service to individuals. When this system is in place, it should be possible to measure changes of impairment level over time and to link the rates of those changes with the provision of comparable units of service; it will also be possible to examine natural rates of changes in impairment that occur in the absence of any particular service (60). The disaggregation of services currently breaks out 25 functions in three general categories: (*a*) basic living components (such as living quarters, transportation, unprepared foodstuffs), (*b*) supportive care elements (such as periodic checking, continuous supervision, meal preparation), and (*c*) remedial care components (physical therapy, nursing, counseling, retraining).

The widespread concern over the cost of nursing home care and its deficiencies led to the series of demonstration projects funded in 1972 under the authority of Section 222 of Public Law 92–603. These projects were intended to produce comparative data about the relative cost effectiveness of covering day care and homemaker programs under Medicare in six sites.

Unfortunately, the wide variation in the program activities, program costs, and program participants across the several sites made summative evaluation difficult. Mortality rates were generally lower among those receiving expanded benefits than those who did not use them. At the same time, those with extended benefits coverage received fewer traditional services than did control group members who were not offered the extended benefits; however, the net costs were greater for those receiving home care and day care than for the control groups (61). It must be recognized that all of these findings cannot be readily generalized in view of the potential for self-selection in utilization of the expanded benefits.

Some research has been done on the housing preferences of elderly persons and the correlation of personal adjustment and housing patterns. For example, preliminary data associate age-segregated housing with higher survival rates compared to age-integrated housing (62). Brody and her colleagues are conducting a multifaceted project to examine the effects of various community housing arrangements; an intriguing early observation from this work is that individuals who decide not to move from their former housing have an increased mortality rate compared to those who follow through with moves to the sheltered housing and those who make other independent moves (63). In a very careful study of sheltered housing, Sherwood and her colleagues used a quasi-experimental design to compare the effects of admission to a medically oriented housing project among physically impaired elderly with a carefully matched group of applicants who were not admitted (64). Results indicate that significantly fewer of the experimental group were admitted to LTC facilities during the follow-up period. At the same time, the mortality rate for the experimental group was also lower. Conversely, the experimental group experienced more hospitalizations and incurred more acute hospital days than did the control group. This decreased mortality rate among movers was also found in Carp's 8-year follow-up of a San Antonio housing project, but she also noted better health indices among the experimental group (65).

These findings offer cause for both caution and optimism. Caution is needed for those hoping to find community-based panaceas that can simultaneously save money and improve client welfare. Optimism is justified by data that suggest that even minimal interventions can have a large effect in promoting independence that will preserve functional ability in nursing home patients (43) and help those in the community to cope with stress (66). Sheltered housing seems particularly promising. Perhaps home care and day care may prove more feasible if combined with sheltered housing to achieve greater efficiency of scale.

FUTURE OF LONG-TERM CARE

In many ways long-term care has begun to replace primary care as a major focus of interest in addition to hospital-based care. If LTC is to improve, there is a need for (*a*) a cadre of better trained personnel for both medical and social services, (*b*) better ability to measure the health status of LTC patients, (*c*) a more rational payment system that provides incentives for the type of care desired, and (*d*) more research on the efficacy of various modes of LTC delivery.

Geriatric Personnel

Major revisions in our medical curricula are required to address the implications of the aging of our population. A 1979 report from the National Academy of Sciences' Institute of Medicine recommends against the development of a geriatric specialty per se and favors instead an added emphasis in geriatrics for all physicians who will work with adults (67). The prevalent attitude of many physicians is reflected in their disengagement from elderly patients who need long-term care. In order to effect the necessary changes in attitude among physicians, their education must help them acquire sufficient skills and knowledge to enable them to provide meaningful care for this group of patients.

In 1976, only two medical schools had required undergraduate courses in gerontology or geriatrics and only 15 had separate educational programs of any kind (18); in April 1979, 71 schools reported having developed or to be developing such programs. Spurred by an analysis of the medical needs of aging veterans (68), the Veterans Administration has undertaken the lead in providing financial support for education and research on aging in academically affiliated VA medical centers.

The answer to the geriatric personnel shortage may lie in nonphysician personnel such as the geriatric nurse practitioner, the social worker, and other care-givers. Geriatric nurse practitioners, for example, have shown the ability to provide first-rate primary care. At the same time they have worked effectively with the staffs of nursing homes (and similar community-based institutions) to upgrade organizational performance. Part of the failure to gain widespread acceptance for nonphysician care deliverers can be traced to the legal and regulatory barriers to their use. Their services are not yet reimbursible under Medicare (Part B), the major source of payment for physician care (as opposed to nursing home services) for the elderly. Then, too, schools of nursing and social work also must develop the curricula to support a geriatrics emphasis if their graduates are to have an important role in care-giving.

Measurement

Manpower reform will require the further development and testing of techniques to assess the functional status of the elderly, particularly the chronically ill elderly. A compilation of such measurements is presently being developed at the University of Missouri, Kansas City, to compile the multitude of measures that have been developed.

An earlier review prepared by Bloom is illustrative of the enormous number of instruments that have been used at some time or another, often without validation or reliability checks (69). A few instruments have been fielded sufficiently frequently that a body of knowledge has been developed; in this category we include Katz' scale for the measurement of ability to perform ADL functions (70) and Lawton's Geriatric Morale Scale (71), which is probably the most prominent measure in the difficult psychosocial area. Several instruments tapping multidimensional aspects of functioning deserve mention: (a) PACE II, a comprehensive model for nursing home assessment and care planning developed by DHEW (72); (b) OARS, a well-tested battery developed at Duke University, which yields an assessment of ADL functioning, physical functioning, mental functioning, economic functioning, and social resources (73); and (c) CARE, an instrument emphasizing psychiatric elements that is being used in a cross-national study (74). OARS is perhaps the most promising screening device yet developed; its problems are that it depends somewhat on implicit judgments and that it does not make distinctions at the lower end of the functional status spectrum.

Incentives

The current system of payment for LTC creates a number of anomalies that plague the institution as well as the professional care-giver. Financial support for long-term care is scarce outside nursing homes. Home care (especially that portion provided by homemakers as contrasted with nursing personnel) is scarcely covered except by special waivers for demonstration projects. Day care services are similarly uncovered by federal funds.

The payments for nursing home care are at once too much for the federal budgets and too little to support the quality of care sought. The mandatory shift to cost-based reimbursement for nursing homes will not ease the problem. The differences between levels of care (i.e. between skilled and intermediate) become less meaningful in the face of such reimbursement, but the budgetary ceilings imposed simultaneously with regulations mandating the way in which care should be rendered leave the nursing home caught in a squeeze with little room to maneuver.

Perhaps worst of all, both cost reimbursement and fee-for-service provide a set of perverse incentives. At a time when we are learning that the chronically ill can improve along a number of dimensions, our incentive system rewards their getting sicker.

One proposal to counter this perverse tendency is the outcome-based reimbursement system noted earlier (14). Such an approach offers at least one means by which the incentives can be corrected to encourage providers of care to help their clients improve. It, or something like it, seems especially needed in LTC today and tomorrow.

Research

Before an outcome-based reimbursement system can be implemented, however, much preliminary work is required. The natural history of patients getting good long-term care needs to be documented. We presently lack the benchmarks against which to compare the results of a variety of ways of delivering LTC. Such an approach underlies the need to test the relative efficacy of alternative methods of LTC, especially when controlled clinical trials will not be feasible. As already indicated, a set of measurement tools must be refined for use by practitioners and program evaluators. After measurements are developed, value preferences would need to be studied and discussed to identify how different clusters of potential outcomes could be ranked. Inevitably, treatment choices will maximize certain ends at the cost of others.

Basic biomedical research is also important. Only recently have such investigators focused significant attention on the problems common to the elderly. Major breakthroughs in the control and prevention of conditions like dementia and osteoporosis could substantially change the way LTC is rendered, redefine its necessity, and generally change the future of long-term care.

THE ROLE OF PUBLIC HEALTH

The essential values of public health with its broad perspective emphasizing social and mental as well as physical well-being are perhaps nowhere better epitomized than in long-term care. Public health has played an important role in upgrading the quality of nursing homes. Health departments carry out a majority of the inspections for Medicare and Medicaid certification of facilities and often conduct the ongoing review of care in those facilities mandated by federal regulations.

In some areas, public health departments sponsor direct services in LTC in the community, often as part of a comprehensive home care program. One area in which health departments could play a vital role in assuring that those in need of LTC receive the necessary care is through organized programs of case-finding and case management. Elderly at-risk populations merit the same attention from public health nurses as do those presently targeted by maternal and infant health programs.

The epidemiological approach, the hallmark of public health, has never been so needed as in this problem area. Public health can contribute to definitions of populations at risk and to development of basic information about the incidence and prevalence of various physical and social conditions in the elderly. Presently the problem of the elderly and the nursing home problem have converged. The challenge is to separate the strands and to develop a real " system" of long-term care than can meet multiple needs.

Literature Cited

1. Weissert, W. G. 1978. Long-term care: An overview. In *Health United States 1978.* Publ. # PHS 78-1232. Hyattsville, Md: DHEW
2. Kovar, M. G. 1977. Elderly people: The population 65 years and over. In *Health United States 1976–1977.* Publ. # HRA 77-1232. Hyattsville, Md: DHEW
3. Kastenbaum, R., Candy, S. E. 1973. The 4% fallacy: A methodological and empirical critique of extended care facility population statistics. *Aging Hum. Dev.* 4:15–21
4. Eggert, G. M., Granger, C. V., Morris, R., Pendleton, S. F. 1977. Caring for the patient with long-term disability. *Geriatrics* 32:102
5. Thomas, W. C. Jr. 1969. *Nursing Homes and Public Policy Drift and Decision in New York State.* Ithaca: Cornell Univ. Press
6. Schmidt, L. J., Reinhardt, A. M., Kane, R. L., Olsen, D. M. 1977. The mentally ill in nursing homes: New back wards in the community. *Arch. Gen. Psychiatr.* 34:687–91
7. Dunlop, B. D. 1979. *The Growth of Nursing Home Care.* Lexington, Mass: Lexington
8. Vladek, B. C. 1980. *Unloving Care: The Nursing Home Tragedy.* New York: Basic. In press

9. US Gen. Account. Off. 1978. *Problems in Auditing Medicaid Nursing Home Chains.* Publ. # HRD 78–158. Washington DC: GPO
10. US Nat. Cent. Health Stat. 1977. *Characteristics, Social Contacts and Activities of Nursing Home Residents United States: 1973–74 National Nursing Home Survey. Vital and Health Statistics,* Ser. 13, No. 27. DHEW Publ. # HRA 77–1778. Washington DC: GPO
11. McCaffree, K. 1977. *Returns to Equity Capital in Nursing Homes.* Seattle: Univ. Washington (mimeo)
12. Ruchlin, H. S., Levey, S., Muller, C. 1975. The long-term care marketplace: An analysis of deficiencies and potential reform by means of incentive reimbursement. *Med. Care* 13:979–91
13. Ruchlin, H., Levey, S. 1975. An economic perspective of long-term care. In *Long-term Care: A Handbook for Researchers,* ed. S. Sherwood. New York: Spectrum Publ.
14. Kane, R. L. 1976. Paying nursing homes for better care. *J. Community Health* 2:1–4
15. Solon, J. A., Greenwalt, L. F. 1974. Physicians' participation in nursing homes. *Med. Care* 12:486–95
16. US Special Comm. on Aging. 1975. Doctors in nursing homes: The shunned responsibility. In *Nursing Home Care in*

the United States: Failure in Public Policy. Washington DC: GPO

17. Kane, R. L., Hammer, D., Byrnes, N. 1977. Getting care to nursing home patients: A problem and a proposal. *Med. Care* 15:174–80

18. Akpom, C. A., Mayer, S. 1978. A Survey of geriatric education in United States medical schools. *J. Med. Ed.* 53:66–68

19. Pepper, G., Kane, R. L., Teteberg, B. 1976. Geriatric nurse practitioner in nursing homes. *Am. J. Nurs.* 76:62–64

20. Kane, R. L., Jorgensen, L. A., Teteberg, B., Kuwahara, J. 1976. Is good nursing home care feasible? *J. Am. Med. Assoc.* 235:516–19

21. Mark, R. G., Willemain, R., Malcolm, T., Master, R. J., Clarkson, T. 1976. *Final Report of the Nursing Home Telemedicine Project,* Vol. 1. Springfield, Va: US Dep. Commer.

22. US Congressional Budget Off. 1977. *Long-term Care for the Elderly and Disabled.* Washington DC: GPO

23. Holmberg, R. H., Anderson, N. D. 1968. Implications of ownership for nursing home care. *Med. Care* 6:300–7

24. Winn, S. 1974. Analysis of selected characteristics of a matched sample of nonprofit and proprietary nursing homes in the State of Washington. *Med. Care* 12:221–28

25. Kosberg, J. I., Tobin, S. S. 1972. Variability among nursing homes. *Gerontologist* 12:214–19

26. Miller, W. R., Hurley, S. J., Wharton, E. 1976. External peer review of skilled nursing care in Minnesota. *Am. J. Public Health* 66:278–83

27. Zimmer, J. G. 1979. Medical care evaluation studies in long-term care facilities. *J. Am. Geriatr. Soc.* 27:62–72

28. Chekryn, J., Roos, L. L. 1979. Auditing the process of care in a new geriatric unit. *J. Am. Geriatr. Soc.* 27:107–11

29. Allison-Cooke, S., Ellis, S. E. n.d. *An Assessment of the Impact of SJPSRO Concurrent Quality Assurance Review on Quality of Care in LTC Facilities. A Final Report.* Providence, RI: SEARCH

30. Kane, R. A., Kane, R. L., Kleffel, D., Brook, R. H., Eby, C., Goldberg, G., Rubenstein, L. Z., Van Ryzin, J. 1979. *The PSRO and the Nursing Home,* Vol. 1. *An Assessment of PSRO LTC Review.* Santa Monica, Ca: Rand Corp. (R-2459/1)

31. US Special Comm. on Aging 1975. Drugs in nursing homes: Misuse, high costs, and kickbacks. In *Nursing Home*

Care in the United States: Failure in Public Policy. Washington DC: GPO

32. Howard, J. B., Strong, K. Sr., Strong, K. Jr. 1977. Medication procedures in a nursing home: Abuse of PRN orders. *Am. Geriatr. Soc.* 25:83–84

33. Gottesman, L. E., Bourestom, N. C. 1974. Why nursing homes do what they do. *Gerontologist* 14:501–6

34. Linn, M. W. 1977. Patient outcome as a measure of quality of nursing home care. *Am. J. Public Health* 67:337–44

35. Kane, R. L., Olsen, D. M., Thetford, C., Byrnes, N. 1976. The use of utilization review records as a source of data on nursing home care. *Am. J. Public Health* 66:778–82

36. Sarton, M. 1973. *As We Are Now.* New York: Norton

37. Tulloch, J. 1975. *A House is Not a Home.* New York: Seabury

38. Gubrium, J. F. 1975. *Living and Dying at Murray Manor.* New York: St. Martin's

39. Brody, E. 1973. A million procrustean beds. *Gerontologist* 13:430–35

40. Seligman, M. 1975. *Helplessness: On Depression, Development and Death.* San Francisco: W. H. Freeman

41. Schulz, R. 1976. Effects of control and predictability on the physical and psychological well-being of the institutionalized aged. *J. Pers. Soc. Psychol.* 33:563–73

42. Langer, E. J., Rodin, J. 1976. Effects of choice and enhanced personal responsibility for the aged. *J. Pers. Soc. Psychol.* 34:191–98

43. Mercer, S. O., Kane, R. A. 1979. Helplessness and hopelessness in the institutionalized aged: A field experiment. *Health Soc. Work* 4:90–116

44. Ogren, E. H., Linn, M. W. 1971. Male nursing home patients: Relocation and mortality. *J. Am. Geriatr. Soc.* 19:229–39

45. Jorgensen, L. A., Kane, R. A. 1976. Social work in the nursing home: A need and an opportunity. *Soc. Work Health Care* 1:471–82

46. Silverstone, B., Wynter, L. 1975. The effects of introducing a heterosexual living space. *Gerontologist* 15:83–87

47. Abdo, E., Dills, J., Shectman, H., Yanish, M. 1973. Elderly women in institutions vs. those in public housing: Comparison of personal and social adjustments. *J. Am. Geriatr. Soc.* 21:81–87

48. Schonfield, D., Hooper, A. 1973. Future commitments and successful aging. *J. Gerontol.* 28:197–201

49. Jones, D. C. 1975. Spatial proximity, interpersonal conflict and friendship formation in the intermediate care facility. *Gerontologist* 15:150–54

50. Kane, R. L., Kane, R. A. 1976. *Long-term Care in Six Countries: Implications for the United States.* Washington DC: GPO

51. Kane, R. L., Kane, R. A., 1980. Alternatives to institutional care of the elderly: Beyond the dichotomy. *Gerontologist.* In press

52. Doherty, N. J. G., Hicks, B. C. 1975. The use of cost-effectiveness analysis in geriatric day care. *Gerontologist* 15: 412–17

53. Rachlin, S. 1978. When schizophrenia comes marching home. *Psychiatr. Q.* 50:202–10

54. Donahue, W. T. 1978. What about our responsibility toward the abandoned elderly? *Gerontologist* 18:102–11

55. Williams, T. F., Hill, J. G., Fairbank, M. E. 1973. Appropriate placement of the chronically ill and aged: A successful approach by evaluation. *J. Am. Med. Assoc.* 26:1332–35

56. Katz, S., Ford, A. B., Downs, T. D., Adams, M., Rusby, D. I. 1972. *Effects of Continued Care: A Study of Chronic Illness in the Home.* DHEW Publ. # HSM 73-3010. Washington DC: GPO

57. Mitchell, J. B. 1978. Patient outcomes in alternative long-term care settings. *Med. Care* 16:439–52

58. Weissert, W. G. 1978. Costs of adult day care: A comparison to nursing homes. *Inquiry* 15:10–19

59. US Comptroller General. 1977. *The Well-Being of Older People in Cleveland, Ohio.* Publ. # HRD 77–70. Washington DC: GPO

60. Maddox, G. L., Dellinger, D. C. 1978. Assessment of functional status in a program evaluation and resource allocation mode. *Ann. Am. Acad. Polit. Soc. Sci.* 438:59–70

61. Weissert, W. G., Wan, T. T. H., Livieratos, B. B. 1979. *Effects and Costs of Day Care and Homemaker Services for the Chronically Ill: A Randomized Experiment.* Hyattsville, Md:DHEW

62. Harel, Z., Harel, B. B. 1978. On-site coordinated services in age-segregated and age-integrated public housing. *Gerontologist* 18:153–58

63. Brody, E. M. 1978. Community housing for the elderly: The program, the people, the decision-making process, and the research. *Gerontologist* 18: 121–29

64. Sherwood, S., Greer, D. S., Morris, J. N. 1978. A study of the Highland Heights apartments for the physically impaired and elderly in Fall River. In *Gerontological Monographs,* Vol. 1, ed. S. Howell, L. Pastalan, T. Byerts. New York: Garland Publ. Corp.

65. Carp, F. M. 1977. Impact of improved living environment on health and life expectancy. *Gerontologist* 17:242–49

66. Sherwood, S., Morris, J. N. 1974. *A Study of Aged Applicants to a Long-Term Care Facility: A Final Report.* Boston: Hebrew Rehabil. Cent. for Aged

67. Inst. of Med. 1978. *Aging and Medical Education.* Washington DC: Nat. Acad. Sci.

68. Veterans Admin. 1977. *The Aging Veteran: Present and Future Medical Needs.* Washington DC: VA Publ.

69. Bloom, M. 1975. Evaluation instruments: Tests and measurements in long-term care. In *Long-Term Care: A Handbook for Researchers, Planners, and Providers,* ed. S. Sherwood. New York: Wiley

70. Katz, S., Ford, A., Moskowitz, R., Jackson, B., Jaffe, M., Cleveland, M. A. 1963. The index of ADL: A standardized measure of biological and psychosocial function. *J. Am. Med. Assoc.* 185:914–19

71. Lawton, M. P. 1975. The Philadelphia geriatric morale scale: A revision. *J. Gerontol.* 30:85–89

72. US Dep. HEW 1978. *Patient Care Management: Theory to Practice.* Washington DC: GPO

73. Duke Univ. Study of Aging and Human Development 1978. *Multidimensional Functional Assessment: The OARS Methodology. 2nd ed.* Durham, NC

74. Gurland, B., Kuriansky, J., Sharpe, L., Simon, R., Stiles, P., Birkett, P. 1977. The comprehensive assessment and referral evaluation (CARE): Rationale, development, and reliability. *Int. J. Aging Hum. Dev.* 8:9–42

Ann. Rev. Public Health 1980. 1:255–76
Copyright © 1980 by Annual Reviews Inc. All rights reserved

ECONOMIC EVALUATION OF PUBLIC HEALTH PROGRAMS

◆12509

Lester B. Lave

The Brookings Institution, Washington DC 20036

INTRODUCTION

Judging from expenditures and publications, economic evaluation of public health programs is a growth sector. These evaluations make use of more traditional aspects of public health (1–4), such as analysis of facilities and manpower for planning (5, 6); of reimbursement such as hospital cost containment (7, 8); and of consumer demand, including the role of private and public insurance and such attributes as co-pay and deductible provisions (3, 9–12).

This paper is focused on economic evaluation of health care, particularly public health care programs. I begin with a discussion of the role of this evaluation, especially in the management of government programs. I then discuss medical evaluation; focus on the tools used for economic evaluation, listing the basic tools and the difficulties associated with their application; compare these frameworks; and summarize some of the recent applications of these tools. I close with a summary of the role of economic evaluation in public health and the difficulties in implementing the analysis and programs under consideration.

ROLE OF ECONOMIC EVALUATION

The vast majority of goods and services in the economy are produced and sold through the marketplace with little government intervention. Aside from attempting to insure that the environment is not polluted, that the workplace is safe, and that products are correctly labeled and generally safe, the government leaves to the private market the determination of what to produce, how much to produce, what price to charge, where to sell it, and how to produce it (13).

255

Health is different. Individuals have an interest not only in protecting their own health, but in protecting the health of others. Society has determined that people shall receive health care even when they cannot afford to pay for it. Furthermore, society guarantees an income to the dependents of someone who is disabled or dies. These guarantees of medical care and of payment to dependents put the government in a position of being interested in the way that individuals behave, insofar as their behavior affects their health, and in the way that medical care is delivered and the costs reimbursed.

Another way of saying this is that medical care is considered to be a fourth right, after food, clothing, and shelter. Clearly, a government that pays for this fourth right is going to be interested in the conditions under which medical care is supplied and in the health behavior of individuals that affects their need for care. Evaluation generally, and economic evaluation in particular, will be instrumental in shaping the government role.

Actually there are three separate roles that analysis can undertake to help the medical care sector to perform its mission better.

1. Evaluation of the efficacy of particular treatment techniques or facilities. Evaluation studies demonstrate that many drugs and procedures, long assumed to be highly effective, in fact are ineffective or pernicious. Scientific disciplines are subject to fads; medicine is no exception. To realize the potentials of innovation, one must evaluate each proposal to determine whether it is effective (14, 15).

2. Setting priorities among procedures shown to be effective. Many modern procedures require vast resources, such as physicians, other health professionals, ancillary workers, facilities, and supplies. It is not possible to offer all of the potentially effective procedures to all people who might benefit. Even after time has been allowed for more people to be trained and more facilities to be constructed, the costs are high enough so that society probably wouldn't choose to devote all of these resources to care (16). Thus, there must be some way of sorting among the available effective procedures to determine which have the highest priority. By identifying the effectiveness of each procedure, evaluation has an instrumental role in helping to set priorities.

3. Identifying future resource needs and implicit problems on the basis of the set of procedures shown to be effective and the prevalence of disease (a role that ventures increasingly away from medical evaluation and into economic analysis). This function is crucial because of the long lead times associated with training new health professionals, midcareer training, and the construction of new equipment and facilities. If we were to wait until there was an acute shortage of some professional manpower, equipment, or facilities, it would be as long as a decade before there could be relief.

None of these three roles would be unique to the government if health care were purely a nongovernmental function. Some combination of the government, medical societies, and foundations would perform the first function. Precedence would come from market demand interacting with the preferences of individual physicians. The marketplace would have to handle shortages of equipment and personnel.

A vast literature has appeared on each of these roles, which is reviewed below.

MEDICAL EVALUATION

A number of recent studies have examined the efficacy of current and past medical procedures (14, 17–20). If ever one were inclined to believe that all surgical procedures were helpful, or at least not harmful, the studies dispel the notion. Indeed, the myriad evaluations make it clear that many medical procedures, even many of those generally regarded as highly effective, are ineffective or pernicious.

In a classic book, Cochrane (14) displays general skepticism regarding the efficacy of medical procedures. He argues that virtually all procedures ought to be formally evaluated before being allowed to become part of the standard set of procedures. Furthermore, this formal evaluation ought to take the form of a clinical trial, rather than some quasi-experiment or time series of observations. In seeking to get the attention of his colleagues and make his point, Cochrane overstated the desirability of clinical trials. Clinical trials are terribly expensive; it is easy to conceive of the British National Health Service spending all of its resources on clinical trials and devoting none to general patient care. However, there is no quarreling with the general point that far too little attention and resources are devoted to evaluation, to the detriment both of patients and the quality of medical care.

Whatever the role of evaluation in a purely private medical care system, that role is greater and more important in a system in which the government, or some other third party, pays virtually all of the cost. For example, under the National Health Service or under many insurance plans, neither the patient nor the physician feel any financial pressures in making decisions about treatment. There are few barriers to rapid increase in costs, as has been demonstrated for hospital care in the US in the past decade. Evaluation serves to rule out procedures that aren't efficacious.

There is a longer and more important tradition in evaluation of preventive health care (21, 22). Presumably this care is advised by a physician or other health professional. Because the initiative rests with health professionals, a higher standard is required. The care must not be harmful and there must be more than a suspicion that it is helpful. Thus, there are many more formal studies of screening, innoculations, and asymptomatic checkups than of acute care.

Even after rejecting procedures shown to be ineffective, a large set still remains. Given the complexity and level of resources required for modern medical procedures, there are too many to be given to all who might benefit.

For example, consider the resources required for maximal preventive care, the services that could be provided to prolong life by a few days for elderly patients, and the services alleged to increase comfort for chronic disease patients. If the level of care currently given to the "best treated" (really, most treated) 5% of the population were given to everyone, we would require many times the current levels of health professionals, facilities, and supplies at many times the current cost. There is no indication that health indices would improve in a way commensurate with these additional expenditures (23, 24).

There then follows the even more difficult choice of deciding which care should be made available to everyone, i.e. paid for by governmental programs and insurance. Making this choice requires the second role, priority setting using economic analysis in conjunction with the medical evaluation.

A PRIMER ON BENEFIT-COST ANALYSIS

Deciding which of a set of efficacious procedures to permit is inherently controversal. A series of economic frameworks have been proposed, including a rough balancing of benefits and costs, the regulatory budget, and formal benefit-cost analysis (25–31).

Quantitative analysis begins with an enumeration of the effects of some treatment (32–34). In benefit-cost analysis this listing is meant to be encyclopedic, encompassing all effects that are nontrivial; in other frameworks, a narrower purview is adopted. The second step is to relate the level of effect to the scope of the treatment, e.g. relate the cost of a preventive procedure to its utilization and thence to improvements in health status.

The information gleaned in these first two stages is interesting in itself and should always be presented in the results of the analysis. One framework chooses to stop at this point, assuming that any further aggregation and analysis will be so controversial as to be dysfunctional, or at least irrelevant (34). However, stopping here means that the results of the analysis will consist of many disparate effects. For example, the effects of abating sulfur oxides air pollution would be described in terms of the number of tons of steel lost to production, man-hours for construction and maintenance, various other materials, land needed for abatement, firms made bankrupt, and workers losing their jobs; the benefits would be described by estimated effects on disease and mortality rates, on visibility, odors, plants, animals etc. Perhaps some people can make sense out of this laundry list, but it is not readily reduced to sense.

All the other frameworks go on, at least partially, to aggregate effects into categories, finding some sort of common metric. Thus, the inputs required to carry out a public health project are aggregated by finding the cost of purchasing each in the market. However, as the example demonstrates, this step is not without controversy. For example, acquiring land for a sanitary landfill often stirs controversy over its location and market value.

Aggregating the effects on health is even more difficult. Often, aggregating effects requires a sort of grisly calculus. For example, a worsening of air pollution is estimated to increase the number of illnesses, the number of sick days, the amount of disability, and the mortality rate. Finding a metric to make disabilities and premature deaths comparable so they can be aggregated into a health effects category is inherently difficult (35–37).

Risk-benefit and cost-effectiveness (regulatory budget) analysis stop when effects have been aggregated into major categories. The former framework attempts to place an estimate of the risks (to health) associated with a project on one side of the scale and the estimated benefits of the project on the other. The cost of the project is neglected, as are other types of risk, such as the danger of exterminating a species of plant or animal. Cost-effectiveness analysis attempts to estimate the benefit per dollar of cost for all possible projects so as to choose the one(s) giving "the most bang for the buck," the greatest level of benefit per dollar expended (16, 19, 25, 28a, b, 38).

Risk-benefit analysis runs afoul of two conundrums. First, there is no unique measure of risk. For example, a risk averse person will not perceive the expected value of the probability distribution concerning risk to be a fair representation of the level of risk. Risk averse people will want to take account of the second and third moments of the distribution, and may want information on the maximum risk. In any case, there is no accepted method to get a scalar, or any common, measure of risk across different projects (39–43).

The second conundrum is the difficulty of estimating benefits. For example, what is the benefit to the nation of greater longevity, less disability, or less morbidity? It would be fair to say that there is no accepted theory of risk-benefit analysis that specifies how it is to be done and what are the resource allocation properties of the solution (26, 44, 45).

If the risks are aggregated, costs are included, benefits are estimated, and the information is arrayed so that the benefits per unit of cost or risk are estimated, risk-benefit analysis is transformed into cost-effectiveness analysis. The basic assumption is that it is not currently possible to translate costs and benefits into comparable units; thus, the problem is set up as a constrained optimization in which the greatest benefits are sought for a given level of expenditure (or of risk).

Benefit-cost analysis assumes that all effects can be translated into the same metric. Thus, rather than ending with estimates of the risk-benefit ratio or benefit per dollar of expenditure per project, the analysis produces an estimate of the relationship of benefits to costs or of the internal rate of return on invested capital. The most comprehensive of the frameworks, benefit-cost analysis is the focus of the criticism of quantitative analysis. However, the major problems are common to all of these frameworks, as elaborated below.

COMPARISON OF FRAMEWORKS

In applying these frameworks, a series of concerns are ubiquitous; they relate to the ability to do quantitative analysis at all, and if so, to the desirability of attempting to apply the more general framework. I begin with the general issues applying to all frameworks and then go on to the more specific problems.

The first step is enumeration of the effects of a project or regulation. This seemingly trivial step has often led to difficulties. For example, the Army Corps of Engineers has been doing benefit-cost analysis of waterway projects since the 1930s; environmental effects were not considered until the late 1960s. But not all effects can be listed. Because the world is interdependent, one action will eventually have ripple effects throughout a wide range of phenomena. Insisting on listing all effects would require a near infinite list. Instead, trivial effects must be excluded. But, which effects are trivial is the heart of the controversy. The corps believed that environmental effects were trivial until the late 1960s. Most people would think that threatening extinction of an obscure and not very desirable type of plant would be a trivial effect, but a vocal minority disagrees emphatically.

The greatest difficulty in applying quantitative frameworks is in the quantification of effects. Some effects cannot be quantified with current techniques. Unfortunately, there is a sort of Gresham's law of decision-making: Quantified effects tend to dominate consideration, even if the unquantified effects are believed to be more important. Thus, quantification can be pernicious if important aspects are left unquantified, if the quantification isn't evenhanded for benefits and costs, or if the quantification is inadequate.

The first problem can be alleviated in part by educating decision makers about the bias. Important aspects are certain to be unquantified and so these frameworks will be helpful to decision makers only if they are educated about the nature of the biases and the ways in which quantification has been done. A particular problem is the universal quantification of costs, and absence of, or inadequate estimation of benefits (46). For many public health programs, the costs are calculated in detail and benefits are alluded to in only a vague fashion. Benefit-cost and other quantitative analysis will be unable to quantify some effects that are important or of potential importance. There is no alternative to the education of decision makers about this problem.

Having to estimate the quantitative relationship between the effects and scope of a project means that data must be collected and analyzed. For some effects, such as the cost of constructing a new hospital, techniques for quantifying the effect are well defined, accepted, and involve little controversy; the data are readily available and the techniques for collection are well defined. However, as the example suggests, defined techniques are not synonymous with confident estimates. At the opposite extreme are possible improvements in health, where data are difficult to gather, privacy issues arise, and estimation of effects is difficult.

To collect good data and to perform meaningful analyses requires a modicum of understanding of the underlying theory of the effect. Without this understanding, the data and analysis can merely present empirical regularities; this problem is particularly acute in extrapolating from animal bioassays at high doses to humans at low doses (47–50). However, mechanisms, such as the effects of long-term exposure to low levels of some toxic substance, are not understood very well (51). Health effects are only one example of effects for which the underlying theoretical knowledge is missing; so one cannot specify precisely what data ought to be collected and how it ought to be analyzed.

Even when one knows what data to collect, it is often difficult to get it. For example, air pollution effects research requires data on the quantities of various air pollutants breathed by an individual over his lifetime, specifying the size of the particulates and their composition and the quantities of each gas (52, 53). These data are difficult to obtain, both because of measurement problems and because of the time span involved. Typically, available data are only a remote approximation to what is desired.

Rarely does theory or knowledge of the underlying mechanisms result in a sharp hypothesis to be tested. Instead, only vague statements of possible relationships are possible. This puts a premium on robust estimation procedures, rather than ones that have spurious power based on arbitrary assumptions (54–57).

This triple set of problems, consisting of only vague knowledge of the theory or underlying mechanisms, poor data, and imprecise estimates, almost inevitably gives rise to the charge that a statistically significant relationship is no proof of a cause and effect relationship. Even when one can rule out the possibility of reverse causation (increased mortality causes air pollution) and of this relationship happening by chance, there remains the possibility of spurious correlation, i.e. the existence of some other factor or set of factors that causes the observed association. The less known about theory and the more vague the data, the more doubt scientists will have about whether the observed association is a causal one (47, 48).

This problem of spurious correlation also extends to the estimation of the quantitative effect. If other factors, known to effect the phenomenon being explored, are missing from the analysis, and if they are correlated with the factors being analyzed, the latter will have biased parameter estimates.

A special case of the general notion that some effects are easier to quantify than others is the general case of costs versus health benefits. There are well-established methods of estimating the former, and it is extremely difficult to estimate the latter. As a result, analysts tend to estimate costs to be somewhat higher than they would actually expect, because their estimates do not take account of technological change or economies of scale (58). At the same time, the controversy surrounding the estimation of benefits leads to choosing a "conservative" value, one below the median effect. A careful analyst would quantify benefits and costs in this fashion, with a resulting upward bias in estimated costs and a downward bias in estimated benefits. Thus, this type of uncertainty will tend to lead to the rejection of good programs, i.e. the estimated benefits will be less than estimated costs for programs for which the true benefits are greater than the true costs.

Two issues have occupied much of the economic literature on benefit-cost analysis: the valuation of nontraded goods and services (25–31, 33, 59) and the social rate of discount (60, 61). When some good is regularly bought and sold in the market and one can expect to be able to purchase the needed quantity without raising price, valuation is simple. But, when the effect is not a good or service traded regularly, such as premature death or severe injury, valuation is difficult and fraught with controversy (62, 69). Four options are possible in such cases.

1. One can refuse to value these effects and instead go to a cost-effectiveness framework.
2. One can adopt entirely subjective judgments and produce an analysis that is likely to be helpful only to the people making the judgments.
3. One can attempt to find some traded good that is very similar to that which is untraded. For example, in choosing their occupation, sports, and other activities, people are implicitly equating dollars and premature death.
4. One can attempt to get people to think about the issue and rely on their stated judgments. This area is controversial and there is little resolution of the proper way of valuing such untraded effects, particularly when emotion enters, as with health.

The single most controversial aspect of benefit-cost analysis is the attempt to place a dollar value on averting a premature death. The valuation may call to mind the cold-blooded sacrifice of some individual, whose death will grieve his relatives and friends. However, an individual is rarely if ever identified. Rather, it is the change in some mortality rate, such as the number of people dying in traffic accidents, that is at issue; even after the untoward event, one could not identify which individual was saved or killed by the decision (62).

An alternative to valuing premature death is to estimate the cost to society of prolonging life via various public health programs (69, 70). This and other attempts to better define goals have shifted the discussion to more fruitful channels.

Enough has been written about this subject that detailed review is not possible. One can, however, review some particular values of life that are often used in decision making. For example, the Department of Defense and State Workers Compensation pay the heirs of a victim a sum of money. Although there is no notion that this payment is full compensation for the death, it nonetheless serves as one dollar estimate of the cost to society of premature death. In both cases, the dollar values are quite low.

The Federal Aviation Administration (FAA) uses an explicit value of life of $300,000 in its various analyses (71, 72). They report that this figure results from recent court awards (see 62–69). The Nuclear Regulatory Commission places an implicit value of premature death in terms of their regulations concerning routine releases of radiation from nuclear power plants: that amount is $1 million (73–75). A large number of analyses have used values ranging from $40,000 to $80,000 based on the present discounted value of future earnings (62–69). A number of studies of wage premia in risky occupations have been done, with the inference that the premium can be ascribed to the additional risk (63, 64, 76). These studies estimate that workers require payments that imply the expected value of their lives is between $260,000 and $1.5 million.

At this time there is an agreement in principle that the proper concept is the amount the individual would be willing to pay (or have to be paid for increased risk) to lower his probability of death by the prescribed amount. However, this individual payment must be supplemented with the additional loss that society suffers from the demise of this individual, e.g. the loss of his earning capacity to his family and the general loss to his family, employer, and community represented by his demise. There is no agreement on what dollar value best implements these concepts; however, estimates in the range from $250,000 to $500,000 seem to be commonly used and defended.

When effects accrue over a period of time, something must be done to make them commensurate in time (62, 69). This is done by choosing a discount rate (not necessarily constant over time). Economists have managed to resolve the theoretical issue as to what discount rate to use: the opportunity cost of the funds invested in the project. There is less agreement, however, as to the precise numerical value to use, as this depends in part on expectations concerning the future.

These issues affect not only the way that analysis is conducted, but also the framework to be chosen for analysis. For example, if one decided that untraded effects couldn't be valued, cost-benefit analysis would be ruled out. Indeed, one might decide that quantification wasn't possible at all in a particular case, which would rule out all these frameworks.

A REVIEW OF RELEVANT LITERATURE

Literature focused on quantitative analysis of health-related programs has been growing exponentially. For example, recent bibliographies show a rapidly expanding number of scholarly papers (78, 79). The relevant literature is far too large for a comprehensive review. Thus, in what follows, I pick and choose, attempting to get at representative studies.

Personal Health Services

With the nationalization of health services after World War II, Great Britain put stringent budget limitations on health care expenditures. This caused the National Health Service to resist new techniques that were extraordinarily expensive. It also allowed the administration of many randomized clinical trials in order to gain information about existing or proposed treatments. A. L. Cochrane (14) describes the results of a number of these clinical trials, arguing that purely observational data are of little value, because of the confounding factors.

Randomized clinical trials have been done all over the world (14, 17–20). They have provided good quantitative estimates of the efficacy of these techniques including the costs and quantitative degree of improvement. Going from these data to a benefit-cost analysis is simple and straightforward.

Lest one have more confidence in personal health services than is warranted, Bunker et al examine the efficacy of surgical procedures and engender a profound skepticism of past and present techniques (15, 18–20). Unlike Cochrane's study, the Bunker studies focus on the qualitative question of whether the surgical procedure helps. Although one must grant that the focus is on bankrupt procedures, the reader carries away a general sense of skepticism about surgical procedures.

For most of the procedures examined, the issue is whether the procedure helps. Because it does not, there is no further question for quantitative analysis. However, several studies consider a series of disease/treatments that do prove effective, although at vast differences in the cost per additional year of life expectancy. For example, Bendixen (80) describes a range of cases involving intensive care, from barbituate overdose (95% survival, young patients, four days of hospitalization at $600 per day) in which life expectancy is prolonged at $84 per year, to hepato-renal failure in chronic alcoholics (20% survival, short life expectancy among those surviving, 30 days hospitalization at $1,200 per day) in which life expectancy is prolonged at a cost of $180,000 per year. By chance, the two extremes in Bendixon's study are defined by patients with drug abuse; both crises result from self-inflicted damage. The assumed increase in life expectancy for the barbituate overdose patient may be too high if the individual is determined to attempt suicide again.

A major goal of the Bunker et al studies is to demystify the use of quantitative evaluation and decision techniques in medical care. They show that these techniques are extremely helpful and not terribly difficult to apply. Thus, there is no doubt that quantitative evaluation techniques can be and are being applied to personal health services. Ethical considerations mean that some well-established techniques will never be evaluated and that some new techniques are likely to be adopted without evaluation. However, there are no good ethical or financial reasons for not evaluating the vast majority of new treatments. Several reviews of the literature using these quantitative techniques show a vast number of studies are now being done and published (8, 32, 78, 79a,b, 81a,b).

Prevention

Preventive health measures have a longer history of formal evaluation. A large literature evaluates innoculations, screening, and asymptomatic exams. In addition, a literature is accumulating of attempts to change health habits and to educate people about how to achieve better health (82).

Much of the literature in the past half decade goes beyond the usual evaluation of efficacy to do a benefit-cost analysis or at least estimate the cost of prolonging life or avoiding an untoward event (70). Many of the analyses are self-serving in the sense that the qualitative outcome was known in advance—that was what prompted the benefit-cost analysis. Thus, quantitative analysis has been used to argue that preventive care generally ought to receive more resources (83, 84), that innoculations ought to receive more (81a,b), and that various disease programs of the National Institutes of Health ought to get more. The technique is conspicuously almost absent in care for children or in other programs in which more is spent than would be justified by a benefit-cost analysis [a notable exception is screening for phenylketonuria (85a,b).]

Occupational Health

The creation of the National Institute of Occupational Safety and Health (NIOSH) and the Occupational Safety and Health Administration (OSHA) in 1969 gave a large push to the field of occupational health. Prognostic studies that quantify the health experience of workers have been done on such industries as steel, nuclear energy, rubber, mining, and textiles (51, 86). Excess risks are calculated in an attempt to identify the overall level of risk and to isolate hazardous substances or working conditions. The quantitative estimates of risk have been used in formulating and defending OSHA standards on coke ovens, cotton dust, and benzene, among others. These risk estimates provide an important component of the estimated benefit of a regulation.

Occupational studies are immersed in controversy for a number of reasons. Generally, exposure to a toxic substance occurs over many years. Thus it is difficult to "prove" that exposure to a particular substance caused the excess risk found. Furthermore, estimating the magnitude of the response is difficult because exposure to one substance is confounded with exposure to many other substances and with the personal habits (e.g. smoking) of the individual. Finally, dose is difficult to estimate because ambient levels of each substance vary over time and among locations in the plant. Estimating an integrated dose for an individual is nearly impossible (aside from a crude estimate of exposure to radiation) (51, 87). However, these objections generally apply to subtle effects; large effects are more easily isolated and there is less dispute concerning causality, e.g. angiosarcoma from vinyl chloride.

OSHA was created, in part, in response to an increase in occupational accidents in the 1960s. Initially, OSHA focused its efforts on reducing occupational accidents, focusing on a target set of industries. The experience of these regulations is analyzed by Smith (64, 76, 77). Unfortunately, the legislation that created OSHA also changed the accident reporting system; injury data before 1970 are not comparable to that for 1971 and later years. Thus, no powerful tests of the hypothesis that OSHA lowered accident rates are possible. A series of weak tests, however, could uncover a substantial effect, if one had occurred.

Smith focuses on the relationship between injury rates before and after OSHA in each industry, hypothesizing that OSHA should have had the most effect on industries targeted for the greatest attention. He finds that injury rates tended to rise in these targeted industries, relative to all others, although the result is not significant statistically. An additional model gives the correct sign, but the effect is still insignificant.

Mendeloff used a slightly different model and more recent data, but also got insignificant results (88); by using California data and focussing on preventable accidents, Mendeloff got significant results. However, the viability of this finding is in question, as California had a strong OSH program prior to OSHA and would not be expected to have had much of an improvement.

DiPietro used data on individual firms (by firm size, by industry) to investigate whether recent inspections tended to lower accident rates (89). Most results are insignificant; those that are significant have at least as many positive as negative signs. Although one can propound plausible explanations for why OSHA inspections should be found to increase the accident rate, the fact is that the analysis fails to uncover evidence that OSHA has succeeded in lowering the accident rate (76, 90).

Taken together, these evaluations of OSHA's accident prevention activities indicate that either they were unsuccessful or at least that they were not very effective. This is not evidence that quantitative evaluation cannot be done for occupational health. It is evidence that under adverse conditions quantitative analysis is difficult and that conclusions necessarily will be crude. Changing the data base so that previous data are not comparable to future data will tend to nullify efforts at evaluation. Yet, care could have been taken to assemble a data base on specific firms that would have allowed evaluation. This area illustrates the need for care in the gathering of data if analysis is to be possible. Clever analysts are able to extract crude estimates even in the face of formidible obstacles, but it would have been far better to have gathered the proper data in the first place.

Transportation Safety

Many of the difficulties arising in the analysis of health also arise in the analysis of accidents. Identifying the immediate and contributory causes is controversial, as is attempting to infer what actions might lower the accident rate or the severity of the consequences of accidents. Perhaps the major difference is that a highway accident is associated with a highway, whereas one can't trace a lung cancer back to any individual activity or location. Even if they aren't the immediate cause, contributors to accidents include the use of psychoactive drugs, fatigue, negligence, and ignorance. It is tempting to seek easy solutions by changing the design or construction of some product, such as an automobile, rather than attempting to deal with the more important factors of personal behavior.

The number of serious accidents and deaths occurring in transportation is public information and is widely disseminated. Individual accidents, especially those involving the deaths of more than one person, are widely publicized. Such specific events, especially air crashes, combine with annual statistics to create pressure for regulatory actions to make transportation safer. The safety of each of the major modes is regulated by a specific agency, each of which is charged with improving the safety of its particular mode. Two agencies, the FAA and National Highway Traffic and Safety Administration (NHTSA), have been especially active in preparing quantitative analyses of new designs, safety features, and operating procedures that would enhance safety (38, 71, 91). Each agency prepares a careful analysis of the extent to which risks would be lowered and property damage and injury averted, as well as the estimated costs of a proposed new regulation. Although controversy is inevitable, these two agencies have established firmly the tradition of careful analyses of proposed regulations.

The principal difference between the analyses of the FAA and NHTSA is that FAA makes use of an explicit cost to society of a premature death ($300,000 based on recent court cases) to achieve a full dollar estimate of benefits (38, 71, 91), whereas NHTSA is content to estimate the number of premature deaths, severe injuries, minor injuries, and property damage that would be averted by a proposed action (thus costs are estimated fully and translated into dollars, but benefits are stated as a vector of health and property damage attributes). However, there is no difficulty in taking the NHTSA analysis all the way to full dollar benefit estimates by using the same assumed dollar cost to society of premature death such as that employed by FAA.

Environmental Health: Air Pollution

A great amount of work has been focused on the health effects of air pollution. Major controversy has not been focused on the value of a life or of other nontraded goods, but instead on establishing that air pollutants in specified concentrations cause increases in morbidity and mortality (47, 48, 92–100). This controversy erupted in part because of the 1970 Clean Air Act Amendments, which essentially directed the Environmental Protection Agency (EPA) to establish the levels of air quality at which no adverse health effects would result. Thus, there was no need to establish the quantitative relationship between air quality and ill health, but only that ill health resulted from a given concentration. The controversy, however, would have erupted even if the Congress had directed the EPA to apply benefit-cost analysis. For air pollution abatement, the health effects appear to be so large that, if they are caused by polluted air, a benefit-cost analysis would call for stringent abatement (47).

The older literature takes two approaches in identifying the health effects of air pollution: (a) analyses of air pollution episodes, such as occurred in London in 1952 when more than 4,000 excess deaths resulted from a prolonged inversion (47, 53, 101) and (b) analyses of workers who were exposed to high levels of air pollution on the job. Both sets of research demonstrate that very high levels of air pollution can be shown to lead to excess morbidity and mortality. However, neither set is relevant to levels of ambient air quality that are typical in cities; they suggest that society ought to avoid severe episodes and high occupational exposure, but do not address usual levels of air quality.

To estimate the health implications of long-term exposure to lower levels of pollution requires one of two approaches. If one knows the physiological mechanisms by which air pollution damages health, the effects of exposures at high concentrations may be sufficient to calibrate the functions and provide estimates of the effects at lower concentrations (102). Unfortunately, little is known of the theoretical mechanisms. The other approach consists of epidemiological studies of people exposed to lower levels of air pollution in an attempt to isolate the more subtle effects of exposure to these lower concentrations.

Until more is learned about the physiological mechanisms (from laboratory studies with lower animals and human volunteers or from analysis of natural experiments such as episodes of air pollution, there is no alternative to the epidemiological studies. Unfortunately, these studies are fraught with controversy because the observed association between pollution and health might be spurious, i.e. due to some unobserved factors that cause both the air pollution and ill health (48, 103, 104). A more subtle consequence of possible spurious correlation, as well as the difficulties with the quality of the data, is that the estimated association might be biased.

These difficulties have been recognized in reviewing work since the 1930s. However, a full scale debate has begun in the last several years, catalysed in part by the work of Lave & Seskin (47, 48, 92–100). Their finding that air pollution is consistently and significantly associated with increases in the mortality rate led them to conclude that there is a cause and effect relationship and that abating air pollution would lead to important reductions in the mortality rate (and hence improvements in life expectancy). A series of critics have questioned the quality of the data used in the analysis and have charged that the results were due, in whole or in part, to the omission of important variables, which led to a spurious correlation.

The controversy is akin to that of whether cigarette smoking causes lung cancer or the correlation is spurious (105). In this case, critics have had their resistance worn down as new studies appeared with results supporting causality. There was no single dramatic study that settled the issue, but rather a handful of important studies; many hundreds of supporting studies have convinced most scientists.

Epidemiological analysis of natural experiments involving long-term, low level exposure to some pollutant represents one of the most difficult analytic problems. No single piece of analysis or result serves either to prove causality or to estimate the quantitative association, assuming causality. Whether the air pollution-mortality association will eventually be accepted as a cause and effect relationship, the analysis has sharpened the debate. Physiologists, toxicologists, and clinicians have been stimulated to look more closely at existing data and to collect new data to examine hypotheses in order to deepen our understanding of the underlying mechanisms by which air pollution might lead to ill health. There has emerged a set of specific hypotheses regarding which pollutants are the culprits (small particles have a much easier time reaching the lower airways and acid sulfates are particularly irritating) and which seem benign (large particles are filtered out in the upper airways and sulfur dioxide is absorbed by fluid in the upper airways and the resulting acid buffered). Hypotheses have been sharpened concerning the particular variables not present in the analysis that might cause a spurious correlation between measured air pollutants and mortality. The attention in the area has resulted in additional research by new investigators. Finally, the work has served to influence the Congress in passing air pollution legislation and the EPA in creating specific regulations.

Environmental Health: Water Pollution

Estimating the costs of water pollution control is comparable to estimating the costs for air pollution control (28a,b, 33, 106–108). The same sorts of uncertainties appear concerning the speed of introduction of control and discoveries concerning new control technologies. The EPA has produced cost estimates for both media.

The categories of benefits from controlling water pollution are almost identical to those for controlling air pollution: health, plants, animals, materials damage, recreation, and aesthetics. The central difference is that central water treatment filters out virtually all of the pollution and therefore estimated health effects are quite small.

A controversy has arisen concerning the byproducts of chlorine used in treatment (109, 110a,b). Health effects are possible for pollutants that aren't treated and for people drawing water directly from a river or well, or being supplied with water from a system too small to have central treatment.

In spite of the difficulties in getting estimates of benefits or costs in which one can have confidence, the quantitative analyses have contributed both to our understanding of the issues and to policy formulation. They have served to rule out some proposed policies, as being either insufficiently stringent or too stringent, have narrowed the set of pollutants that are of primary concern, and have served to give a crude priority ordering among issues, pollutants, and geographical areas. The lesson is that, even though a formal benefit-cost analysis wasn't possible (or one in which one could have confidence wasn't possible), quantitative analysis can be used to gain insights and provide policy advice. Some early analysts pushed through formal benefit-cost analyses, making assumptions as necessary. At the time and subsequently, these analyses have been of limited utility. A more sensitive treatment of the problems, using the analysis where possible, has more to contribute. That is, one gains little by pushing the quantitative analysis further than one can have confidence in the data and estimates, but the range of techniques permits methods of lesser power to be selected whose results are worthy of confidence.

Environmental Health: Other Environmental Pollutants

A series of other environmental pollutants don't fit into the general categories of air and water. Some, like mercury, lead, and radiation, are ingested via a number of pathways so that the focus must be on the total dose, rather than on the pathway (51, 111, 112). Others, such as flourocarbons or carbon dioxide, are in one medium but aren't themselves harmful; they pose a threat because of the secondary effects they produce (113, 114).

The effects of radiation have been studied more intensively than those of virtually any other hazard (87). The effects of radiation are known and the dose-response relationships, both acute and chronic, are known with a high degree of certainty, even though there are still controversies concerning the effects of low-level, chronic doses whose predicted effects are generally too small to be detected empirically.

A series of analyses point out the implied cost per millirem of reducing human exposure and, by implication, the implicit value to society of preventing a premature death due to radiation exposure (74, 75). Analyses also point out the inconsistent policies for reducing exposure by contrasting the highly stringent standards for emissions from nuclear power plants with standards for exposure to X rays. If the total concern were for reducing total exposure, it would cost 200 to 600 times less to improve X-ray equipment and film sensitivity as to reduce routine releases from nuclear power plants.

But public understanding of the effects of radiation and suspicion of the technology has meant that the analyses have had little effect on policy. Scientific analysis simply hasn't been accepted in this area.

There is a great deal of evidence about the effects of exposures to very high levels of lead, mercury, and other substances. The devastating effects both in humans and in lower animals are well documented (51, 111, 112). However, there is much less evidence about the effects on humans of low level, long-term exposure. This is an area ripe for quantitative analysis precisely because there has been so little attempt to perform these analyses to date.

THE APPLICABILITY OF QUANTITATIVE
ANALYSIS TO PUBLIC HEALTH PROGRAMS

People who develop a technique or receive graduate training in applying it often become advocates who overstate the usefulness of their brainchild. Certainly, there are advocates of benefit-cost analysis and similar techniques who have claimed that it would solve the difficulties of formulating public policy, even in such a value-laden area as health policy.

Such advocates fail to acknowledge that the world is a terribly complicated place in which no generalizations are totally legitimate. Case studies of social decisions (such as that to have controls on air pollution emissions) reveal the complexity of the decision process and the diverse influences. Furthermore, a decision has myriad consequences, few of which can be forecast. It is easy to overstate the applicability and usefulness of analytic techniques such as benefit-cost analysis (115, 116).

Indeed, failing to recognize the complexity of decision processes and the implementation of new programs or hubris concerning the contribution of benefit-cost analysis is certain to lead to bad decisions that have little chance of being implemented.

The literature reviewed suggests that benefit-cost analysis does not provide a sufficient basis for making decisions concerning public health programs but that it is a highly useful tool for informing decisions. Values, uncertainties, and public interpretation of uncertainties are highly important in making decisions of public health programs. It should not be expected that the outputs of quantitative analysis will be unequivocal or uncontroversial; however, significant improvements in health have resulted from evaluations that led to the rejection of some services, the identification of hazards, and the adoption of effective services. The difficulty and controversy is centered in the medical evaluation of a program; once agreement has been reached on the physical inputs and cause and effect relationships, translating these into risk-benefit, cost effectiveness, or benefit-cost analysis is relatively straightforward, although additional controversy is certain to be added.

More important than deciding whether dollar benefits exceed dollar costs is the questioning approach inherent in these frameworks. One cannot assume that a program is efficacious without evidence, even though prestigious experts may "feel" that it is. One cannot begin with the notion that resources are plentiful so that one need make only some emotional plea in order to be able to mount a major health program. More attention to defining goals and to evaluating efficacy should be combined with benefit-cost analysis if we are to improve the health of the nation.

Literature Cited

1. Klarman, H. E., ed. 1970. *Empirical Studies in Health Economics.* Baltimore: Johns Hopkins Univ. Press
2. Perlman, M., ed. 1974. *The Economics of Health and Medical Care.* New York: Wiley
3. Sorkin, A. A. 1975. *Health Economics.* Lexington: Lexington Books
4. Univ. Michigan. 1969. *The Economics of Health and Medical Care.* Ann Arbor: Univ. Michigan
5. Bice, T. W. 1980. Health planning and regulation effects on hospital costs. *Ann. Rev. Public Health* 1: 137–61
6. Lave, J., Lave, L. B., Leinhardt, S. 1975. Medical manpower models: Need, demand, and supply. *Inquiry* 12(2):97–125
7. Watts, C. A., Dowling, W. L., Richardson, W. C. 1980. Strategies for the reimbursement of short-term hospitals. *Ann. Rev. Public Health* 1: 95–119
8. Lave, J., Lave, L. B. 1979. Hospital reimbursement under national health insurance. *Health Commun. Inf.* In press
9. Grossman, M. 1972. *The Demand for Health.* New York: Columbia Univ. Press
10. Newhouse, J. P., Phelps, C. E. 1974. Price and income elasticities for medical care services. See Ref. 2, pp. 139–61
11. Scitovsky, A. A., McCall, N. 1979. Impact of coinsurance on the demand for physician services. In *Health Handbook,* ed. G. Chacko. New York: North-Holland
12. Rosett, R. N., Huang, L. F. 1973. The effect of health insurance on the demand for medical care. *J. Polit. Econ.* 81(2):281–302
13. Baumol, W. J., Oates, W. E. 1975. *The Theory of Environmental Policy.* Englewood Cliffs, NJ: Prentice-Hall
14. Cochrane, A. L. 1972. *Effectiveness and Efficiency: Random Reflections on Health Services.* London: Nuffield Prov. Hosp. Trust
15. Bunker, J. P., Barnes, B. A., Mosteller, F. 1977. *Costs, Risks, and Benefits of Surgery.* New York: Oxford Univ. Press
16. Lave, J., Lave, L. B. 1970. Medical care and its delivery: An economic appraisal. *Law Contemp. Probl.* 35(2):252–66
17. Barnes, B. A. 1977. Discarded operations: Surgical innovation by trial and error. See Ref. 15, pp. 109–24
18. Bunker, J. P., Hinkley, D., McDermott,

W. V. 1978. Surgical innovation and its evaluation. *Science* 200:937–41
19. Barnes, B. A., Barnes, A. B. 1977. Evaluation of surgical therapy by cost-benefit analysis. *Surgery* 82:21–33
20. Wenneberg, J. E., Bunker, J. P., Barnes, B. 1980. The need for assessing the outcome of common medical practices. *Ann. Rev. Public Health* 1: 277–95
21. Rosen, G. 1976. Preventive medicine in the United States, 1900–1975. See Ref. 84, pp. 715–808
22. Shapiro, S. 1977. Measuring the effectiveness of prevention, II. *Milbank Mem. Fund Q.* 55(2):291–306
23. Fuchs, V. 1979. Economics, health, and post industrial society. *Milbank Mem. Fund Q.* 57(2):153–82
24. Belloc, N. B. 1973. Relationship of health practices and mortality. *Prev. Med.* 2:67–81
25. Natl. Res. Counc. 1977. *Decision Making in the Environmental Protection Agency,* Appendix D. Washington DC: GPO
26. Natl. Acad. Engineering. 1971. *Perspectives on Benefit Risk Decision Making.* Washington, DC: GPO
27. Niskanen, W. A., Harberger, A. C., Haveman, R. H., Turvey, R., Zeckhauser, R., eds. 1973. *Benefit-Cost Policy Analysis, 1972.* Chicago: Aldine
28a. Peskin, H. M., Seskin, E. P., eds. 1975. *Cost Benefit Analysis and Water Pollution Policy.* Washington DC: Urban Institute
28b. Peskin, H. M., Seskin, E. P. 1975. Introduction and overview. See Ref. 28a, pp. 1–33
29. Dasgupta, A. K., Pearce, D. W. 1972. *Cost-Benefit Analysis; Theory and Practice.* New York: Barnes & Noble
30a. Haveman, R. H., Harberger, A. C., Lynn, L. Jr., Niskanen, W. A., Turvey, R., Zeckhauser, R., eds. 1974. *Benefit Cost Analysis and Water Pollution Policy.* Chicago: Aldine
30b. Zeckhauser, R., Harberger, A., Haveman, R., Lynn, L. E. Jr., Niskanen, W. A. 1975. *Benefit-Cost and Policy Analysis 1974.* Chicago: Aldine
31. Mishan, E. J. 1971. *Cost Benefit Analysis.* New York: Praeger
32a. Klarman, H. E. 1974. Application of cost-benefit analysis to health systems technology. *J. Occup. Med.* 16:3–74
32b. Klarman, H. E. 1974. Application of cost-benefit analysis to the health ser-

vices and the special case of technological innovation. *Int. J. Health Serv.* 4(2):325–52

33. Freeman, A. M. III. 1979. *The Benefits of Environmental Improvement.* Washington DC: Resources for the Future

34. Raiffa, H., Schwartz, W., Weinstein, M. 1977. On evaluating health effects of societal programs. In *Decision Making in the Environmental Protection Agency: Selected Working Papers,* Vol. 2. Washington DC: Natl. Res. Counc.

35. Berg, R. L., ed. 1973. *Health Status Indexes.* Chicago: Hospital Res. and Educ. Trust

36. Fanshel, S., Bush, J. W. 1970. A health-status index and its applications to health services outcomes. *Oper. Res.* 28:1021–66

37. Hopkins, C. E. 1979. Patient outcome measures. In *Health Handbook,* ed. G. Chacko. New York: North-Holland

38. Trilling, D. R. 1978. A cost-effectiveness evaluation of highway safety countermeasures. *Traffic Q.* 32:41–66

39. Fischoff, B., Slovic, P., Lichtenstein, S., Read, S., Combs, B. 1978. How safe is safe enough? A psychometric study of attitudes toward technological risk and benefits. *Policy Sci.* 8:128–52

40. Fischoff, B., Slovic, P., Lichtenstein, S. 1979. Weighing the risks. *Environment* 21(4):17–38

41. Tverski, A., Kahneman, D. 1974. Judgement under uncertainty: Heuristics and biases. *Science* 185:1124

42. Kunreuther, H. 1976. Limited knowledge and insurance protection. *Public Policy* 24:227–61

43. Kunreuther, H., Slovic, P. 1978. Economics, psychology, and protective behavior. *Am. Econ. Rev.* 68:64–69

44. Starr, C. 1969. Social benefit versus technological risk. *Science* 165:1232

45. Lowrance, W. W. 1976. *Of Acceptable Risk.* Los Altos, Ca: William Kaufmann

46. Environmental Protection Agency 1972. *The Economics of Clean Air.* Washington DC: GPO

47. Lave, L. B., Seskin, E. P. 1977. *Air Pollution and Human Health.* Resources for the Future. Baltimore/London: Johns Hopkins Univ. Press

48. Lave, L. B., Seskin, E. P. 1979. Epidemiology, causality, and public policy. *Am. Sci.* 67(2)178–86

49. Crump, K. S. 1977. Estimating human risks from drug feed additives. Office of Technology Assessment, US Congress, working paper

50. Rai, K., Van Ryzin, J. 1979. Risk assessment of toxic environmental substances using a generalized multi-hit dose response model. In *Energy and Health,* ed. N. Breslow, A. Whittemore. Philadelphia: Soc. Ind. Appl. Math.

51. Natl. Inst. of Environ. Health Sci. 1977. *Human Health and the Environment— Some Research Needs,* DHEW Publication No. NIG 77–1277. Washington DC: GPO

52. Levenstein, M. J., Bishop, Y. M., Ferris, B. G. Jr., Speizer, F. E. 1979. Six city study. In *Energy and Health,* ed. N. Breslow, A. Whittemore. Philadelphia: SIAM

53. Ferris, B. G. Jr. 1980. Sulfur dioxide and particulates: Human exposure-response relationships. In *Scientific Basis of Health, Safety, and Environmental Regulation,* ed. R. Crandall, L. B. Lave. Washington DC: Brookings Inst. In press

54. McDonald, G. C., Schwing, R. C. 1973. Instabilities of regression estimates relating air pollution to mortality. *Technometrics* 15:463–81

55. Schwing, R. C., McDonald, G. C. 1976. Measures of association of some air pollutants, national ionizing radiation and cigarette smoking with mortality rates. *Sci. Total Environ.* 5:139–69

56. Mosteller, F., Tukey, J. 1978. *Exploratory Data Analysis.* Reading, Mass: Addison-Wesley

57. Pratt, J., ed. 1974. *Statistical and Mathematical Aspects of Pollution Problems.* New York: Dekker

58. Lave, L. B. 1971. Air pollution damage. In *Research on Environmental Quality,* ed. A. Kneese. Baltimore: Johns Hopkins Univ. Press

59. Bishop, J., Cichetti, C. 1975. Some institutional and conceptual thoughts on the measurement of indirect and intangible benefits and costs. See Ref. 28a, pp. 105–25

60. Arrow, K. J. 1966. Discounting and public investment criteria. In *Water Research,* ed. A. Kneese, S. Smith. Baltimore: Johns Hopkins Univ. Press

61. Baumol, W. J. 1970. On the discount rate for public projects. In *Public Expenditures and Policy Analysis,* ed. R. Haveman, J. Margolis. Chicago: Markham

62. Schelling, T. C. 1968. The life you save may be your own. In *Problems in Public Expenditure Analysis,* ed S. B. Chase. Washington DC: Brookings Inst.

63. Thaler, R. H., Rosen, S. 1976. The value of saving a life: evidence from the labor market. In *Household Production and Consumption*, ed. N. E. Terleckyj. New York: Columbia Univ. Press

64. Smith, R. S. 1976. *The Occupational Safety and Health Act.* Washington DC: Enterprise Inst. Public Policy Res.

65. Linnerooth, J. 1975. The evaluation of life-saving: A survey. RR-75-21. Laxenburg, Austria: Int. Inst. Appl. Syst. Anal.

66. Cooper, B. S., Rice, D. P. 1976. The economic cost of illness revisited. *Soc. Secur. Bull.* 39(2):21–36

67. Conley, B. C. 1976. The value of human life in the demand for safety. *Am. Econ. Rev.* 66:45–55

68. Jones-Lee, M. W. 1976. *The Value of Life: An Economic Analysis.* Chicago: Univ. Chicago Press

69. Acton, J. P. 1973. *Evaluating Public Programs to Save Lives: The Case of Heart Attacks.* Santa Monica, Calif: Rand Corp.

70. Schwing, R. C. 1978. Expenditures to reduce mortality risk and increase longevity. Working Paper, GMR-2353-A. General Motors Res. Lab., February, 1978

71. Federal Aviation Administration 1978. *Establishment of Criteria for Distance Measurement Equipment with Instrument Landing System and/or Localizer Approach Aids.* Washington DC: GPO. 77 pp.

72. Fromm, G. 1968. Civil aviation expenditures. In *Measuring the Benefits of Government Investments*, ed. R. Dorfman. Washington DC: Brookings Inst.

73. Cohen, B. L. 1979. Society valuation of life saving in radiation protection and other contexts. Working paper, Univ. Pittsburgh and Argonne Natl. Lab.

74. Cohen, B. L., Lee, I-S. 1979. Catalog of risks. Working paper, Univ. Pittsburgh

75. Terrill, J. G. Jr. 1972. Cost-benefit estimates for the major sources of radiation exposure. *Am. J. Public Health* 62(7):1008–13

76. Zeckhauser, R., Nichols, A. 1978. The occupational safety and health administration—An overview. In *Committee on Governmental Affairs, United States Senate, Study on Federal Regulation*, Appendix to *Framework for Regulation*, 6:163–248. Washington DC: GPO

77. Smith, R. 1978. Compensatory wage differentials and public policy: A review. Working paper, Cornell Univ.,

prepared under NSF grant Soc 77–15800

78. Warner, K. E., Hutton, R. C. 1979. *Benefit-Cost and Cost-Effectiveness Analysis in Health Care.* Ann Arbor: Univ. Michigan, Sch. Public Health

79. Clark, E. M., Van Horn, A. J. 1978. *Risk-Benefit Analysis and Public Policy: A Bibliography.* Cambridge, Massachusetts, Energy and Environ. Policy Cent. Cambridge: Harvard Univ. Press

80. Bendixen, H. H. 1977. The cost of intensive care. See Ref. 15, pp. 372–86

81a. Axnick, N. W., Shavell, S. M., Wittee, J. J. 1969. Benefits due to immunization against measles. *Public Health Rep.* 84(8):673–80

81b. Albritton, R. B. 1978. Cost-benefits of measles eradication: Effects of a federal intervention. *Policy Anal.* 4:1–21

82. Rosenman, R. H. 1979. The heart you save may be your own. See Ref. 11, pp. 403–27

83. LaLonde, M. 1974. *A New Perspective on the Health of Canadians.* Ottawa, Canada: Dep. Natl. Health and Welfare

84. Fogarty International Center. 1976. *Preventive Medicine USA.* New York: Prodist

85a. Starfield, B., Holtzman, N. 1975. A comparison of effectiveness screening for phynylketonuria in the United States. *N. Engl. J. Med.* 293(3):118–21

85b. Steiner, K. C., Smith, H. A. 1973. Application of cost benefit analysis to a PKU screening program. *Inquiry* 10: 34–40

86. Merchant, J. A. 1980. Byssinosis. See Ref. 53. In press

87. Biological Effects of Ionizing Radiation Advisory Committee. 1972. *The Effects of Populations of Exposures to Low Levels of Ionizing Radiation.* Washington DC: GPO

88. Mendeloff, J. 1976. *An Evaluation of the OSHA Program's Effect on Workplace Injury Rates.* Washington DC: ASPER, US Dep. Labor. 232 pp.

89. DiPietro, A. 1975. Data needs for the evaluation of OSHA's net impact. Office of Evaluation, Assistant Secretary for Policy, Evaluation and Research, US Dep. Labor. 16 pp.

90. Ashford, N. A. 1976. *Crisis in the Workplace.* Cambridge, Massachusetts: MIT Press

91. Natl. Highway Traffic Safety Admin. 1976. *Societal Costs of Motor Vehicle Accidents.* Washington DC: US Dep. Transportation

92. Landau, E. 1978. The danger in statistics. *Nation's Health* 6(3):1

93. Viren, J. R. 1979. *Cross-Sectional Estimates of Mortality Due to Fossil Fuel Pollutants: A Case of Apurious Association.* Washington DC: Dept. Energy
94. Cooper, D. E., Hamilton, W. C. 1979. Atmospheric sulfates and mortality—The phantom connection. *Am. Min. Congr.* 64:44–56
95. Lipfert, F. W. 1978. *The Association of Air Pollution with Human Mortality.* New York: Long Island Lighting Co.
96. Haveman, R. H. 1979. Review of *Air Pollution and Human Health. J. Econ. Lit.* 17:141–43
97. Thibodeau, L., Reed, R., Bishop, Y. 1979. A review of *Air Pollution and Human Health. Environ. Health Perspect.* In press
98. Natl. Res. Counc. 1978. *Sulfur Oxides.* Washington DC: GPO
99. NY Acad. Med. 1978. *Symposium on Environmental Effects of Sulfur Oxides and Related Particulates-1978.* New York: NY Acad. Med.
100. Lave, L. B., Seskin, E. P. 1977. Air pollution and human health. *Science* 169:723–33
101. Goldsmith, J. R., Friberg, L. T. 1976. Effects on human health. In *The Effects of Air Pollution,* Vol. 2, ed. A. Stern. New York: Academic
102. Amdur, M. O. 1977. Toxicological guidelines for research on sulfur oxides and particulates. *Proc. Symp. Stat. Environ., ASA, 4th,* Washington DC, p. 48
103. Simon, H. 1954. Spurious correlations: A causal interpretation. *J. Am. Stat. Assoc.* 49:467–79
104. Hill, A. B. 1965. The environment and diseases: Associations and causations. *Proc. Royal Soc. Med.* 58:295–300
105. Sterling, T. D. 1975. A critical reassessment of the evidence bearing on smoking as the cause of lung cancer. *Am. J. Public Health* 65(9):939–53
106. Gianessi, L. P., Peskin, H. M. 1977. *Water pollution discharges: A comparison of recent national estimates.* Resources for the Future Discussion Paper, D-2
107. Tihansky, D. 1975. A survey of empirical benefit studies. See Ref. 28a, pp. 127–72
108. Hanke, S., Gutmanis, I. 1975. Estimates of industrial water-borne residuals control costs: A review of concepts, methodology, and empirical results. See Ref. 28a, pp. 231–68
109. Hoel, D., Crump, K. 1980. Scientific evidence of risks from water-borne carcinogens. See Ref. 53. In press
110a. Harris, R., Page, T., Reiches, N. 1977. Carcinogenic hazards of organic chemicals in drinking water. In *Origins of Human Cancer,* ed. H. Hiatt, J. Watson, J. Winsten, pp. 308–30
110b. Page, T., Harris, R. H., Epstein, S. S. 1976. Drinking water and cancer mortality in Louisiana. *Science* 193:55–57
111. Natl. Acad. Sci. 1977. *Drinking Water and Health,* Washington DC: GPO
112. Natl. Acad. Sci. 1977. *Effects of a Polluted Environment.* Natl. Res. Counc. Comm. on Natural Resources. Washington DC: GPO
113. Natl. Acad. Sci. 1979. *Protection Against Depletion of Stratospheric Ozone by Chlorofluorcarbons.* Washington DC: NAS. In press
114. US Dep. Energy. 1979. *Carbon Dioxide Effects Research and Assessment Program: Workshop on the Global Effects of Carbon Dioxide From Fossil Fuels.* Conf 770385. Washington DC: GPO
115. Fischoff, B. 1977. Cost benefit analysis and the art of motorcycle maintenance. *Policy Sci.* 8:177–202
116. Rowen, R. 1975. The role of cost-benefit analysis in policy making. See Ref. 28a, pp. 361–69

Ann. Rev. Public Health 1980. 1:277–95
Copyright © 1980 by Annual Reviews Inc. All rights reserved

THE NEED FOR ASSESSING THE OUTCOME OF COMMON MEDICAL PRACTICES

♦12510

*John E. Wennberg**

Department of Community Medicine, Dartmouth Medical School, Hanover, New Hampshire 03755

*John P. Bunker**

Stanford University School of Medicine, Stanford, California 94305

*Benjamin Barnes**

Harvard Medical School, Boston, Massachusetts 02115

INTRODUCTION

Medical innovations have not generally been subjected to rigorous evaluation prior to their widespread use by the medical community (1, 2). As a result, a good deal of uncertainty and disagreement exists among physicians concerning the value of many common practices in all fields of medicine—uncertainty and disagreement which is in turn reflected in the large variations in therapeutic practices among physicians and among groups of physicians and in the large variations in the frequency with which therapeutic procedures are prescribed for one population or another.

In this chapter we summarize the controversies concerning surgery for the treatment of common, noncancerous conditions. Based on epidemiologic data, we estimate the costs associated with different frequencies of prescribing surgery. The varying probabilities that patients will undergo specific procedures, when summed across the populations living in geographically defined medical market areas (3, 4) [or counties (5), states (6),

*Partially supported by a grant (18T97192/1-02) from the Health Care Financing Administration, DHEW.

277

0163-7525/80/0510-0277$01.00

and nations (7)], translate into costs that vary strikingly from area to area. The significance of the different levels of population exposure to the procedures cannot be fully assessed because of incomplete evidence on outcomes. However, data on the average dollar costs and on the immediate risk of death associated with exposure to a unit of service are available, and we use them to estimate the per capita dollar cost and per capita death rates associated with different exposure rates as recorded in the United States and elsewhere. We argue that the cost implications of professional uncertainty justify a substantial investment to clarify the advantages and disadvantages of the various approaches to common medical problems.

CONTROVERSIES CONCERNING THE VALUE OF COMMON SURGICAL PROCEDURES

Our intention is to indicate the nature of current controversies concerning the value of selected surgical procedures and to call attention to recent articles that discuss the issues in greater depth. We make no attempt to review the entire literature but, rather, we illustrate the issues through selected articles. Using National Center for Health Statistics data for 1975, we identify the nine most common surgical procedures that result in organ repair, organectomy, or organotomy (8). We consider their use for treatment of common, noncancerous conditions. The procedures are discussed in order of their frequency in the United States in 1975.

Hysterectomy for Sterilization

Hysterectomy goes without challenge when performed for cancer of the uterine cervix or endometrium, for prolapse, or for a large, bleeding fibroid tumor. Controversy arises over elective hysterectomy for sterilization or for cancer prophylaxis, with the medical profession sharply divided. How often hysterectomy is performed for these reasons is difficult to say; because of the controversy and because reimbursement may be denied, other diagnoses, such as stress incontinence or pelvic relaxation, may be listed in the hospital record. Some idea of the magnitude of hysterectomy for sterilization can be gained, however, from the fact that the total number of hysterectomies performed nationally rose from 525,000 in 1970 to 725,000 in 1975, an increase of 38%. The sharpest increase in rates occurred between 1970 and 1973 (30%), during the years in which the earlier strong proscription against sterilization was being relaxed.

Hysterectomy as a method of sterilization is less cost effective than tubal ligation (9). To justify hysterectomy for this purpose, it is necessary to invoke some additional indication. Prevention of future cancer of the cervix and endometrium (and of the ovaries if they, too, are removed) is the usual second indication. Hysterectomy in a good risk young woman probably does increase life-expectancy, and, on the average, by as much as 2.5 months (10).

For most women, however, there is no gain at all, because all of the increase is received by the 1.3% of women otherwise destined to die of cancer of the cervix or endometrium and, therefore, it is by no means clear that this gain is worth the risks of hysterectomy. The risk of anesthetic or surgical death is relatively small—probably between 0.05% and 0.1% in a 30-year-old woman in good general health—but the morbidity is substantial, and post-operative recovery is apt to be prolonged when compared to other major surgery such as cholecystectomy and appendectomy (11.9 months in one survey of patients as compared to 3.0 months) (11). Forty days after hysterectomy, 5% of women report they feel "worse" or "much worse" than they did prior to surgery and 35% still have one or more problems related to their surgery (12). In the year following hysterectomy, there are fewer hospitalizations than in the year preceding surgery, and there are a smaller number of visits to physicians and to hospital outpatient and emergency rooms (N. Roos and L. Roos, work in progress, University of Manitoba, 1979); however, although the number of women making visits for uterine-related diagnoses such as prolapse, disturbances of menstruation, and endometriosis is decreased, there are more visits for urinary tract infections, psychiatric problems, menopausal symptoms, skin infections and inflammations, and back problems. Although the majority of women who have undergone hysterectomy report that they are glad they had the surgery, and many report feeling better emotionally (13), more hysterectomy patients are referred for psychiatric care than are women who have undergone cholecystectomy or appendectomy (11, 14).

Whether the benefits of elective hysterectomy for sterilization and/or for cancer prophylaxis are worth these risks is a highly personal matter. The very high hysterectomy rates for physicians' wives (15) suggest that the "informed consumer" places a high value on this operation. On the other hand, there are reasons to doubt that the average risk-averse individual would wish to undertake even a small risk of death or serious injury in the hope for uncertain benefits far in the future (16). The decision should clearly be made by the patient, herself, on the basis of reliable data on potential risks and benefits. Unfortunately, there are no comprehensive data on the quality-of-life benefits of hysterectomy (17) or on patient preferences and, therefore, the issue is for the moment unresolvable.

Tonsillectomy for Hypertrophy of the Tonsil

Although tonsillectomy for hypertrophy of the tonsil may have been beneficial before the availability of antibiotics, there is no evidence for its effectiveness in the vast majority of cases today. The parents of many children do report fewer episodes of sore throats following tonsillectomy, but it is not clear whether this is the result of the operation or simply of growing older (18). The variability in professional judgment concerning the indication for this procedure was dramatically illustrated in a classic study reported in 1934: In a sample of 1000 New York school children 11 years of age, 60% were already tonsillectomized. The remaining 40% were examined by school physicians who selected 45% for T & A. The children not selected for tonsillectomy were reexamined by a second group of physicians who recommended that 45% undergo the procedure. The third examination of the twice-rejected children by yet another group of physicians produced recommendations for the operation in 44%; only 65 children of the original 1000 survived the screening examination without a recommendation for tonsillectomy (19).

In more recent years, the climate of clinical opinion is swinging against the widespread use of tonsillectomy. The rate peaked in earlier decades of this century and is declining in popularity, the numbers dropping by 50% between 1965 and 1975. The increase of the controversy, along with pediatricians' antipathy for the procedure, appears to have played an important role in its decline (20). One article in the *New England Journal of Medicine* labeled the procedure as "ritualistic surgery" (21). Presumably, a well-designed randomized clinical trial could have clarified this controversy long ago, but no such studies have been undertaken for the use of tonsillectomy for hypertrophy of the tonsil. [In an extensive randomized clinical trial currently underway, uncomplicated hypertrophy of the tonsil is not considered a valid reason for entry into the study (J. Bluestone, personal communication).] Nevertheless, despite evidence of the loss of popularity of tonsillectomy, the tonsil was the second most frequently removed organ in the United States in 1975.

Repair of Inguinal Hernia

Inguinal herniorrhaphy, when performed to correct a definite hernia, with or without localized pain and with or without episodes of incarceration, is a classical surgical procedure that virtually every physician recommends, excluding only premature infants and patients that have associated disease that substantially increases the risk of morbid or mortal complications (22). Among the procedures reviewed for this chapter, its use appears to be the least controversial. However, the diagnosis of an inguinal hernia, although straightforward in a young person with a thin abdominal wall, may be more difficult in older patients, particularly the obese, in whom a general weakness of muscles and connective tissue of the lower abdomen may be confused with a hernia. The possibility thus exists that some patients undergo "unnecessary" inguinal herniorrhaphies because of uncertainty of some surgeons in establishing the diagnosis. If the surgical teaching in a certain community is in favor of interpreting physical signs broadly, the diagnosis will be more common than in medical communities where the surgical tradition and teaching has been more rigorous and exacting.

Some controversy does exist concerning the use of the procedure in the elderly. Neuhauser compared the impact on life expectancy of 65-year-old men under two alternative methods of treating inguinal hernia: an operation and a supportive truss (23). Although he found the data for making estimates weak, he concluded that the immediate risk of death associated with the surgical procedure exceeds the future risk of death associated with a possible emergency obstruction when a truss is worn; thus, the decision to undertake the procedure on patients greater than 65 years of age can probably not be justified on the basis of extending life but must be based on its effect on the quality of life. In the patient's mind, the quality of life improvements may easily justify the risks involved, but the choice must be made by the patient and not all informed patients will make the same choice. Neuhauser compares the choices made by two surgeons as patients: One, who once used a truss, complained that they are "dirty, tight, uncomfortable, hot, and smelly"; another surgeon, 69 years of age, "had a painless hernia and preferred to avoid an operation. For him, the truss was the preferred choice" (23). Beyond the anecdotal, there is little evidence concerning the quality of life implications of the use of a truss or on the complication rates associated with either approach; as with many operations, informed choice based on probable outcomes is, for the patient, exceedingly difficult.

Cholecystectomy for Silent Gallstones

There is substantial agreement within the profession that cholecystectomy, when undertaken for obstructive jaundice and/or biliary colic secondary to cholelithiasis, for a severe attack of acute cholecystitis, for cancer of the gallbladder, and for a few other less frequent conditions, can provide substantial symptomatic relief and is sometimes lifesaving. Cholecystectomy for patients with asymptomatic, "silent," or minimally symptomatic gallstones, however, provokes widespread disagreement among clinicians (24).

At the extremes, some physicians pursue the aggressive surgical policy that all gallstones should be removed together with the gallbladder unless the patient is an unacceptable operative risk; others are noninterventionist, promoting the medical point of view that patients may be safely buried with their gallstones and not because of them. The latter point of view is buttressed by the repeated autopsy findings that indicate a high incidence of gallstones in patients expiring from other diseases (25).

In an attempt to resolve this continuing professional dilemma, Fitzpatrick and his associates have examined the impact of elective cholecystectomy for minimally symptomatic gallstones on the life expectancy of good
and poor risk middle-aged patients (26). "The most striking finding is that
the losses and gains are small, the largest being of the order of a month
saved" (for low risk patients who accept the procedure); poor risk patients
stand to lose two weeks of life expectancy if they elect the procedure. The
authors conclude, "The decision to operate on a silent gallstone ought not
to be based solely on life expectancy, but should be heavily influenced by
other considerations such as risk of morbidity and patient's peace of mind."
Unfortunately, the quality of life aspects of outcome are poorly documented
and there is little objective information on which to base an analysis of the
trade-off. The importance of the problem is indicated by estimates that
9.6% (27) to 12% (24) of the adult population carry silent gallstones.

Extraction of Lens for Cataract

The use of lens extractions doubled on a per capita basis in the United States
between 1965 and 1975 and an intense debate is occurring concerning the
indications for the procedure. A 1978 editorial in the *Archives of Ophthalmology* quipped that this increase in rate of use of the procedure has "placed
ophthalmology in the eye of a surgical storm" (28). Jaffe has recently
reviewed the major controversies (29). Removal of the cataract is only the
first step in restoring vision. The traditional means of postoperative refrac-
tion involves cataract spectacles that cause reduction in peripheral vision
and distort objects through magnification. A more recent technique uses a
contact lens, which reduces distortion but cannot be used in many patients,
particularly the elderly (the population most likely to receive the procedure). A third technique, lens extraction followed by lens implantation, is
considered the treatment of choice in the elderly and infirm, but it is a
procedure with greater risk of complications. Jaffe states his perspective on
the decision to operate:

> Faced with a patient whose cataracts have lessened his vision . . . the only pertinent
> question is whether the operation will benefit the patient. The surgeon's ability to achieve
> a satisfactory anatomic result is of lesser importance. It may not be fully appreciated how
> disabled a person can be after a perfectly executed uniocular cataract operation. There
> are countless patients who have corrected visual acuity of 20/20 in one eye after cataract
> operation but who find it impossible to use the eye because the opposite eye, not operated
> on, still has useful vision. A cataract spectacle lens cannot be worn unilaterally because
> there is a 30% difference in retinal image size between the unoperated eye and the
> optically corrected aphakic eye. It is not unusual for patients to prefer to perform most
> manual and physical activities with the help of the eye not operated on even though it
> may have 20/60 to 20/80 vision because of an incipient cataract. This situation fre-

quently causes the surgeon to recommend cataract surgical removal in the eye with an incipient cataract to achieve binocularity. This step will improve the situation, but in the end the patient may be little better off after two cataract operations than he was before the first operation. Many patients are sorely disillusioned after a "perfect cataract operation" has made them functionally more disabled.

Caesarian Section

Between 1965 and 1975 the percentage of deliveries in the United States performed by Caesarian section more than doubled, with most of the increase occurring after 1970 (8). Since 1970, clinical strategies have been greatly influenced by changing opinion on the use of Caesarian sections for breech presentation (30, 31) and by use of electronic fetal monitoring (EFM) to detect fetal distress. In both cases, the changes have occurred without benefit of a randomized clinical trial (RCT). Subsequent RCTs have challenged the claims for the efficacy of routine Caesarian section for breech delivery (32) and of the routine use of fetal monitoring for low-risk deliveries (33). Haverkamp's RCT on high-risk deliveries indicates that EFM produces no more favorable results than traditional auscultation techniques but is associated with an increase in risk of use of Caesarean section (34). A recent exhaustive review of the EFM literature by Banta & Thacker concludes that EFM provides little increased benefit when compared with older techniques of detecting fetal distress: "The risk from EFM is substantial, especially but not wholly through the increased Caesarian section rate that its use apparently engenders" (35).

Routine use of EFM is the conventional wisdom of contemporary obstetrics. Banta & Thacker's critique of the scientific basis of that practice ignited an intense (36–39), sometimes *ad hominem* (40–43) controversy within the profession. The importance for the public health of the increased use of Caesarians includes increased risk of material morbidity and death associated with increased Caesarian sections (44), risk of respiratory distress syndrome in the infant (45) and risk imposed to subsequent infants who are likely to be delivered by Caesarian section (because of the rule, "Once a Caesarian always a Caesarian") (46).

Appendectomy

For over 90 years, the solution to acute appendicitis has been the surgical removal of the inflamed appendix. There is little controversy that the classic progression of the disease—from minimal abdominal pain, nausea, and vomiting to a full-fledged mass in the right lower quadrant followed by appendiceal perforation, general peritonitis, malfunction of the bowel and likely death—should be interrupted as soon as possible by surgery. The controversies concern when to operate: Other causes of abdominal pain, nausea, and vomiting are commonly confused with appendicitis, leading to appendectomy in patients who do not have appendicitis. Neutra (47) has analyzed the circumstances associated with making a diagnosis of appendicitis. His analysis makes explicit the weights that physicians attach to the costs of various outcomes: the true positive, the false positive, the true negative, the false negative. In the equivocal case, the judgment of the physician will be influenced by the subjective weight he gives to (a) missing the early false negative case and delaying intervention (with the possible complication of an abscess or perforation) and (b) operating on the false positive patient. deDombal and his associates (48) and Graham (49) have shown that computer-assisted diagnosis can improve clinical judgment, helping the physician to reduce the number of false positive cases that receive appendectomy.

Alternative therapeutic approaches to acute appendicitis involving the use of antibiotics have occasionally been proposed but never seriously tested (50). Considering its antiquity, it is not surprising that appendectomy has never been subjected to a randomized clinical trial. This, however, may soon change, at least for one indication for use of the procedure: A recent editorial in the *Lancet* (51) suggests that a randomized prospective trial is needed to test the value of appendectomy in the treatment of appendiceal abscess, a complication of acute appendicitis that is usually treated in the United Kingdom by simple drainage followed by appendectomy two or three months later. The suggestion is based on the apparent good outcomes of patients with appendiceal abscesses who did not undergo the conventional treatment (52).

Prostatectomy for Prostatic Hypertrophy

Prostatectomy for benign prostatic hypertrophy has largely escaped the furor of the unnecessary surgery debate, despite the fact that variations in prostatectomy rates are approximately as great as for hysterectomy, and greater than for cholecystectomy or appendectomy. In estimated total costs, prostatectomy is exceeded only by hysterectomy and cholecystectomy (Table 2) and in expected number of surgery-related deaths is exceeded only by cholecystectomy (Table 3). Why, then, has there been no concern expressed? The principal reason seems to be that neither the urologists, themselves, nor the referring physicians have broken rank to question the indications for prostatectomy. This is in marked contrast to the sharp professional disagreements surrounding hysterectomy, cholecystectomy, and tonsillectomy. Nevertheless, it is apparent that there are two distinct camps: (a) the early-interventionists, who believe that prostatic resection should be carried out when early symptoms of urinary obstruction are first apparent, while the patient is relatively young and in reasonably good physical condition and (b) members of the conservative school, who believe that early symptoms may not be relieved by surgery and that symptoms may remain mild to moderate for many years without surgery.

The issue and the arguments are the same as those for many other surgical diseases. Note the similarity to the controversy over cholecystectomy for minimally symptomatic gallstones: Surgery will entail lower risks if carried out electively today than later as an emergency. On the other hand, elective surgery does carry significant risk and, if it can be deferred, may never become necessary. The question of the impact on life expectancy is straightforward and, using currently available risk data for prostatectomy, should be amenable to quantitative analysis (2).

Ultimately, as for other primarily elective operations, the decision concerning whether to operate should rest on the preferences and values of the individual patient. Little has been published on the preferences of patients suffering from benign prostatic hypertrophy, but the personal observations of Dr. Maurice Root, a retired physician, recounted in a recent letter to the editor of the *New England Journal of Medicine* (53) (July 5, 1979), offer at least a hint of a possible alternative to surgery:

> Benign prostatic hypertrophy has awakened me several times a night for years. This past winter my loss of water through perspiration was reduced; I began to wake up every hour or two with visions of an impending transurethral resection. There was always more urine that could be voided by pushing and pumping after I had seemingly emptied my bladder. I thought that there was probably a considerable volume of residual urine that would sooner or later cause infection and necessitate an operation. I began to spend a minute or more voiding, but carefully not straining, until no more spurts could be obtained. The results were immediate and dramatic. I now sleep three or four hours at a time and occasionally get up only once in eight hours, even in warm weather. If I am lazy and fail to take plenty of time to void, there is a prompt return of the frequency. It may be that this technique will preclude unnecessary surgery, even without a second opinion.

Hemorrhoidectomy

In contrast to the rather discrete pathological anatomy associated with an inguinal hernia, the abnormality in patients with hemorrhoids is more diffuse; its severity is frequently not easy to assess and the interpretation depends almost entirely on the physician's evaluation of the patient's history and physical findings. The problem can be handled in a variety of ways: sclerosing injections, rubber banding, maximal dilatation of the anal canal, cryotherapy (freezing), and the more traditional surgical excision with plastic repairs of varying degrees of complexity. One authority states, "In general, hemorrhoids need no treatment at all" (54). An editorial in the *British Medical Journal* calls for the cessation of surgical approaches to the problem in most patients (55). A similar editorial in the *Lancet* ("To Tie, To Stab; Perchance to Freeze") states that the "aim should be to avoid hospital admission and operation if possible" (56).

IDENTIFIED COSTS ASSOCIATED WITH VARIOUS STRATEGIES FOR USING COMMON SURGICAL PROCEDURES

In the foregoing section we have seen that the benefits of common procedures for many conditions are poorly defined. We address the cost side of the ledger in this section, looking at cost in terms of dollars and lives under various rates of use of seven of the nine procedures. Because of the lack of comparative data, cost estimates have not been made for variations in the rate of use of Caesarian sections and lens extractions.

Methods for Estimating Costs

The two aspects of cost we estimate are per capita death rates and hospitalization dollar costs associated with surgery. To estimate these costs under various strategies for using common procedures, we have reviewed the literature on population exposure to surgery. We have based our estimates on the range of exposure to surgery reported among health regions in the United Kingdom and among Canadian provinces for 1974 by K. McPherson and A. M. Epstein (unpublished); among states or major metropolitan areas in the United States for 1971 reported in the American College of Surgeons study on surgical services for the United States (57); and among medical market areas in Vermont and Maine for 1975 reported by the Codman Research Groups.[1] We have also used the estimated rate of surgery for the United States in 1975 provided by the National Center for Health Statistics (8). The extent of variation in population exposure rates to surgery reported in these studies is given in Table 1.

Estimates for average cost per hospitalization include surgeon's fees and are based on data provided by the Maine Health Data Service.[2] The data are for Maine in 1975. Case fatality rates (proportion of cases having undergone surgery who are discharged dead from hospital) have been obtained from the Commission on Professional and Hospital Activities (58). The estimates for expenditures and surgery associated deaths for each area are linear extrapolations from the area's exposure rates:

Expected cost =   Surgical exposure X Average cost
per capita   per capita   per case

Expected deaths = Surgical exposure X Average case
per capita   per capita   fatality

---

[1]*Final Report, Year 1: The Impact of Health Planning and Regulation on the Patterns of Hospital Utilization in New England,* Contract #291760003, Codman Research Group, Washington DC, September 1, 1977.

[2]Maine Health Data Service, 110 Free Street, Portland, Maine 04101.

Table 1 Surgical procedure rates per capita in various geographic areas: Rates expressed as ratio to US national rates, 1975

Procedure	United Kingdom regional health authorities		SOSSUS[a] areas		Canadian province		Maine & Vermont hospital service areas		Ratio high to low
	Low	High	Low	High	Low	High	Low	High	
Hysterectomy	.23	.39	.59	1.26	.77	1.11	.49	1.43	6.20
Tonsillectomy	.52	.94	.79	2.06	.77	1.88	.33	1.83	6.19
Inguinal hernia	.40	.63	.81	1.16	.60	1.04	.69	1.19	2.95
Cholecystectomy	.26	.49	.48	.90	1.27	2.42	.67	1.57	9.09
Appendectomy	.87	1.38	.67	1.13	.83	1.35	.40	1.40	3.45
Prostatectomy	.24	.55	.46	.85	.34	.95	.54	1.92	8.06
Hemorrhoidectomy	.23	.39	.60	.80	.52	1.14	.20	1.00	7.55
All listed	.32	.59	.54	.97	.83	1.62	.58	1.59	5.00

[a]*Study on Surgical Services for the United States* (57).

The expenditure estimates are thus based on the assumption that mean cost in dollars and in fatalities per case within areas (regions, states, counties, or hospital service areas) is not proportional to the per capita rate of surgery. Studies within Maine indicate that this is a reasonable assumption (59).

Use of an estimate for the national case fatality rate (58) to estimate case fatality rates in populations exposed to differing rates of surgery deserves some further explanation. The problem is to know whether areas with higher rates of surgery have higher or lower case fatality rates. If the selection criteria in high rate areas favor candidates with, on the average, fewer risk factors than members selected for surgery in low rate populations, then the assumption would be incorrect and the method would over-predict the range of per capita deaths. However, if the trend is in the reverse direction—toward the selection of more risky cases in the high rate areas —then the assumption would also be wrong, but in the opposite direction: It would underestimate the number of surgical associated deaths in high rate areas. In the absence of evidence on the direction of the bias, we have selected the estimate for the national average case fatality rate as the best available estimate.

It is important also to point out that, at least for some of the nine operations, fewer operations and fewer surgical deaths will presumably mean more deaths among those who are not selected for surgery. It is our hypothesis that the lives saved as a result of fewer operations will be greater in number than those lost, as we are concerned with patients presenting minimal indications for surgery. Available data for many of the cases summarized above are consistent with this hypothesis, and for at least three procedures (lens extraction, tonsillectomy, hemorrhoidectomy), the disease itself is never fatal. Nevertheless, it should be recognized that the calculations do not take into account the possibility of an increase in non-surgical deaths.

In the following analysis, dollars and deaths associated with various strategies of use of the seven procedures are estimated for the US population in 1975.

Dollar Costs

The estimated expenditures for care under the various strategies for allocating the seven surgical procedures are listed in Table 2. If the surgery rates used in the low rate health region in the United Kingdom were the norm for the United States, the dollar investment in the procedures in 1975 would be $1.5 billion; under the high rate strategies in the Canadian provinces and in the Vermont/Maine study, the investment would be over $6.7 billion; the low Vermont/Maine strategy results in an estimated expenditure of $2.4

Table 2 Estimated expenditures (1975, in millions of dollars) for surgical care under various strategies for allocating common surgical technology to populations

Procedure	United Kingdom		SOSSUS[a]		Canada		Vermont/Maine		USA
	Low	High	Low	High	Low	High	Low	High	
Hysterectomy	308	523	791	1,690	1,033	1,489	657	1,918	1,341
Tonsillectomy	191	345	290	756	283	690	180	525	367
Inguinal hernia	234	369	474	679	351	608	404	696	585
Cholecystectomy	245	461	452	847	1,195	2,276	630	1,477	941
Appendectomy	360	570	277	467	343	558	165	579	413
Prostatectomy	149	342	286	529	212	840	336	1,195	622
Hemorrhoidectomy	57	97	149	199	129	284	50	249	249
All listed	1,544	2,707	2,719	5,167	3,546	6,745	2,422	6,639	4,527

[a]Study on Surgical Services for the United States (57).

billion. The Table also gives the differences in expenditures between the extreme examples of rates of use. For the seven procedures, the difference in expenditures between a US national rate of surgery based on the low example of use in the United Kingdom and one based on the high example of use seen in the Canadian study is over $5 billion. Among the individual procedures, strategies for use of hysterectomies, cholecystectomies, and prostatectomies result in the greatest net differences in expenditures: For hysterectomies, the difference between high and low use strategies projected to the US population is $1.5 billion; for cholecystectomy it is $2.0 billion; and for prostatectomy it is $1.0 billion.

These costs do not, of course, reflect the alternative costs for nonsurgical management of the condition. These costs are large and certainly important, but for most operations there are no reliable data on which to estimate them. An important consideration in attempting to compare the costs, however, is the fact that surgical costs are incurred at the present time, whereas nonsurgical costs are incurred as a stream into the future and, therefore, are subject to an appropriate discount rate. Thus, Cole & Berlin, in their study of the cost effectiveness of elective hysterectomy, estimated an average cost for hysterectomy of $2,900, an average undiscounted cost of nonoperative gynecological care of $1,417, and an average cost of nonoperative gynecological care of $570 at a discount rate of 6% (10). In making comparisons of surgical and nonsurgical management, it is also necessary to include the future disease-related costs of the care of patients following surgery, including, of course, the costs of the treatment of surgery-related complications. In the absence of complete data on which to make such comparisons, we postulate that for comparable populations and for the common conditions examined here the aggregate costs of surgical care for patients presenting marginal indications for these nine operations are greater than the costs of alternatives because of the higher initial investment and the occurrence of expensive complications after surgery.

Expected Numbers of Surgery-Associated Deaths

The estimated numbers of surgery-associated deaths that would occur in the United States in 1975 under the various strategies for allocating the seven procedures is given in Table 3. The Table also gives the percentage of all deaths in the United States in 1975 represented by each estimate. Under the high rate use strategy that is observed in the Canadian province study, the number of expected deaths exceeds 20,000; this number is equal to 1.07% of all deaths in the United States in that year. The high Vermont/Maine strategy results in nearly the same estimate. The United Kingdom low strategy predicts about 4000 deaths, which is equal to .21% of all deaths in the United States in that year (60). The estimates thus indicate a five-fold difference in the probability of deaths associated with surgery in the jurisdictions selected for this study. (These estimates do not take into account the possible increase in nonsurgical deaths, as discussed in the previous section.)

Among the individual procedures, cholecystectomy and prostatectomy stand out as the most significant contributors to the death rate. For cholecystectomy, generalizing the high area rates for Canadian provinces to the United States population predicts over 12,000 deaths; generalizing the low rate (United Kingdom) predicts less than 1400. The difference—over 10,000 deaths—is greater than the annual number of deaths from automobile accidents in the United States for persons aged 55 years and older. Prostatectomies show a somewhat less extensive range with a low estimate of 840 deaths associated with the United Kingdom low strategy and 6768 deaths associated with the Vermont/Maine high strategy. Most of these deaths are in males over the age of 65. There were 615,000 deaths among males over 65, which suggests that under the high strategy, about 1% of United States males over 65 could expect to die following prostatectomy.

As with dollar costs, we need to know the savings in lives as well as the costs in lives. For elective hysterectomy among low risk patients, the savings in lives may be substantial, but they are deferred far into the future and restricted to the 1.3% of those who would otherwise develop cancer of the uterine cervix or fundus. For patients with minimally symptomatic gallstones, the balance of gains and losses of life expectancy between surgical and expectant management depend on patient risk status. For asymptomatic inguinal hernia in the elderly, and perhaps for appendectomy for minimal symptoms, there may be a loss of life expectancy with surgical management. For prostatectomy, a similar situation may exist. For lens extraction, hemorrhoidectomy, and for tonsillectomy, there are, of course, no gains in life expectancy as a result of surgery.

Table 3 Expected number of deaths associated with surgery in United States under various strategies for allocating surgical technology to population[a]

Procedure	United Kingdom		SOSSUS[b]		Canada		Vermont/Maine		USA
	Low	High	Low	High	Low	High	Low	High	
Hysterectomy	241	407 (1.7)[c]	623	1,326 (2.1)	808	1,172 (1.5)	512	1,506 (2.9)	1,055
Tonsillectomy	33	59 (1.8)	50	130 (2.6)	49	119 (2.4)	21	115 (5.5)	63
Inguinal hernia	562	873 (1.6)	1,124	1,606 (1.4)	830	1,445 (1.7)	963	1,659 (1.7)	1,389
Cholecystectomy	1,367	2,490 (1.8)	2,440	4,639 (1.9)	6,495	12,427 (1.9)	3,414	8,053 (2.4)	5,132
Appendectomy	956	1,522 (1.6)	738	1,250 (1.7)	926	1,485 (1.6)	440	1,544 (3.5)	1,104
Prostatectomy	840	1,949 (2.3)	1,624	2,979 (1.8)	1,192	3,358 (2.8)	1,895	6,768 (3.6)	3,521
Hemorrhoidectomy	46	78 (1.7)	121	161 (1.3)	105	229 (2.2)	40	201 (5.0)	201
All listed	4,045	7,378 (1.8)	6,720	12,091 (1.8)	10,405	20,235 (1.9)	7,285	19,846 (2.7)	12,465
% of all US deaths (1975)	.21	.39	.36	.64	.55	1.07	.38	1.05	.66

[a] Standardized to US population, 1975.
[b] Study on Surgical Services for the United States (57).
[c] Figures in parentheses denote high to low ratios.

DISCUSSIONS AND CONCLUSIONS

The foregoing review of the controversies concerning the effectiveness of surgery as one approach to the treatment of common conditions shows that clear information on the risks and the expected gains of alternative methods of treatment does not exist as part of a systematic, accepted body of scientific knowledge. Variations in rates of use of surgery occur, in part, because professional consensus on the value of specific uses of surgical technology is lacking. There are, however, substantial nonmonetary costs associated with the use of surgery: the pain and discomfort of hospitalization; the mortality and morbidity associated with surgery. These costs are greater among populations receiving greater amounts of surgery per capita: we estimate in this chapter, using reports on rates of surgery, a four-fold difference in surgery-associated deaths per capita and expenditures per capita between populations experiencing high and low rates of exposure to seven common procedures. We also cite evidence suggesting that the choice of treatment will vary among informed patients, some relying on surgery, others preferring nonsurgical modalities of care. The expected outcomes of such medical choices are unclear, however, and therefore can be anticipated with certainty by neither patients nor doctors. The full implications of this uncertainty for public policy cannot be addressed within this paper; however, two implications are discussed briefly to emphasize the need for improving knowledge about medical care outcomes through assessing existing treatment alternatives.

1. The limits on informed decision-making in medical markets are more severe than is generally realized, a fact that affects physicians as well as patients. If the outcomes of alternative treatments are not understood, how is it possible to make informed decisions or give informed consent? Informed decision-making is particularly problematic when an intervention is undertaken to improve in some uncertain way the quality of life, when the trade-off demonstrably involves an increased risk of immediate death or iatrogenic complication, and when there is little or no expected increase in life expectancy. Such is the case for many of the surgical applications reviewed in this paper. When decisions are made, whose values are being expressed, the patient's or the physician's? The geographic variations in exposure rates are consistent with the thesis that medical care choices are highly dependent on the preferences of physicians. When professional disagreement is strong and patients delegate decision-making to physicians, the probability of exposure to specific interventions will often depend on the style of practice of the physician or clinic selected for care rather than the nature and severity of illness.

2. The second implication is for public regulatory policy: Much of current policy is based on the belief that an underlying professional consensus exists on the optimum methods for allocating medical technology. For example, such programs as the Professional Standards Review Organization assume that meaningful consensus exists on which standards of care can be developed that will promote the public health by insuring that only necessary hospitalizations and procedures are undertaken. Similarly, the development of national standards for health resources—physicians per capita and facilities per capita—rests on the assumption that there is a determined relationship between resource input and health care outcomes. However, the existing evidence is usually insufficient to settle controversies on the value of common medical practices. Therefore, consensus standards represent weighted averages of those selected to establish them and cannot serve as a basis for the rational allocation of medical care technology. Indeed, without more direct information on the outcomes of alternative approaches, rational allocation is not possible if the criterion for rationality is the maximization of health through the efficient use of health care.

The most widely accepted method for acquiring systematic descriptions of clinical outcomes associated with alternative therapeutic modalities is probably the randomized clinical trial (1). However, case control studies that take advantage of natural experiments generated by the various rates of exposure to medical or surgical intervention should be useful for characterizing major outcome differences. In the design of protocols to measure the quality of life gains subsequent to medical care, special attention must be paid to measures of patient utility: What dimensions of outcome are to be included, how are they to be measured, and how are the results to be communicated to individual patients so that when patient and physician values diverge, choices may be rational from the point of view of the patient? The importance of these questions is emphasized by the recent study by McNeil and her colleagues (16), which demonstrated that patient preferences for treatment of cancer were different from the choices their physicians had recommended for them: The patients tended to prefer less risky therapies with higher short-term probability of survival; their physicians preferred more risky therapies with higher long-term (five year) probabilities of survival.

We believe that there is a persuasive need to make a substantial public investment in the assessment of the outcome of common medical and surgical practices; this need should influence research priorities for programs to assess the value of health care technology. Although the agenda for the newly established National Center for Health Technology remains to be established, much of the discussion concerning its mandate has focused on the assessment of new technology prior to its implementation.

Although this is clearly important, the dollar and mortality implications of uncertainties concerning the value of existing services warrant a substantial investment in studies to learn more about their outcomes so that the trade-offs under their various patterns of use can be understood by physicians, patients, and those responsible for public policy.

Literature Cited

1. Cochrane, A. L. 1972. *Effectiveness and Efficiency: Random Reflections on Health Services.* Nuffield Prov. Hosp. Trust. 92 pp.
2. Bunker, J. P., Barnes, B. A., Mosteller, F., eds. 1977. *Costs, Risks, and Benefits of Surgery.* New York: Oxford Univ. Press. 401 pp.
3. Wennberg, J. E., Gittelsohn, A. 1973. Small area variations in health care delivery. *Science* 182:1102–7
4. Wennberg, J. E., Gittelsohn, A. 1975. Health care delivery in Maine. I. Patterns of use of common surgical procedures. *J. Maine Med. Assoc.* 66:123–30 149
5. Lewis, C. E. 1969. Variations in the incidence of surgery. *N. Engl. J. Med.* 218:880–84
6. Vayda, E., Anderson, G. D. 1965. Comparison of provincial surgical rates in 1968. *Can. J. Surg.* 18:18–26
7. Bunker, J. P. 1970. Surgical manpower: A comparison of operations and surgeons in the United States, England, and Wales. *N. Engl. J. Med.* 282(3):135–44
8. Ranofsky, A. L. 1978. Surgical operations in short-stay hospitals, United States, 1975. *Vital and Health Statistics:* Ser. 13, No. 34, Natl. Health Surv., DHEW publ. No. (PHS) 78–1785. Washington DC: GPO
9. Deane, R. T., Ulene, A. 1977. Hysterectomy or tubal ligation for sterilization: A cost-effectiveness analysis. *Inquiry* 14:73
10. Cole, P., Berlin, J. 1977. Elective hysterectomy *Obstet. Gynecol.* 129:117–23
11. Richards, D. H. 1974. A post-hysterectomy syndrome. *Lancet* 2:983–85
12. Stanford Cent. For Health Care Res. 1978. *Impact of hospital characteristics of surgical outcomes and length of stay.* A final report to the National Center for Health Services Research, DHEW, Washington DC
13. Richards, B. C. 1978. Hysterectomy: From women to women. *Am. J. Obstet. Gynecol.* 131:446
14. Barker, M. G. 1968. Psychiatric illness after hysterectomy. *Br. Med. J.* 2:91–95
15. Bunker, J. P., Brown, B. W. 1974. The physician-patient as an informed consumer of surgical services. *N. Engl. J. Med.* 290:1051–55
16. McNeil, B. J., Weichselbaum, R., Pauker, S. G. 1978. Fallacy of the five-year survival in lung cancer. *N. Engl. J. Med.* 299:1397–1401
17. Bunker, J. P., McPherson, K., Henneman, P. L. 1977. Elective hysterectomy. See Ref. 2, pp. 262–76
18. Harper, P. 1962. *Preventive Pediatrics: Child Health and Development.* New York: Appleton-Century-Crofts. 798 pp.
19. American Child Health Association. 1934. *Physical Defects: The Pathway to Correction,* p. 80. New York: Res. Div. Am. Child Health Assoc. 171 pp.
20. Wennberg, J. E. 1977. Commentary: Physician uncertainty, specialty ideology, and a second opinion prior to tonsillectomy. *Pediatrics* 59(6):952
21. Bolande, R. P. 1969. Ritualistic surgery-circumcision and tonsillectomy. *N. Engl. J. Med.* 280:591
22. Koontz, A. R. 1963. *Hernia.* New York: Appleton-Century-Crofts. 227 pp.
23. Neuhauser, D. 1977. Elective inguinal herniorrhaphy versus truss in the elderly. See Ref. 2, pp. 223–39
24. Ingelfinger, F. J. 1968. Digestive disease as a national problem. V. Gallstones. *Gastroenterology* 55:102
25. Hogan, J., Lonergan, M., Holland, P. D. J. 1977. The incidence of cholelithiasis in an autopsy series. *Ir. Med. J.* 70:608–11
26. Fitzpatrick, G., Neutra, R., Gilbert, J. P. 1977. Cost-effectiveness of cholecystectomy for silent gallstones. See Ref. 2, pp. 246–61
27. Bainton, D., Davies, G. T., Evans, K. T., Gravelle, I. H. 1976. Gallbladder disease prevalence in a South Wales industrial town. *N. Engl. J. Med.* 294:1147–49
28. Blodi, F. C. 1978. A surgical storm. *Arch. Ophthalmol.* 94:427
29. Jaffe, N. S. 1978. Cataract surgery-A modern attitude toward a technologic

explosion. *N. Engl. J. Med.* 299(5): 235–37

30. Kauppila, O. 1975. The perinatal mortality in breech deliveries and observations on affecting factors. *Acta Obstet. Gynecol. Scand.* 1975: Suppl. 39. pp. 9–79

31. Niswander, K. R. 1978. *Am. J. Obstet. Gynecol.* 131(2)

32. Collea, J. V., Rabin, S. C., Weghorst, G. R., Quilligan, E. J. 1978. The randomized management of term frank breech presentation: Vaginal delivery vs. cesarian section. *Am. J. Obstet. Gynecol.* 131(2):186–95

33. Kelson, I. M., Parsons, R. J., Lawrence, G. F., Arora, S. S., Edmonds, D. K., Cooke, I. D. 1978. An assessment of continuous fetal heart rate monitoring in labor. *Am. J. Obstet. Gynecol.* 131:526–32

34. Haverkamp, A. D., Thompson, H. E., McFee, J. G., Cetrulo, C. 1976. The evaluation of continuous fetal heart rate monitoring in high risk pregnancy. *Am. J. Obstet. Gynecol.* 125:310–20

35. Banta, H. D., Thacker, S. B. 1979. Costs and benefits of electronic fetal monitoring: A review of the literature. NCHRS Publ. No. (PHS) 79–3245. Hyattsville, Md: US DHEW

36. Hobbins, J. C., Freeman, R., Queenan, J. T. 1979. The fetal monitoring debate. *Pediatrics.* 63(6):942–51

37. Queenan, J. T. 1979. EFM revisited. *Contemp. OB/GYN* 14:9

38. Schifrin, B. S. 1979. Perils of perinatology. *Contemp. OB/GYN* 13:13–19

39. Goodlin, R. C. 1979. Rebutting Dr. Schifrin. *Contemp. OB/GYN* 14:21

40. Bolton, R. M., Mark, C., Neilson, D. R., Prins, R. 1979. Defending EFM. *Contemp. OB/GYN* 14:13, 14, 21

41. Queenan, J. T. 1979. Who's evaluating the efficacy of your monitoring? *Contemp. OB/GYN* 13:9–10

42. Goldstein, P. J. 1979. Replying to Dr. Queenan. *Contemp. OB/GYN* 14:2304

43. Caire, J. B. 1979. Equal time. *Contemp. OB/GYN* 14:25

44. Evrard, J. R., Gold, E. M. 1977. Cesarean section and maternal morbidity in Rhode Island: Incidence and risk factors, 1965–1975. *Obstet. Gynecol.* 50:394–97

45. Goldenberg, R. L., Nelson, K. 1975. Iatrogenic respiratory distress syndrome: An analysis of obstetric events preceding delivery of infants who develop respiratory distress syndrome. *Am. J. Obstet. Gynecol.* 123(6):617–20

46. Fons, J. W., Brennan, J. J. 1967. Views and reviews: Multiple cesarean section. *Obstet. Gynecol.* 29:287–94

47. Neutra, R. 1977. Indications for the surgical treatment of suspected acute appendicitis: A cost-effectiveness approach. See Ref. 2, pp. 277–307

48. deDombal, F. T., Leaper, D. J., Horrocks, J. C. Straniland, J. R., McCann, A. P. 1974. Human and computer-aided diagnosis of abdominal pain: Further report with emphasis on performance of clinicians. *Br. Med. J.* 1:376–80

49. Graham, D. F. 1977. Computer-aided prediction of gangrenous and perforating appendicitis. *Br. Med. J.* 2:1375–77

50. Coldrey, E. 1959. Five years of conservative treatment of acute appendicitis. *J. Int. Coll. Surg.* 32:255

51. *Lancet* 2:618, 1978. Appendix abscess: Time for a trial?

52. Bradley, E. L., Isaacs, J. 1978. Appendiceal abscess revisited. *Arch. Surg.* 113:130

53. Root, M. T. 1979. Living with benign prostatic hypertrophy. (Letter to the editor.) *N. Engl. J. Med.* 301(1):52

54. Ferguson, J. A. MacKeigan, J. M. 1978. Hemorrhoids, fistulae, and fissures: Office and hospital management—A critical review. *Adv. Surg.* 12:111–15

55. 1975 Outpatient treatment of haemorrhoids. *Br. Med. J.* 2(5972):651

56. Editorial 1975. To tie; to stab; to stretch; perchance to freeze. *Lancet* 2:645–46

57. American College of Surgeons 1975. Surgery in the United States: A summary report of the study on surgical services for the United States. Baltimore: Am. Coll. Surg. & Am. Surg. Assoc. 207 pp.

58. Commission on Professional and Hospital Activities. 1977. *Hospital Mortality. Professional Activity Study of Hospitals in the United States, 1974–75.* Ann Arbor: CPHA. 400 pp.

59. Wennberg, J. E., Gittelsohn, A., Shapiro, N. 1975. Health care delivery in Maine. III. Evaluating the level of hospital performance. *J. Maine Med. Assoc.* 66:11, 298–306

60. US DHEW. NCHS 1975. *Vital Statistics of the United States, 1975,* 2: P. B, 134–51. Washington DC: US DHEW

Ann. Rev. Public Health 1980. 1:297–321

THE FUTURE OF HEALTH DEPARTMENTS: The Governmental Presence

♦12511

G. Pickett

West Virginia Department of Health, Charleston, West Virginia 25305

INTRODUCTION

In the study of public institutions, health departments remain in the forefront of confusion. In 1976, Milton Terris wrote (1):

> In the 30 years preceding the end of World War II, local and state health departments and the U.S. Public Health Service grew and flourished as guardians of the people's health. In the subsequent 30 years, health departments have lost much of their momentum. The traditional U.S. Public Health Service has disappeared and its replacements have been transitory both in leadership and composition. Public health programs have been handed over to private interests and agencies lacking public health competence. The result has been confusion and pessimism about the future role of health departments.

In spite of this gloomy outlook, two years later Terris predicted that health departments in the future would be much more important and responsible for all aspects of the environment, including roads, auto design, housing, air, water, and pharmaceuticals as well as the administration of a National Health Service (2). Glogow (3) wrote, "A combination of external forces, such as elected public health officials, appointed health commissioners, and private interests—together with cautious, survival-oriented health department professionals—have contributed to the present state of conditions of public health." Hanlon reflected the professional agonizing in an article titled, "Is there a Future for Local Health Departments?" (4).

The American Public Health Association (APHA) adopted a major new policy paper on local health departments in 1974 (5) that called for active and extensive involvement of local health departments in virtually all aspects of community life. That document was delayed for two years as

297

several sections within the APHA struggled over some aspects of the hegemony expressed in the final paper. Some doubted that local health departments were useful. Shonick & Price (6) said, "Internal differences in ... the American Public Health Association, have hindered the realization of the potential of the (public health) movement." In that same article, they stated that, whereas many have criticized public health departments for their failures, "Closer study of history suggests ... that the local public health department, while being accused of inaction, was simultaneously being denied sufficient means to take action."

In the US Department of Health, Education and Welfare's (DHEW) *Forward Plan for Health, FY 1978–82* (7), no mention of state or local health departments appears under the topics of health manpower, health services integration efforts, prevention, or environmental health. In their 488 page report to the Congress in 1978, HEW makes no reference to state or local health departments (8). Yet Miller and his associates (9) said, "Official public health agencies are far too extensive to be consistently overlooked in development of the nation's health policies."

The recent pattern of ignoring the very existence of health departments when wrestling with such problems as health insurance for the aged and the poor, comprehensive health planning, the formation of health maintenance organizations, quality control, and the development of primary care centers is in sharp contrast to the illumination cast on official health agencies during the decades prior to the 1960s (10–13). Looking at what has actually happened, analysts of the 1970s have portrayed a decline in prominence, yet have forecast an important future for public health (1–4, 6, 9).

In the pages that follow, the structure and role of state and local health departments are examined and information is presented that suggests that the public health movement, often described as characterizing the earlier decades of this century, may have been more an expression of wishes than of reality. The changing federal influence is examined. The need for what some have called a "governmental presence at the local level" (14) is described. Finally, three basic, and, to some extent, uniquely American issues are explored to see whether some sensible directions out of the present state of confusion can be detected: (*a*) the organizational boundaries of the health sphere of interest, (*b*) the private sector/public sector controversy, and (*c*) the conflict of interest issue involved when government mixes service roles and regulatory roles in one agency. This exploration results in a description of a health department much like that portrayed by Glogow (3), characterized by a centrality of focus with more dynamic acceptance of heterogeneity and shifting array of coalitions rather than a prescription for an organizational structure.

THE CURRENT SCENE

State Health Agencies

Information about the roles of state health departments is surprisingly sketchy. Most of the available information has been collected to prove a point rather than to understand the true scope and function of government in the field of public health.

The state health agencies are relatively easy to count. The Association of State and Territorial Health Officials (ASTHO, formed in March 1942) lists 57 state health agencies (SHAs) (15). The ASTHO established the National Public Health Program Reporting System in 1970 "to provide comprehensive and uniform data concerning public health programs of SHA's on a national basis" (16). The program has been of considerable value, but its auspices meant that it would report what its members were doing, not necessarily what state government was doing in public health, as many health functions are served by other public agencies. A more serious shortcoming is the association's admission that it has very little information about the programs and expenditures of local health departments.

The reporting system classifies programs so that costs and services can be counted, although the attempt to count services is in an earlier stage of development. According to the association's report for fiscal year 1977, the official state health agencies spent a total of $2.8 billion with 70.6% of that amount going for "personal health services" (15). The category of "personal health services" includes institutions operated by the agencies. It does not include the Medicaid programs of any of the states, even the eight states in which the health agency is the administering department, but does include those crippled children's services and mental health services that are under the supervision of the state health agency. The categorization used by the association is shown in Table 1 along with expenditure efforts and personnel estimates.

The emphasis of the reporting system on the identification of state health agency expenditures to justify federal appropriations for basic public health services administered by those agencies results in an incomplete picture. For example, only 16 of the reporting state health agencies had mental health programs, only 10 had mental retardation programs, and only 19 were involved in air pollution control or could claim designation as their state's "lead" environmental agency. In the others, the lead agency was either a state environmental protection agency or a natural resources department.

The deficiencies in the National Public Health Program Reporting System can be realized by examining data published in the *Statistical Abstract of the United States, 1978* (17). Table 489 in that document shows that

Table 1 Public health expenditures of state health agencies by program area and category and employees by program area, fiscal year 1977 (15)

Program area and selected program category	Total expenditures	Employees
Personal health[a]	$1,387,548,000	35,440
General and supporting	229,207,000	
Maternal and child health	596,183,000	
Crippled children	157,025,000	
Communicable disease	130,990,000	
Dental health	25,854,000	
Chronic disease	57,106,000	
Mental health and related programs	129,575,000	
Other personal health	61,608,000	
State health agency operated institutions	597,633,000	40,740
Environmental health	211,860,000	10,883
Consumer protection and sanitation	80,111,000	
Water quality control	44,775,000	
Air quality control	19,667,000	
Waste management	13,323,000	
Occupational health and safety and related areas	8,989,000	
Radiation control	9,873,000	
General environmental health	35,122,000	
Health resources	263,183,000	8,640
Planning	15,398,000	
Development	14,669,000	
Regulation	152,513,000	
Statistics	40,765,000	
General health resources	39,839,000	
Laboratory	116,580,000	6,208
General administration and services	176,048,000	9,217
Funds to local health departments not allocated to program areas	58,760,000	
Total	$2,811,611,000	112,096

[a] Excluding state health agency operated institutions.

states reported expenditures for health and hospitals (not including Medicaid) totaling $11.1 billion in 1976 as contrasted with ASTHO's total of only $3.2 billion (16). Some of the disparity is due to such programs as mental health, mental retardation, and substance abuse, which are often in agencies other than those directed by the designated state health official. Although the "official" state health agencies reported that they had spent $130 million on mental health, mental retardation, alcoholism, and drug abuse, the President's Commission on Mental Health (18) reported that $3.91 billion had been spent in 1977 in public mental health hospitals alone and that at least $680 million had been spent on the programs of community mental health centers. Still more important, the commission found that Medicaid actually represented the biggest mental health "program" in the country with 1977 expenditures of $4.1 billion. The disparities in environmental health are just as significant. For example, although the ASTHO reported that state and territorial health agencies spent $16.9 million on air quality control in 1976, the census bureau (see 17, Table 353) reported expenditures amounting to $157 million. The ASTHO report shows $39.4 million spent for water quality control in 1976 whereas the states reported $939 million (see 17, Table 353). The disparities in estimates of the state health work force are likewise severe. Although the ASTHO report shows a total of approximately 105,000 workers employed in state health agency programs in 1976, the states have separately reported that they employed 614,000 workers in health programs (see 17, Table 505). Estimates of expenditures prepared by state budget analysts differ sharply from those provided by public health practitioners because they define the subject and the object differently.

The fractionation of health programs among different agencies has been a source of concern to public health workers for years. In a 1954 policy statement, the APHA (19) noted that there was evidence that "administrative experts" were placing some traditional inspectional functions of health departments in other agencies and strongly opposed such action. In an elaborate policy paper in 1965 (20), the association identified the states as the principal agencies for public health programs and urged that all federal funds for health programs be funneled through the state health departments. (This was at the beginning of the era of community action programs and direct federal grants to nontraditional agencies.) The statement seemed to recognize that the channels of communication needed broadening beyond the traditional lines that existed between the surgeon general, the state health officer, and the local health officer, but in other respects the statement was highly traditional. By 1968, federal grant strategies had continued to unfold in such a way that the association adopted another resolution (21), which described the proliferation of grants outside of the health department as a "clear challenge" to public health.

Much of the concern was focused on new community action programs. Concern about mental health and mental retardation separatism has been traditionally less troublesome to public health professionals. The increase in the release of patients from state mental hospitals had begun in 1955 and the American Public Health Association adopted a resolution in 1961 (22) that urged public health agencies to become more involved in mental health programs, but did not insist on health department hegemony. Following the passage of P.L. 88–164 (The Mental Retardation Facilities and Community Mental Health Centers Construction Act of 1963), the APHA rather mildly urged that the isolation of mental health and mental retardation services be ended and that integrated planning take place (23).

More noticeable was the lack of public health involvement in medical care issues. Congress appeared not to know about health departments when Medicare and Medicaid were adopted. Management of the former went largely to private insurance carriers and the latter, generally, to state welfare agencies. Although some analysts have described the extensive involvement of public health agencies in the provision of personal health care services (24, 10, 25), most public health agency directors have been reluctant to become involved aggressively in such activities. The Association of State and Territorial Health Officials has not adopted a strong position on such issues as national health insurance or recent efforts to put a lid on hospital costs. State associations of local health officers have been equally reticent about their responsibility for the provision of medical care services except in limited situations. Because most health officers, at least at the local level, are physicians (9) and most boards of health are dominated by physicians in private practice (26), the long-standing opposition of organized medicine to public medical care programs has had a significant influence on public health agencies. This apparent lack of involvement by official public health agencies and their directors has resulted in considerable criticism of health departments (6) and a long-standing problem for the membership of the American Public Health Association (27, 28).

At the state level, only eight health agencies (as distinct from welfare departments) were assigned responsibility for the management of the Medicaid program. That program, along with the Medicare program, was drafted by the secretary of the Department of Health, Education and Welfare without the involvement of the US Public Health Service or its surgeon general (29). Its welfare-oriented authorship and management assured that it would encourage the development of insurance style, vendor-payment programs rather than public health service systems.

Although each state has an "official" health focus, health programs and functions are carried out by many agencies of state government. Traditional public health programs such as communicable disease control and maternal and child health services are most often found in the health agency. Program areas or functions that developed outside of that tradition or that were developed for mixed purposes—such as mental health programs, rehabilitation programs, and medical care payment mechanisms, as well as large area environmental health initiatives—tend to be more distant from the central focus of the official agency and more often in separate organizations. They are less consistently identified or counted as part of a state's public health effort.

Many state health agencies have been reorganized in recent years, either by becoming parts of larger human resource agencies, or by forming aggregations with other state agencies such as mental health. In many states, environmental health programs have been separated from the health agencies and new environmental protection agencies have been formed. Some, such as California, have done both by effecting a major consolidation and then a subsequent separation when legislative leaders found that they were unable to obtain satisfactory accounting for state programs from the leaders of the conglomerate. In many states, what was once an independent health officer reporting to a semiautonomous board of health has become a deputy or assistant director for some aspects of a larger health and environment agency or human services organization. As indicated by the succession of APHA resolutions and policy papers mentioned above, changes that affected the core, traditional programs of public health, such as maternal and child health, communicable disease control, and neighborhood sanitation efforts, were resisted strongly by public health directors. In the meantime, new and less traditional programs involving the development of primary care centers, the major national health insurance programs for the aged and the indigent, the development of community mental health centers, the organization of area-wide and state level comprehensive health planning processes, and the broad field of rehabilitation and developmental disabilities were not zealously pursued by state health agencies because they did not fit the traditional models taught in textbooks and sanctioned by organized medicine. In the eyes of many, at the state and national as well as the local level, health departments became irrelevant.

Local Health Departments

The numbers and functions of local health departments are even more difficult to define than are the programs of state health agencies. Kratz (12) had counted 1669 counties with full-time public health departments in

1942: 633 single county units, 426 "local-district" units involving two or more counties, and 580 state controlled districts involving one or more counties. The Subcommittee on Administrative Practice of the American Public Health Association, under the chairmanship of Haven Emerson in 1945, proposed 1197 local health units for the United States with 318 single county units, 821 multicounty units, 36 county-district units, and 22 city units with a population range from 10,200 to 7,455,000 (11). The subcommittee clearly saw a need to consolidate many small, county health departments. Terris (10) in 1949 said that there were 1385 full-time local health units in the country. More recently, Miller and his associates (9) collected information from 1345 local health units and estimated that they represented 68% of the total. They classified local health units as those with a "central organization" (local health units run directly by the state), a "decentralized organization" (local health units operating under substate area governmental jurisdiction), and those operating with "shared organizational control" (local health units operated by local government but under the authority of the state health department). Of the units surveyed, 47.4% were single county units (as contrasted with the 27% recommended by Emerson), 14.1% were city units, 8.4% were units serving two or more counties (in contrast to Emerson's recommended 68.6%), and 15.2% of the units were consolidated city-county units.

The ASTHO said that 44 of the state and territorial agencies reported a total of 3264 local health departments (15). The year before, the association concluded that the difference between their estimate and that of Miller and his associates was due to the definitions used (16). The association defined a local health department "as an official (governmental) public health agency which is in whole or in part responsible to a sub-state governmental entity or entities" and that it had to have a staff of one or more full-time professional public health employees, deliver public services, serve a definable geographic area, and have an identifiable budget to qualify. Miller and his associates seem to have used the same working definition.

All of the reports suggest that there are a large number of small health departments in spite of repeated recommendations that health departments not be formed in jurisdictions with less than 50,000 people. Consolidations have been attempted and recommended as a way to achieve greater effectiveness and efficiency, yet that effort has achieved little success. It has been very difficult to join two or more counties together to form one public health department even though the entire country has been covered with approximately 200 health planning agencies—about one tenth the number of local health departments.

The city-county consolidation effort has been only a little more successful. In most states, counties serve as the administrative unit for carrying out state functions. Cities are often authorized to establish health departments but are not required to do so. As fiscal pressures on cities have increased, city officials have realized that the county is responsible for public health services within the city as well as in the surrounding county area. However, the effort to force the county to either provide or pay for municipal health services has run into weak county property tax systems resulting in no merger or in agreements whereby the city continues to pay an extra share of the cost of services. The effort has also occurred at a time when inner city minority groups have begun to wield real political power; they have seen the effort to move public services to the county level as an attempt to deprive them of the control over public programs that they have struggled so long to acquire.

Another form of merger is that which combines agencies, such as health and hospitals or mental health. In their analysis of the situation, Shonick & Price (30) have concluded that this merger trend is continuing, even though some of them have been reversed. The human service agency mergers involving health departments with hospitals or social service agencies seem particularly prone to subsequent separation because some of the responsible officials were not sufficiently aware of the sharp differences in opinion and background that have characterized these agencies.

Miller and his associates (9) collected information about programs in local health departments (Table 2). As was noted for state health agencies, the programs that had their origins within the traditions of public health during the earlier part of the twentieth century tend to have adhered to the official public health focus at the local level. Programs that developed in another tradition, such as the public hospital or public mental health programs, tend to be less often a part of that central focus. Although the consistent performance of the more highly traditional functions is apparent in the data shown, it is also apparent that local health departments are extensively involved in providing direct medical care services despite the generally reported belief to the contrary.

The average local health department, according to Miller et al, had 34.4 employees in 1974. The questionnaires returned included data that would enable an analysis to be made of the frequency distribution of local health departments by size, but this information has not yet been reported. If it is assumed that a relatively small number of large health departments account for a relatively large proportion of the total work force, it would not be difficult to imagine that many of the reporting units had only 8 to 15 employees. It is also apparent, both from Miller's work and earlier studies (11, 12, 30), that a substantial number of the units counted as local health departments are actually state health department operated district offices. Although textbooks repeat the thesis that a population base of

Table 2 Percent of health departments providing selected services, 1974 (9)

Services	Percentage providing each service
Immunization programs	96.3
Environmental surveillance	96.0
Tuberculosis control	93.9
Maternal and child health	89.4
School health program	89.2
Venereal disease control	88.0
Chronic disease programs	84.3
Home care	76.7
Family planning	63.3
Ambulatory care	50.3
Mental health	47.4
Chronic institutional care	11.8
Acute institutional care	8.4

50,000 is the minimum necessary to support a local public health unit, the services recommended in the APHA's 1974 policy paper could not be provided by an agency drawn from so small a population. It is known that many of those units counted in the reports noted above are found in counties with a much smaller population. Many local health departments consist of one or two sanitarians, clerks, and nurses (rarely with baccalaureate level or public health training), and a local practicing physician who serves as the part-time health officer.

Textbook descriptions of local health agencies tend to describe a larger and better trained unit. Mountin & Flook (13), the APHA (5), and Hanlon and Pickett (31) describe a health department that may rarely if ever have existed. The functions and organizational structures described or recommended seem to be at variance with the more individualized patterns actually observed. Moreover, although most people live in areas that may be served by reasonably proficient, locally governed health departments, at least one third of the nation's counties do not have such an agency and many of those that do could not have enough staff or money to meet the expectations or recommendations of the American Public Health Association's 1974 policy paper. When the units counted represent such diverse ecological and political systems, statistical analyses that result in a portrait of the "average" unit tend to increase rather than decrease distortions of reality. Thus, despite the models described and advocated, it seems likely that the public health movement in the United States as it has often been portrayed represents an exaggerated description of what actually happened, and the recommendations for what should happen represent an equally unrealistic appraisal of what is probable or artfully possible given the resistance to merger and the adherence to tradition.

The Federal Influence

The authority and responsibility for public health programs and services are generally reserved to the states except in matters involving interstate commerce. The federal government, however, is not without influence. The Children's Bureau was created in 1912 but could only study problems until the Sheppard-Towner Act was passed in 1921 (31). This began the pattern of stimulating state and local health agency action through federal grants. The Public Health Service Act subsequently authorized the distribution of formula grant funds to the states for basic public health programs and numerous other acts of Congress have authorized both project grants and formula grants for public health programs at the state and local level. Taken as a whole, according to the Advisory Commission on Intergovernmental Relations, these federal initiatives have been stimulative, i.e. they have resulted in state and local expenditures of more than one dollar for every federal dollar provided (32).

It is clear that the way federal grants are distributed has had a significant effect on the structure as well as the programs of state and local government. The Sheppard-Towner Act stimulated the establishment of maternal and child health divisions in most state health departments within the first year of its enactment (31). Later efforts were aimed at different outcomes.

Shonick & Price (6) found during the 1960s:

Wherever feasible, federal policy . . . favored the use of private providers or suppliers over public ones to achieve public goals. The political utility of this approach . . . serves several purposes. It provides benefits to the supplier industries who then are motivated to support the federal bureaucracy and elected incumbents. In addition, in the health field, use of private providers is presented as being of particularly high quality because it is "main stream" and not "government issue," a rhetoric that enhances the symbolic value of meager or quite modest tangible benefits to the poor. Finally, it markedly simplifies the task of limiting the duration and magnitude of the real or tangible benefits being given. If local public agencies were used, it would prove difficult to avoid mounting widespread programs across the country and the pressures from local governments would be for guarantees of long-term funding distributed among them according to need.

State and local public health officials would prefer that all federal grant monies be funneled through their official agencies. In 1965 the American Public Health Association adopted a resolution (33) that acknowledged that federal initiatives in vocational rehabilitation and Medicaid had leaned toward state departments of education, vocational rehabilitation, and welfare and urged that the health departments be relied upon for their medical direction and leadership. The same theme, played against a background of ten more years of federal initiatives, was adopted in a 1977 resolution that noted that professional standards review organizations, health systems agencies, renal dialysis projects, and health maintenance organizations were being established without the mandatory involvement of state and local health agencies, and the association urged that no federal health dollars go to such organizations without going through state and local health departments (34).

During the last 14 years there has been a continuing erosion in the relationship of state and local health departments with the federal health establishment, as Congress and a succession of presidents and officials of DHEW (now DHHS—the Department of Health and Human Services) have worked with new and nontraditional state and community agencies and focused increasing concern on the economic aspects of medical care, an issue that has not been seen as one of primary concern to public health officials. The picture that emerges is one in which traditional relationships and concepts were largely destroyed (in reality if not always in rhetoric) and most of the important new health initiatives of the federal government were launched without depending on official state and local health agencies for either leadership or, often, participation. Medicaid and Medicare, Comprehensive Health Planning, Comprehensive Health Centers, the OEO programs, cost containment efforts, air pollution and water quality control programs, rural health initiatives, and efforts to monitor the quality of medical care have all been initiated by statutes that persistently refused to include the existing official health agencies of the country. Because the real strengths of those agencies did not match the expectations or the mythical portraits drawn by public health's practitioners and supporters, they were ignored altogether; as Miller and his associates pointed out (9), in spite of their shortcomings, they are far too extensive and too effective to be ignored. They may still represent the strongest institutions available to bring about needed progress and change.

In 1977, the ASTHO, together with representatives of county and city health departments and the APHA, was successful in obtaining passage of the Health Services Extension Act (P.L. 95–83), which increased the authorization for federal formula grant funds to state and local health departments. Consistent with the commitment contained in the APHA's 1974 policy paper on local health departments (5), the new law required that standards be developed for community preventive health services within two years. Bergheim (35) found that 32 states had already developed standards for local health departments but most of them dealt with procedures and "input" requirements. In order to focus on objectives and results, a working group was formed involving the United States Conference of City Health Officers, the National Association of County Health Officials, the Association of State and Territorial Health Officials, the American Public Health Association, and the Center for Disease Control of the US Public

Health Service. The group quoted from the congressional conference committee report on the bill (Health Services Extension Act of 1977) in their draft report of August 1978 (14):

> By requiring the development of model standards for community public health programs, the conferees intend to emphasize their commitment to the continuing need for such programs and services, and to the benefits which accrue to the entire population. It is apparent that cost-effective public health programs, including preventive health services and those environmental control measures directed at protecting human health will need to assume even greater significance in any program of National Health Insurance. Accordingly, standards need to be developed now to assure that public health programming is maintained as a crucial element of, or an equal partner to, any National Health Insurance Plan.

The working group quickly realized that it was very difficult to define a local health department given the wide array of agencies involved in various aspects of public health at all levels of government. The group then formulated the concept of a "governmental presence at the local level," which recognized the confounding heterogeneity that necessarily existed, but adopted the concept that "every community must be served by a governmental entity" charged with the responsibility to see that basic standards were met. The group concluded, "Government at the local level has the responsibility for ensuring that a health problem is monitored and that services to correct that problem are available. The state government must monitor the effectiveness of local efforts to control health problems and act as a residual guarantor of services where community resources are inadequate." This statement appears to be the most emphatic and concise agreement achieved to date about the role of state and local health agencies. It accepts the variability of state and local arrangements as inherent in the American system of federalism and reaches for the concept of a centrality of focus and concern rather than any stereotyped organizational structure. It assumes that much of the needed service will be provided by other agencies and institutions, public and private, and that the governmental presence in the health field need not have all of the resources and capabilities within its organizational matrix. Although the authorized appropriation for these new initiatives is not forthcoming—in fact federal dollars for support of state and local public health services are declining rapidly—there are signs from within the office of the secretary of DHHS and the assistant secretary for health, as well as the Center for Disease Control and the Bureau of Community Health Services, that a more cohesive strategy for prevention and the use of state and local health agencies is emerging. Efforts to link primary care centers with public health programs and mental health programs—combining dollars, facilities, and scarce administrative and health professional work force skills—can help to overcome the dollar shortage problem. More importantly, they may encourage the further development of public health programs through negotiation and coalition-building rather than through acquisition of control and resources.

ISSUES IN CONFLICT

A number of issues underlie some of the confusion that exists in trying to describe health departments as they are or as they should be. The problem and theory of boundaries has an inherent ingredient of conflict. Organizational boundaries are always in a state of tension; management of the ensuing conflict is difficult. The public sector/private sector dichotomy is another major issue that causes confusion and has some uniquely American flavor to it. Finally, the "conflict-of-interest" issue confuses efforts to settle on a locus of control for health programs. Can a regulator be a provider of regulated services?

The Theory of Boundaries

As shown above, in every state and in most communities of any size, there is an identifiable health focal point—a governmental presence in the health interest area. Many other agencies also have an interest in issues that affect the public's health: agricultural agencies, welfare departments, natural resources agencies, schools, industrial development and labor departments, etc. Certain highly traditional public health programs adhere tightly and consistently to that health focal point and are a part of that organizational sphere of interest—activities such as immunizations, venereal disease control, and maternal and child health services. Other programs are somewhat more remote from the health focal point, often because they developed in another sphere of interest (such as public hospitals, which came from a welfare background or vocational rehabilitation efforts and programs for the developmentally disabled, which have an education system background). These programs are less often adherent to the health focal point, even though health agencies have an interest in such activities and a contribution to make.

The organization of state and local governments can be viewed as a number of overlapping spheres of interest, each with a core focal point establishing the governmental presence in that particular area of interest. The more proximate a governmental activity is to that core, the more likely it is to adhere to that sphere of interest and that organization. The more remote it is, the less the gravitational pull there is and the more likely it is that the activity will adhere to another interest sphere's focal point. Most of these spheres of interest overlap and, at the interfaces, there is constant tension as a particular activity finds itself part way between two focal points, each with its own gravitational pull. It is at these interfaces that most disputes over organizational hegemony take place and that most reorganization efforts occur. It is also at these points that gaps are most likely to occur and client groups are most likely to find an incomplete and vague response to their needs.

Often a constituency will emerge and consolidate around an interest sphere interface and apply sufficient pressure that that interface becomes a new and separate organizational sphere of interest. This happened in some states when federal funds first became available for the establishment of alcoholism programs in 1970 (P.L. 91–616). This sort of change also has occurred with the passage of national legislation concerning educational services and civil rights for the handicapped (P.L. 93–112 and P.L. 94–142). In some states, seven major organizational units involving as many as five different spheres of interest are involved in providing services for the handicapped: welfare, education, health, mental health, mental retardation, corrections, and rehabilitation. Each state has to develop a plan for serving those with developmental disabilities. This can be done by pulling the involved parts out of their existing organizations and creating a new agency to deal with developmental disabilities or by establishing an interagency coordinating mechanism. The constituent groups usually prefer to have their own organization. It is clear, however, that removal of social workers from a welfare department, teachers from an education department, physical therapists from a rehabilitation agency, and nursing and medical personnel from a health agency or a public hospital will leave gaps in those diminished organizations. Moreover, although the component parts may be drawn together to deal with the developmental disability, the client may again be segmented when some other problem arises, such as a need for the fiscal support of the state's crippled children's services agency. Often those newly created interfaces serve as a fresh source of friction between the different interest spheres, with the result that the client with the need is confronted with new and different gaps and disputes.

As government has become involved in more aspects of community life, the interfaces between interest spheres have become more numerous. This has led to a tendency to reorganize at an increasing rate. Yet the very nature of the governmental presence in so many interest spheres is such that neatly drawn lines around areas of responsibility and authority cannot be drawn —certainly not with any hope of permanence. Interface tension is inherent in the governmental process and the loci and severity of the tension will change, often rapidly, depending on interest group success and legislative initiatives. Although it is desirable to analyze the number and the nature of the separate organizational interest spheres that exist at the state and local level to assure that the central focal point of each interest sphere is discrete, comprehensible, and durable, government agency managers, if they are to be effective rather than immobilized by continuing reorganizations, need to learn the art of ad-hocracy and coalition-building. It should be possible for skillful administrators to develop effective coalitions so that those with developmental disabilities can get needed services as if there were an agency with that sole concern, without creating disabling upheavals in multiple and important spheres of interest such as education, health, and welfare. The professional and technical staff required often can function together effectively if the administrators—those who work at the core of each involved interest sphere—can sanction and support such collaboration. This requires administrators who can agree to give up some control and to support an interagency coordinator so that that individual takes on the semblance of authority customarily reserved for those who are in actual control. That such coalitions are not easily built is obvious; that they require astute, sensitive, and skilled professionals as coordinators is clear; that enforced reorganizations will occur unless such ad hoc coalitions can be formed is apparent. The theory of boundaries in governmental organization and management is that (*a*) tension at the boundary interfaces is inevitable and (*b*) it often can be constructively managed through negotiation rather than acquisition by one agency or partitioning by a superior power.

The Public Sector/Private Sector Dichotomy

Davis (36), in 1937, listed seven reasons for public involvement in the provision of personal health services, such as mental health, communicable diseases, and illnesses that cause permanent and severe dependency. Although it was partly true then, it is even more apparent now that there is virtually no public health activity that does not have or could not have private sector entrepreneurial involvement, and there is virtually no private sector enterprise in which public involvement is forbidden. Arguments about which sector ought to be involved in a particular health endeavor are often couched in theoretical or patriotic terms; however, there are four factors that determine whether or not it is acceptable or necessary for the public sector to become involved: (*a*) whether those who need services have the money to pay for them or whether a money transfer system has been developed to pay a vendor on behalf of the client, (*b*) whether the police powers of government are intimately involved in the activity, (*c*) whether the service is thought to be essential but too high in cost for users to bear the price directly, and (*d*) whether the clients are so severely dependent that they are subject to exploitation.

PAYMENT   Most medical care for the indigent has been purchased by governments from private providers or provided through public hospitals. With the emergence of organized medicine in the United States in the early part of the twentieth century and heightened respect for what well-trained physicians could accomplish by then, additional public incursions into the medical care arena, which was considered a private matter and not necessarily a right, have been vigorously opposed. To the extent that new initiatives have been taken by the federal government, they have relied on vendor payment mechanisms and the private sector.

Mental hospitals were established, in part, because the clients could not pay for their own care and families either could not or would not be relied upon. Moreover, because the disability was considered permanent, the need was for custodial care, not treatment and rehabilitation, and the private sector had not yet developed any interest in organizing and selling custodial care services. Another factor was involved too.

POLICE POWER ROLES   During the late 1800s and continuing to some extent into the present, the separation of the mentally ill from the rest of society was not functionally different from separating criminals from the rest of society. Undesirable people were sorted out (triaged) on the basis of mental illness or the commission of a criminal act and sentenced accordingly. To a substantial extent the mental hospitals served a police power function, not a poor law function.

The practice is more overt and acceptable in coping with dangerous communicable diseases. Private physicians treat a substantial number of patients with venereal diseases and a growing number of patients with tuberculosis. The epidemiologic investigation of a reported case, however, is a public sector responsibility. This is in part due to the fact that the physician has neither the skill nor the time to conduct an epidemiologic investigation and the responsible public agency is not inclined to pay a physician to do so. But it is also due to the fact that implicit in that investigation is the responsibility of the public health agency to protect the public from a dangerous disease and to take such steps, including quarantine, as may be necessary—a police power function. Although the explicit exercise of that police power function is rarely carried out or even mentioned, it is latent in the process and most participants know that it is. The same is true of most environmental health activities. Police power functions of government are rarely delegated even though an entrepreneurial interest might be provoked if a payment mechanism were developed.

ESSENTIAL HIGH-COST SERVICES   Some services are deemed to be essential, yet not well-suited to client payment or insurance mechanisms that might support a private sector involvement. This is true for police and fire protection services, although a supplementary private sector industry has developed. Emergency medical services have become a major new area for public sector involvement in recent years, often with the enthusiastic support of private sector interests that would have been expected to oppose such involvement. Some states have actually declared that the provision of emergency medical services is a governmental responsibility and have taken steps to remove private sector involvement altogether. There are several reasons for this rather sudden emergence of public sector dominance: 1. The services have immense popularity and are now considered to be essential public services. 2. Such services are, in their fullest state of development, very expensive and likely to be used in such a way as to rule out effective budgeting for the service by a client. 3. Like fire protection services, which are also very expensive, emergency medical services are characterized by substantial amounts of inactivity between calls. The amount of inactive time increases as efforts are made to reduce the response time of the unit—the time between the call for help and the arrival on the scene of advanced life support services. In such circumstances, the cost per response is likely to come under frequent scrutiny, if not attack, and public exposure and accountability is necessary if local elected officials are to be in a position to justify the costs and the use of time. These reasons for supporting public sector involvement were met with a lack of opposition in many communities from those who have provided ambulance services in the past, because many of them lacked the expertise and management skills to upgrade their services and equipment to meet the requirements of governmental agencies. The development of public sector involvement was also encouraged rather than opposed by interested physicians, because it heightened the technology of their involvement and their position in the hierarchy of medicine. It also helped to increase substantially the amount of money flowing through the system.

It seems likely that the same sequence of events will unfold in the future management and governance of hospitals and for the same reasons. It will not occur as rapidly, because of the long tradition of private, nonprofit governance. But rising costs, erratic payments, increased public concern for both availability and accountability, the rapid increase in the cost of construction, and the controls on investments in both facilities and services are likely to push hospitals more fully into the form of public utility management and even public governance.

DEPENDENCY AND EXPLOITATION   The dependency of some individuals—whether due to social, physical, or emotional reasons—is so complete that they are essentially defenseless against exploitation. This is true of substantial numbers of people currently housed in nursing homes. It is also true of many of those in community programs and institutions for the developmentally disabled and the mentally ill. Under such circumstances and, in part, because government funds are frequently used to pay for both the lodging costs and whatever treatment and rehabilitation services are provided, public sector involvement in either providing the services or in monitoring their availability and quality is expanding.

Except for state and county mental hospitals and the Veterans Administration Hospitals, the majority of dependent people are cared for in private, proprietary institutions and programs. Private sector interest in this field has grown rapidly with the expansion of public programs to pay for health services provided to the elderly and the indigent. It has been suggested (37) that private sector interest is more in the real estate transactions than in the sale of services and that nursing homes should be publicly rather than privately owned. The essential fear is that dependent and often defenseless individuals may be exploited by an industry that finds that the human service needs of their clients erode their profits. The customary response to this situation, a situation that has been exacerbated by the type of governmental payment mechanisms established for Medicare and Medicaid patients, is to assume that effective regulations governing facilities and services can be developed and enforced by other agencies of government. Thus, one creation of government that supports private sector entrepreneurs has resulted in the creation of another, expanded function of government to regulate the entrepreneurs.

Public scrutiny is clearly necessary, but considerable experimentation is called for to ascertain the best mix of payment mechanisms and regulatory controls. The likely course of events over the next few years will be continued reliance on private sector services, with more public control and oversight. In the longer run, a move toward more direct public governance of such care systems is a possibility.

The continuing public/private sector debate in the United States has some uniquely native qualities to it. There is a deep-seated assumption that private sector management skills are better developed and that the public sector cannot compete in matters in which cost, efficiency, and flexibility are important. To the contrary, there are many examples that indicate that private sector and public sector management techniques are necessarily different and that successful private sector managers often fail in the public sector. Moreover, some of the impassioned defense of private as opposed to public medical care systems in the United States is based more on rhetoric than on fact. Miller and his colleagues have listed many examples that show that public programs are often effective, efficient, and of high quality (9, 25).

The dynamics of a free market do not work effectively to achieve equitable, need-related distribution of health services in the United States; public intervention, if not outright ownership, is required. Medical goods are not distributed, priced, or purchased as are other goods. Some who fear an expanded provider role for the government advocate reliance on private, nonprofit forms of governance as a compromise, but Etzioni & Doty (38) have illustrated the ways in which a nonprofit corporation can circumvent public policy objectives just as readily as can a more overtly entrepreneurial corporation.

The public/private argument will continue in the United States. The basic issues need to be more clearly expressed: 1. A real commitment to the right of access to needed health care has to be made if that is the nation's intention. 2. Rights must be guaranteed by government—that is, the difference between a right and a privilege. The unregulated dynamics of a free market cannot assure that right. 3. The systems or agencies responsible for providing the necessary services must be publicly accountable if the right is to be maintained, and that ultimately requires a public governing board. The board may be elected or appointed by elected officials, but it must be publicly accountable to the community served. 4. Such a governing board can arrange to provide those services either through directly employed workers (who earn a personal "profit" for their labor) or by contracting with a public or private organization that will provide the agreed upon services. The essential feature is public governance and accountability, not whether the individual providers are public or private sector entrepreneurs.

The Conflict of Interest Conflict

Can one agency of government carry out legislative, executive, and judicial functions? Can a city or county own and operate a public hospital and license private hospitals? Can a state build or repair a public hospital while it administers a "certificate of need" program? Can a Health Systems Agency (generally a private corporation) make decisions about the use of public money in a community that has an elected governing body responsible for taxes?

At the federal level, the separation of powers into executive, legislative, and judicial functions has served to avoid macroconflicts. On a smaller scale, however, conflicts are abundant. The US Department of Health and Human Services administers the Medicaid program (which pays bills to providers for services rendered to eligible clients), establishes guidelines for state programs to determine who is an eligible client, administers the certification program (which determines who is an eligible provider), and audits the process. Thus, one agency of the executive branch has several internal conflicts of interest.

The legislative branch has similar problems. When the Congress passed the National Health Planning and Resources Development Act of 1974 (P.L. 93–641), the emphasis was on private corporations that would enter into a contract with the secretary of DHEW to plan for a community. The act gave an obligatory seat on the governing body to a representative of the Veterans Administration if a VA Hospital was in the service area, but the health systems agency was to have no voice in the construction or service

plans of the Veterans Administration. Thus, although Congress made clear
its mistrust of local government when it came to making health planning
decisions, fearing that local, elected officials might make wasteful or unwise
decisions about building hospitals, it demonstrated the problem by removing its own hospitals from the review process.

It is not often understood that, at the local level, the separation of powers
concept does not apply. Most county commissions serve as elected boards
in charge of a diversified conglomerate and they have legislative, executive,
and some judicial powers. They are, of course, rather visible and immediately accountable to the community served. Although such boards may
have made unwise decisions about their hospitals, construction decisions
made by the boards of voluntary hospitals have not been uniformly defensible.

In developing the language of the health planning law and the regulations
and guidelines used to administer it, a great deal of attention has been paid
to possible "conflicts of interest." Those providers on the boards of health
systems agencies who may have such a conflict are expected to be removed
from deliberations in which the conflict may be real. Reduced to its literal
meaning, conflict of interest should be present in every discussion. Those
who serve on health systems agencies should be interested in what they are
doing and, whether they are consumers or providers, that interest will at
times be in conflict with another member's interests. The only way to avoid
that would be to insist that all of the members be disinterested. The test is
deemed to be one of a "fiduciary" interest, i.e. does the member stand to
make money out of the decision. But there are other less direct forms of
interest that can be translated into equally compelling reasons for conflict.
Certainly any business person who has studied the community knows that
a new hospital will support an enormous peripheral economy: restaurants,
drug stores, parking lots, florists, office supplies, the development of doctors
offices, and all of the unrelated businesses that will experience a substantial
increase in trade simply by virtue of the large numbers of visitors, patients,
and workers who circulate around a major hospital. Community pride and
a sense of security can create considerable interest as well.

Public agencies can both provide services and regulate them. Ultimately,
a state health agency and a state health planning and development agency
must report to the same governor. A state health agency has several options
when considering a health facility construction program or a major change
in services. It can ignore the state's certificate of need law, but that would
eventually destroy the law, something that should be of as much concern
to a public health agency as its own programs. Alternatively, it can submit
its proposal to the planning agency for review. If this is done before the
plans are too rigidly formed in the minds of the administrators and the
legislators, they may find that the public review process can improve on the

original idea or perhaps show that another solution to a perceived problem would be better. A conflict is likely to occur when the public agency administrator becomes overcommitted to a particular plan before it has been publicly examined. Legislators, once they understand the process, can be protected also. If their interest is in doing something for their area and they are successful in obtaining an appropriation, local area planning and review may show that the need is not there, that it is different from what it was presumed to be or that another response to the need would be better. In any case, the interested legislator who can avoid premature commitment to a particular project can find the process to be both effective and politically helpful.

The conflict of interest argument is usually used by someone who wants to keep someone else from doing something. It is often raised by private sector rationalists who are trying to prevent incursions into their domain by public sector interests that might either compete with them or attempt to regulate their practices. Yet, given the distributive dynamics of the health system economy in the United States, it is clear that the private sector is as laden with conflict of interest as is the public sector, is much less accountable for its actions, and will not be able to guarantee access without public intervention.

As is suggested above, it is important that the governing body responsible for health programs in a community be accountable to the community served. This accountability cannot be routed through the secretary of DHHS and a community service provider accountable to a state agency cannot be deemed sufficiently accountable to the community served. The state agency's contract should be with an elected governing body for the community (or, if that is not practical, a governing body appointed by elected officials) that can, in turn, contract with a service group if it chooses to do so and if state laws permit that. So long as public health programs, be they service programs or regulatory programs, are accountable to the community served and in compliance with the regulations of the government paying for the activity, then conflicts of interest are basically within the community, where they ought to be. Treated with understanding and without secrecy, conflicts of interest are essential and positive elements in any decision-making process.

CONCLUSIONS

Until recently, attempts to describe what a health agency is or should be have been misleading for two reasons: (a) the agencies keep changing and (b) they are so different from state to state and community to community that statistical averages are not helpful. Recently, Miller and his colleagues (9) have begun to develop a clearer picture of the scope and importance of public health agencies at the local level. The working group on model standards (14) has added greatly to the understanding of the changing yet durable nature of the "governmental presence" in health.

The picture that emerges is one of a core interest in health—the prevention of illnesses and injuries that lead to dependency and death—with a surrounding sphere of interest that, although solid near the core, becomes more amorphous toward the periphery, finally interacting with other spheres of interest, such as education, welfare, and environmental protection. At these interfaces, tension occurs, which may lead to reorganization or to collaborative coalitions. Although the health focal point has been criticized and ignored for its alleged shortcomings in recent years, this seems to be due more to shifting interests external to the traditional core of the health interest sphere and continuing concern about the propriety of public involvement in providing private health services than any inherent weakness in health agencies. Despite the fact that these changing interests and arguments have led to the neglect of local health departments, they remain vigorous, ubiquitous, and important public agencies. Regarded as parts of a system, they are a major provider of traditional medical care as well as many specialized, essential personal and environmental health services.

Many of the issues in conflict that have been partly responsible for curbing the contributions that could be made by health departments can be settled by less traditional approaches toward organization and management. The ability to live with changing spheres of interest rather than sharply demarcated organizational boundaries, a better understanding of the need to make health systems and programs directly accountable to the people served (and of the fact that such accountability does not preclude the enlightened use of private entrepreneurs to produce and even manage needed services), and a realization that public bodies can both produce and regulate services by using conflicts of interest creatively are essential ingredients in the effort to reduce dependency by protecting and improving health. Glogow (3) has said that the demands on the modern administrator will be so enormous as to cause "burn-out" in four to five years. Perhaps so, but "burn-out" is more likely to occur when a machine is ill-designed for the job at hand. Understanding the issues in conflict can make their management easier and more effective. The governmental presence in the health interest sphere is just as important as it is in the education interest sphere and for many of the same reasons. Its influence is likely to increase both as a regulator and a manager of essential health programs and services that cannot otherwise contribute to their ultimate purpose.

Literature Cited

1. Terris, M. 1976. The epidemiologic revolution, national health insurance, and the role of health departments. *Am. J. Public Health* 66:1155–64
2. Terris, M. 1978. Public health in the United States: The next 100 years. *Public Health Rep.* 93:602
3. Glogow, E. 1973. Community participation and sharing in control of public health services. *Health Serv. Rep.* 88:442–48
4. Hanlon, J. J. 1973. Is there a future for local health departments? *Health Serv. Rep.* 88:898–901
5. Am. Public Health Assoc. 1978. *Public Policy Statements of the American Public Health Association*, No. 7434. Washington DC: APHA. 238 pp.[1]
6. Shonick, W., Price, W. 1977. Reorganization of health agencies by local government in American urban centers: What do they portend for "public health?" *Milbank Mem. Fund Q.* 55:233–71
7. US Public Health Service 1976. *Forward Plan for Health: FY 1978–82.* Washington DC: DHEW. 137 pp.
8. US Public Health Serv. 1978. *Health— United States, 1978.* Washington DC: DHEW. 488 pp.
9. Miller, C. A., Brooks, E. F., DeFriese, G. H., Gilbert D., Jain, S. C., Kavaler, F. 1977. A survey of local public health departments and their directors. *Am. J. Public Health* 67:931–39
10. Terris, M. H., Kramer, N. A. 1949. Medical care activities of full-time health departments. *Am. J. Public Health* 39:1129–35
11. Emerson, H. 1945. *Local Health Units for the Nation: Report of the Sub-committee on Administrative Practice.* New York: Commonwealth Fund
12. Kratz, F. W. 1942. The present status of full-time, local health organizations. *Public Health Rep.* 57:194–96
13. Mountin, J. N., Flook, E. 1953. *Guide to Health Organization in the United States.* Publ. no. 196. Washington DC: PHS
14. US Conf. City Health Off., Natl. Assoc. County Health Off., Assoc. State and Territ. Health Off., Am. Public Health Assoc. DHEW 1978. *Model Standards for Community Preventive Health Services* (draft). Atlanta, Ga.: US PHS, Cent. Dis. Control. 114 pp.
15. Assoc. State and Territ. Health Off. 1979. *Services, Expenditures and Programs of State and Territorial Health Agencies, Fiscal Year 1977.* Washington DC: ASTHO. 176 pp.
16. Assoc. State and Territ. Health Off. 1978. *Services, Expenditures and Programs of State and Territorial Health Agencies, Fiscal Year 1976.* Washington DC: ASTHO. 144 pp.
17. US Bureau of the Census 1978. *Statistical Abstract of the United States: 1978.* Washington DC: US Dep. Comm. 1057 pp.
18. Report to the President from the President's Commission on Mental Health, 1978, Vol. II, Append. Washington DC: GPO
19. Am. Public Health Assoc. 1954. See Ref. 5, No. 5405
20. Am. Public Health Assoc. 1965. See Ref. 5, No. 6526
21. Am. Public Health Assoc. 1978. See Ref. 5, No. 6812
22. Am. Public Health Assoc. 1961. See Ref. 5, No. 6112
23. Am. Public Health Assoc. 1964. See Ref. 5, No. 6416
24. Myers, B. A., Steinhardt, B. J., Mosley, M. L., Cashman, J. 1968. The medical care activities of local health units. *Public Health Rep.* 83:757
25. Miller, C. A., Moos, M.-K., Brown, M. L. 1978. *A study of local health departments.* Presented at Ann. Meet. Am. Public Health Assoc., 106th, Los Angeles
26. Gossert, D. J., Miller, C. A. 1973. State boards of health, their members and commitments. *Am. J. Public Health* 63:486–93
27. Viseltear, A. J. 1973. Emergence of the Medical Care Section of the American Public Health Association, 1926–1948. *Am. J. Public Health* 63: 986–1007
28. Roemer, M. I. 1973. The American Public Health Association as a force in medical care. *Med. Care* 11:338

[1]Original publication of APHA policy papers and resolutions can be found in the *Journal of the American Public Health Association.* The first two digits in the number of each cited policy paper or resolution refers to the year of adoption and they are sequentially numbered in the compilation (reference 5).

29. Corning, P. A. 1969. *The Evolution of Medicare . . . From Idea to Law.* Soc. Secur. Admin., Off. Res. Stat. Res. rep. no. 29. Washington DC DHEW 151 pp.
30. Shonick, W., Price, W. 1978. Organization milieus of local health units: Analysis of response to questionnaire. *Public Health Rep.* 93:648–65
31. Hanlon, J. J., Pickett, G. E. 1979. *Public Health: Administration and Practice.* St. Louis, Mo: Mosby. 748 pp.
32. Advis. Comm. on Intergovernmental Relations 1977. *Federal grants: Their Impact on State-local Expenditures, Employment Level, Wage Rates.* Washington DC: Advis. Comm. Intergov. Relat. 77 pp.

33. Am. Public Health Assoc. 1965. See Ref. 5, No. 6523
34. Am. Public Health Assoc. 1977. See Ref. 5, No. 7705
35. Begheim, M. L. 1977. *State Standards for Local Public Health Services, Final Report.* Washington D.C: Georgetown Univ. Health Policy Cent. 150 pp.
36. Davis, M. M. 1937. *Public Medical Services.* Chicago: Univ. Chicago Press
37. Shulman, D., Galanter, R. 1976. Reorganizing the nursing home industry—A proposal. *Milbank Mem. Fund Q.* 53:129–43
38. Etzioni, A., Doty, P. 1976. Profit in not-for-profit corporations: The example of health care. *Polit. Sci. Q.* 91:433–53

Ann. Rev. Public Health 1980. 1:323–44
Copyright © 1980 by Annual Reviews Inc. All rights reserved

EPIGEMIOLOGY AS A GUIDE TO HEALTH POLICY

◆12512

EPIDEMIOLOGY AS A GUIDE TO HEALTH POLICY

Milton Terris

Department of Community & Preventive Medicine, New York Medical College,
New York, NY 10029

There is little doubt that epidemiology should play a major role in the formulation of health policy. A number of factors, however, restrict its influence: (*a*) the failure of the health professions and of society to understand the primacy of prevention, (*b*) the unwillingness to accept the validity of epidemiologic discoveries, and (*c*) the power of private interests. These factors may act singly or more often together.

A great deal of lip service is paid to prevention; in actuality, society does relatively little about it. In 1977, total national health expenditures in the United States were $162,600,000,000, or 8.8% of the Gross National Product. Almost all of these expenditures went for medical care; 5% was spent for research and construction of medical facilities, whereas only 2% was spent on government public health activities (1).

This gross imbalance reflects the almost completely therapeutic orientation of the medical and allied health professions, whose attitudes range, with relatively rare exceptions, from sheer indifference to outright hostility toward epidemiology, preventive medicine, and public health.

The failure to appreciate the primacy of prevention is not limited to the health professions. It is shared, unfortunately, by the general public, which spends vast sums for curative services, building great complexes—the urban medical centers—as monuments to its belief in the importance of treatment. New hospitals have been built in every nook and corner of the land as secondary symbols of this faith.

Large armies of medical workers minister to the demand for medical care. The public's heroes, enshrined in books, magazines, movies, and television programs, are the surgeons and other clinicians who work miracu-

323

0163-7525/80/0510-0323$01.00

lous cures in hospital settings. Those who wield power in health affairs are largely the heads of clinical services, the representatives of medical societies, the directors of hospitals, and the administrators of medical care programs.

If we subject this fervently held public view of medical care to critical analysis, we are forced to more qualified conclusions. The relevance of medical care to the public health is determined primarily by its impact on mortality and morbidity. A hundred years ago medical care was largely ineffectual in these terms, and most of the subsequent progress in diminishing death and illness has resulted from the operation of other factors.

INFECTIOUS DISEASES

According to the 1850 census of mortality, approximately three-fifths of all deaths in the United States were caused by infectious diseases, including (in order of importance) tuberculosis, dysentery and diarrhea, cholera, malaria, typhoid fever, pneumonia, diphtheria, scarlet fever, meningitis, whooping cough, measles, erysipelas, and smallpox. As Smillie states, the great proportion of these deaths were due to "unfavorable environmental factors, to polluted water supplies, indescribable systems of feces disposal, overcrowding, with resultant disreputable housing conditions, bad milk, bad food, flies in millions, poor nutrition, long hours of overwork, and gross ignorance and carelessness" (2).

Cholera, dysentery and diarrhea, and typhoid fever have largely disappeared as a result of environmental control measures directed at water, milk, and food supplies. Infantile diarrhea succumbed because of these environmental measures, the development of well baby clinics independent of medical care services, health education, and the extension of medical care to include preventive care of well infants.

The decline of malaria was primarily a social phenomenon, caused, as Smillie points out, by "a transition from pioneer conditions to improved cultivation of the land, better rural housing, more cattle, more drainage of the bottom land, rapid transportation, replacement of the village mill and its mill pond by centralized milling, and all the other components of an advancing civilization." In more recent years, malaria has been driven from its remaining strongholds by planned measures of environmental control.

Diphtheria, smallpox, whooping cough, and measles have been conquered by public health programs of immunization. Pneumonia, scarlet fever, meningitis, and erysipelas may have receded because of long-term social changes, including improvement in housing with a consequent decline in overcrowding. Medical intervention became effective only with the prophylactic and therapeutic use of antibiotics during the past few decades.

Tuberculosis has declined primarily because of improvement in the standard of living, assisted by public health control measures such as isolation and case-finding programs. Here medical care served a preventive function by isolating infective persons in tuberculosis hospitals. More recently, treatment with new drugs has enabled medical care to be more efficacious in reducing infectivity, morbidity, and mortality.

The treatment of syphilis with effective drugs, likewise, has played a key role in controlling infectivity and thereby preventing disease spread as well as reducing mortality and morbidity. On the other hand, medical care proved to be largely powerless in the face of tetanus and poliomyelitis, diseases that are being virtually eliminated by public health immunization programs. Puerperal fever was conquered primarily by controlling the hospital environment; this was a salient factor, along with the establishment of public health prenatal clinics and improvement in obstetric care, in the reduction of maternal mortality.

In summary, then, the major forces operating to lower morbidity and mortality from infectious diseases during the past 100 years have been economic and social changes, environmental control measures, immunization, health education, and other public health activities. Medical care per se has played a secondary role, limited for the most part to two main functions: the alleviation of suffering, a notable contribution of medical care in all illness and one that cannot be overlooked in any evaluation of the relevance of medical care to the health of the public; and the reduction of severity of illness through supportive measures, a function that medical care performs with varying success in specific diseases. It is only during the past few decades that the advent of the new chemotherapeutic and antibiotic agents has enabled medical care to go beyond these functions and to make a greater contribution to the health of the public by definitive treatment and cure of infectious diseases.

NONINFECTIOUS DISEASES

When we turn our attention to the noninfectious diseases, we find considerably less success in reducing mortality and morbidity, with two outstanding areas of exception: (a) the nutritional deficiency diseases, including scurvy, rickets, pellagra, endemic goiter, and others, which have been largely eliminated in the United States and other industrialized countries by improved living standards, food enrichment and supplementation, and health education of the public and (b) the occupational diseases, which have been substantially reduced by the development of public health programs and the use of workmen's compensation laws to provide a stimulus to prevention.

Medical care has become increasingly efficacious in lowering mortality and morbidity from trauma, whether due to accidents or violence. Yet accidents remain a leading cause of death. The immense carnage wrought by two world wars is a grim reminder that the only definitive answer to the conquest of trauma lies in social means of prevention.

Surgical intervention is of unquestionable value in a variety of diseases including, among others, hyperthyroidism, peptic ulcer, appendicitis, cholecystitis and cholelithiasis, hernia, and hemorrhoids.

Replacement therapy has curtailed mortality and morbidity from such diseases as diabetes mellitus, hypothyroidism, Addison's disease, and pernicious anemia. Diabetes mellitus, however, remains a leading cause of death in the United States.

The value of therapy for cancer varies with the site, histological type, and stage of development of the malignancy. In far too many instances the results of treatment are unsatisfactory. Cancer remains the second leading cause of death.

The efficacy of treatment varies for other major causes of illness. In asthma and other diseases of allergy, the most valuable approach is to prevent contact with antigens, although desensitization therapy may be useful when such avoidance is impossible; however, there is no actual cure. Peptic ulcer, gout, and epilepsy are chronic diseases in which treatment of acute attacks must be followed by preventive therapy in order to reduce the number and severity of recurrences.

Despite the decline in syphilitic and rheumatic heart disease and the contributions of surgery in correcting certain congenital and rheumatic cardiac defects, heart disease remains the most important cause of death and illness. The treatment of coronary heart disease remains only moderately effective despite dramatic advances in the treatment of damaged hearts.

Definitive therapy is still unavailable for major afflictions such as arthritis, cerebral vascular disease, and chronic bronchitis. Preventive treatment with lithium has proved effective in limiting recurrences of manic-depressive psychosis. There are no cures, however, for schizophrenia.

This necessarily brief review indicates that the contribution of medical care in mitigating the burden of noninfectious disease is substantial but limited; although curative in some, it is only partially effective in most of these diseases. This weakness is largely inherent in medical care, for once the pathological changes have reached the stage at which they produce symptoms requiring treatment, reversal of the process may no longer be possible.

As in the infectious diseases, the greatest potential for improving the health of the public lies in prevention. The correctness of this statement is evident from these facts: the elimination of nutritional deficiency diseases and control of occupational diseases, the success of epidemiology and public health in lowering the prevalence of dental caries by fluoridation, and the significant and continuing contributions of epidemiology to an understanding of the causes and means of prevention of the major noninfectious diseases.

THE SECOND EPIDEMIOLOGIC REVOLUTION

During the past few decades, enormous advances have been made through epidemiologic studies of cancer, heart disease, stroke, and other important noninfectious disease entities. The epidemiologists have forged effective weapons for control—weapons that must now be grasped by health departments and wielded for our traditional aims of preventing disease, disability, and death. The significance of these weapons may be understood by reviewing their potential impact on the ten leading causes of death.

The leading cause of death—diseases of the heart—accounts for 38% of all deaths. Ninety percent of cardiac deaths are the result of ischemic heart disease. Epidemiologic research has identified three major risk factors—high serum cholesterol, hypertension, and cigarette smoking—that increase the incidence and mortality rates for ischemic heart disease. Epidemiologic studies have also shown that each of these factors is amenable to change: serum cholesterol can be lowered by the substitution of an unsaturated fatty acid diet, high blood pressure can be brought down by suitable drugs, and cigarette smoking can be reduced under the impact of adequate knowledge. We are now reaching the end of the investigative period and the beginning of the time for action by federal, state, and local health departments.

Cancer accounts for 18% of all deaths, many of which are still unpreventable. For certain sites, however, considerable progress has been achieved by epidemiologic research. We now know that cigarette smoking causes cancer of the lung, mouth, pharynx, and larynx. It is becoming increasingly evident that alcohol consumption is related to cancer of the mouth, pharynx, esophagus, larynx, and liver. The important role of X rays and other sources of radiation in the etiology of leukemia and other forms of cancer has been demonstrated, and the effects of a variety of industrial carcinogens have been ascertained. Effective screening methods have been developed for breast cancer and cancer of the cervix.

Cerebrovascular diseases, which account for 11% of all deaths and comprise the third leading cause of death, were completely unpreventable a quarter of a century ago. Now we know that the incidence of these diseases —caused primarily by hypertension and by atherosclerosis—can be lowered significantly by screening and long-term treatment for hypertension and presumably also by the prevention of atherosclerosis.

Accidents are a particularly tragic cause of mortality because they so often kill children and young people. Indeed, they are the leading cause of death up to the age of 35 years. For all ages, they are fourth in importance; if the attention given to them were on a par with their significance to the nation's health, they undoubtedly could be driven from the list of ten leading causes of death. Epidemiologic research has deepened our understanding of the host, agent, and environmental factors involved in various types of accidents and has indicated the preventive measures that can and should be employed. One major research finding may be cited as an example: the discovery that high blood alcohol levels are found in 50% of the drivers responsible for fatal auto accidents. The implications of this finding are clear, but effective public health action has yet to be taken in the United States.

Influenza and pneumonia, fifth in importance, continue to decline, presumably because of the use of influenza vaccines for high-risk individuals and because of improvements in antibiotic therapy.

Bronchitis, emphysema, and other chronic obstructive lung diseases— now the sixth leading cause of death—result mainly from cigarette smoking and other air pollutants. Most of these deaths could undoubtedly be prevented by effective public health action against these agents. On the other hand, significant declines in the mortality rate for diabetes mellitus, which is seventh on the list, cannot be expected with the knowledge and methods that are currently available.

Cirrhosis of the liver, which did not appear among the ten leading causes of death in 1965, was the tenth leading cause in 1969 and has been the eighth since 1973. This rapidly increasing cause of mortality has been shown by epidemiologists to be a function of alcohol consumption. As alcohol consumption rises in the population, so does the cirrhosis mortality rate, and as the consumption falls, so does the death rate.

Ninth on the list is arteriosclerosis, which is amenable to the measures recommended for ischemic heart disease. Last is birth injury, difficult labor, and other causes of mortality in early infancy, which have continued to decline, presumably as a result of improved obstetrical and pediatric practice.

As one reviews the ten leading causes of death, and the tools for their control that the epidemiologists have fashioned for us, it becomes apparent that large declines in mortality are not only possible but inevitable, given a determined public health onslaught on the vulnerable causes of death. Powerful barriers, however, stand in the way.

"Scientific" Obstacles to Health Policy

Among the significant obstacles to epidemiology as a guide to health policy are the views of clinicians who are unwilling to accept the validity of epidemiologic discoveries. At the turn of the century, for example, when the New York City Health Department declared tuberculosis to be a communicable disease and proposed a series of measures to prevent its transmission, the medical board of the West Side German Dispensary adopted resolutions to the effect that the statement that tuberculosis is a communicable disease "is not entirely correct and is not the opinion of many distinguished clinicians" (3).

One of the major obstacles to the acceptance of epidemiological findings by clinicians relates to the character of the evidence. This was as true during the first epidemiologic revolution, the control of infectious diseases, it is now during the second, when the issues relate to the noninfectious diseases. In the middle of the nineteenth century, John Snow came to remarkably accurate conclusions on the etiology and prevention of cholera by the use of "merely statistical" evidence (which is the layman's and clinician's term of disparagement of epidemiology, i.e. the study of disease in human population groups); only later was there confirmation by so-called real science, i.e., the study of disease in rats, mice, and guinea pigs. Snow's natural experiment in the real world of London had to be validated more than a quarter of a century later by contrived experiments in the laboratory.

And so it is today. Epidemiologists have come to remarkably accurate conclusions on the etiology and prevention of a host of diseases, such as lung cancer, ischemic heart disease, and cerebrovascular disease, long before the laboratory scientists will succeed in discovering the precise pathophysiologic mechanisms that are involved. Because, as in John Snow's time, the latter information is not yet available, epidemiologists have difficulty in obtaining acceptance of their scientific conclusions and recommendations for preventive action. The lung cancer controversy is perhaps the most dramatic example of the struggles that epidemiologists have had to wage in order to overcome this obstacle.

Vested Interests and Health Policy

It is often true that the so-called scientific objections to epidemiologic findings receive powerful support from private interests greatly concerned with the possible use of the findings as a guide to health policy. In 1897, when the New York City Board of Health made tuberculosis a notifiable disease, the medical profession condemned the action—not only the New York County and Kings County medical societies but even the New York Academy of Medicine officially opposed it. The *Medical Record* reacted with an editorial that stated, "The real obnoxiousness of this amendment to the sanitary code is its offensively dictatorial and defiantly compulsory character. . . . The profession as a whole has watched with jealous eye the encroachments of the Board upon many of the previously well-recognized privileges of the medical attendant . . ." In a later editorial, the objections were made more explicit:

> There is no objection to the reports of pulmonary cases for statistical purposes. . . . It is, however, the extra missionary work assumed by the board which is the ominous and threatening quantity in the equation—the desire to assume official control of the cases after they have been reported, thus not only, by means of alarming bacteriological edicts, directly interfering with the physician in the diagnosis and treatment of the patient, but in the end, by the creation of a public suspicion of his ignorance, possibly depriving him of one of the means of a legitimate livelihood. . . . The only basis of a proper understanding in this matter is the guarantee of the board that in case the returns of pulmonary cases are faithfully made, for statistical purposes only, there shall be on its part no direct or indirect interference between patient and physician, either in the way of official inspections, bacteriological diagnosis, forced isolation, suggestions for treatment, or presumptuous instructions to the patient regarding hygienic precaution. If we mistake not, the profession is very much in earnest in thus dividing responsibility with the board and will yet be able to vindicate its rights and demonstrate its power (3).

In our day, perhaps the most blatant example of private interests attempting to prevent acceptance of epidemiologic facts is the establishment of the Tobacco Industry Research Committee. The history of occupational health is replete with such instances. These activities do not stop at the scientific level: Powerful industrial and other private interests are able to exert considerable influence to prevent epidemiology from fulfilling its role as a guide to governmental health policy.

The only antidote to their power is that of an informed and aroused community. As Hermann Biggs wrote in the New York City Health Department's *Monthly Bulletin,* about a decade after his victory in the tuberculosis campaign,

> Disease is largely a removable evil. It continues to afflict humanity, not only because of incomplete knowledge of its causes and lack of adequate individual and public hygiene, but also because it is extensively fostered by harsh economic and industrial conditions and by wretched housing in congested communities. These conditions and consequently the diseases which spring from them can be removed by better social organization. No duty of society, acting through its governmental agencies, is paramount to this obligation to attack the removable causes of disease. The duty of leading this attack and bringing home to public opinion the fact that the community can buy its own health protection is laid upon all health officers, organizations and individuals interested in public health movements. For the provision of more and better facilities for the protection of the public health must come in the last analysis through the education of public opinion so that the community shall vividly realize both its needs and powers (3).

Ideological Obstacles to Health Policy

It is obvious that the second epidemiologic revolution, like the first, will require government action of various kinds in order to protect the health of the public. One such action is the imposition of financial barriers against tobacco, alcohol, and other harmful substances.

Perhaps the most frequent and important question asked about such action concerns its effect on civil liberties. Is this not another example of Big Brother, of governmental interference with personal liberty and the freedom of individuals to do as they wish with their lives?

The reply to this question has a number of facets. One is that the individual will still have freedom of choice; if he really wants to smoke or drink, no one will stop him from doing so. He may think twice about spending more money for these amenities, but whether he buys them or not is really up to him.

Another aspect relates to the fact that when the oil companies sharply increased the price of gasoline, nobody raised the question of civil liberties or the palpable interference with the freedom of individuals to do as they wish with their cars, their weekends, and their lives. Even more serious is the current unprecedented increase in the price of food and other necessities, which threatens the freedom of choice as well as the health of the people of this country—if not all the people, then certainly those in poor or moderate circumstances. Yet there was no outcry against this increase on the basis of interference with the freedom of choice of individuals, even though it was caused in large measure by the policy of the federal government, which has been unwilling to take effective action against inflation.

We must then ask the question: Whose freedom, and to what purpose? Our freedom as a sovereign people to defend ourselves from lung and other cancers, from chronic bronchitis, pulmonary emphysema, and coronary heart disease, and from having literally millions of lives wasted by illness, disability, and death? Or the freedom of the tobacco companies, among others, to continue to make their profits over the corpses of their victims? These victims are not an abstraction. Probably not a single person who reads this review has not had a close relative or friend who died unnecessarily and too soon, often in the prime of life, as a result of cigarette smoking.

If we allow the present situation to continue, giving freedom to the tobacco and other companies to spread their message while refusing to interfere on the grounds of freedom, then we shall be accomplices in the lethal consequences. Further, we shall betray the great tradition of public health, a tradition that destroyed the freedom of water companies to sell polluted water, that prohibited farmers and distributors from selling unpasteurized milk—yes, that even made it compulsory for children to be vaccinated against smallpox.

Our predecessors in public health took away the individual's freedom not only to have smallpox, but also to become ill with cholera, typhoid fever, and other diseases spread by water and milk. They did so by depriving individuals of the freedom to drink polluted water and to enjoy raw milk which, as everyone knew in those days, was much tastier than the pasteurized product. We need to act in our own time with the vision and courage that earlier public health workers demonstrated when they established a greater freedom, the freedom to enjoy health and life, as a major concern of government.

The Lifestyle Approach to Health Policy

One result of the pressures by private interests, and the ideological obstacles that are created by these interests, is the development of an approach to health policy that states, essentially, that there is no need for health policy.

The economist, Victor Fuchs, for example, takes the reasonable position that disease prevention is more important to health than medical care, but carries the argument further in terms of his philosophy:

> Emphasizing social responsibility can increase security, but it may be the security of the "zoo"—purchased at the expense of freedom. . . . The greatest current potential for improving the health of the American people is to be found in what they do and don't do to and for themselves. Individual decisions about diet, exercise, and smoking are of critical importance, and collective decisions affecting pollution and other aspects of the environment are also relevant (4).

To Fuchs, it is the individual decisions that are of critical importance; social decisions are "also relevant" but limited to such problems as pollution.

Fuchs uses the term "life-style" to describe what he believes to be the most important determinant of health and disease. Perhaps the most widely known example of the lifestyle approach is the report by Mark Lalonde, the former Canadian Minister of National Health and Welfare, titled *A New Perspective on the Health of Canadians* (5). In an interesting attempt to broaden the theoretical and practical basis of public health in Canada, Lalonde proposed that the health field be broken up into four broad elements: human biology, environment, lifestyle, and health care organization. After reviewing Canada's major health problems, he concluded that in addition to the health care system and the collective problem of the environment,

> Individual blame must be accepted by many for the deleterious effect on health of their respective lifestyles. Sedentary living, smoking, overeating, driving while impaired by alcohol, drug abuse and failure to wear seat-belts are among the many contributions to

physical or mental illness for which the individual must accept some responsibility and for which he should seek correction (5).

A major weakness of this approach is that it conceives of individual lifestyles as though they exist in a vacuum. Society has nothing to do with the matter. Furthermore, society takes no responsibility; as Lalonde states, "Individual blame must be accepted," or as Fuchs says in closing his book, "The greatest potential for improving health lies in what we do and don't do for and to ourselves. The choice is ours" (4). That is why Fuchs has much to recommend on the social organization of health care, but nothing on social measures to change lifestyles. Lalonde has a long list of recommendations to influence lifestyles, but they seem to consist largely of moderate programs of health education and a few very weak regulatory proposals.

In fact, this lack of a program for effective social measures is inevitable, given the fundamental ideology of the lifestyle approach. This ideology, which places all the blame on the individual and thereby absolves society of responsibility, has enjoyed a good deal of popularity in recent years among those who counsel "benign neglect" of the problems of poverty. In a carefully reasoned refutation of these views, William Ryan characterizes them as *Blaming the Victim* (6).

The technique of "blaming the victim" is not new in American society, it has simply become more sophisticated. Public health in our country has been hampered by various versions of the lifestyle approach from the very beginning. Speaking to the New York State Legislature in 1865, Stephen Smith noted that first among the alleged causes of the high mortality in New York City was the large foreign immigration. He considered the immigrants to be scapegoats, and defended them by quoting the City Inspector's report for 1860:

> Most of the children who arrived in this city from foreign ports, although suffering from the effects of a protracted voyage, bad accommodations, and worse fare, do not bring with them any marked disease beyond those which, with proper care, nursing, and wholesome air, could be easily overcome. The causes of this excessive mortality must be searched for in this city, and are readily traceable to the wretched habitations in which parents and children are forced to take up their abode; in the contracted alleys, the tenement house, with its hundreds of occupants, where each cooks, eats, and sleeps in a single room, without light or ventilation, surrounded with filth, an atmosphere foul, fetid, and deadly, with none to console with or advise them, or to apply for relief when disease invades them (7).

Blaming the victim is as unjustified today as it was 120 years ago. It is difficult to accept the concept that smoking is an individual matter when it is well-known that cigarette advertising, costing more than $300 million a year, transformed smoking from a minor to a major addiction; that the women's market was developed by carefully designed advertising campaigns; and that the youth market was next opened up by systematic advertising directed at college newspapers and youth magazines.

The alcohol industries have improved greatly on the free-cigarettes-on-airplanes and similar routines of the tobacco industry. The following account of how individual lifestyles are created comes from *The New York Times* of December 26, 1974:

> The liquor companies are similarly big clients of CMR (College Marketing and Research Corporation). . . . Now one of CMR's major activities is giving on-campus liquor tasting parties. It gave 400 of them last year, the biggest being for 4,000 at a homecoming at Florida State where the only drink served was a Mexican Sunrise with Jose Cuervo tequila. . . . CMR is now extending tasting parties to 'singles' apartment complexes and to Junior Chamber of Commerce activities, which increases its demographic reach from 18 to 23 up to 18 to 34 (8).

If alcohol consumption is simply a matter of individual choice, it is difficult to explain the fact that in Great Britain the highest death rates from cirrhosis of the liver occur in social class 1, the wealthiest class, whereas in the United States the highest rates are in the poorest group, the unskilled workers in social class 5.

Individual lifestyles cannot explain why drug addiction in the United States is largely confined to the slums and ghettos in which minority groups live. Or why black men have fewer myocardial infarctions than white men. Or why different types of accidents have such clear cut and differing occurrence rates in different segments of the population.

The trouble with the lifestyle approach is that it tends to disregard epidemiology, for it reduces everything to the single factor or habit and its use or nonuse; no thought is given to other variables in the social environment that affect such use. Perhaps this reflects a self-protective reaction, for the social engineering required to change the significant variables is difficult to achieve. The industries whose interests are threatened by preventive programs have large financial resources available to block effective governmental action. Nevertheless, that action can and will be realized in the interest of the health of the population because eventually the public will understand and demand it.

A HEALTH POLICY BASED ON EPIDEMIOLOGY

If epidemiology is used as a guide to health policy, the latter will then be based on the primacy of prevention. As representatives of the public, health departments will have as their major goal the development of programs to prevent the major causes of death. The programs will have three basic components: control of the environment, screening, and health education.

Except for immunization, these are much the same approaches that were used effectively in the campaigns against communicable diseases during the first epidemiologic revolution. It is only the content that will be different.

Control of the Environment

During the first epidemiologic revolution, environmental control was directed primarily against vehicles and vectors of living agents, whereas today the agents are primarily physicochemical in nature. The fundamental strategy, however, remains the same: to create environmental barriers between agent and host. A wide variety of methods were used in the earlier period, such as construction of public water supply and sewage systems, residual spraying of dwellings, regulations requiring pasteurization of milk, and hospitalization of individuals with tuberculosis and other infectious diseases.

During the current period, the available measures for control of the environment may be grouped into those which are regulatory in nature, and those which are based on financial considerations. Among the former would be the following:

1. Laws proscribing all advertising for cigarettes and alcohol and forbidding smoking in public areas.
2. Laws requiring that only unsaturated fats be used in commercial baking, and that labels specify the amount and degree of saturation of the fats contained in packaged foods.
3. Regulations to prevent air and water pollution, accidents, and exposure to radiation, carcinogens, and other toxic substances in industry, in medical care facilities, in the general community, and in the home.
4. Regulations requiring installation of safety features in motor vehicles, lowering the maximum speeds permitted on highways, and revoking driving licenses of motorists found to be driving under the influence of alcohol.

The financial measures are of two kinds: those which create a financial barrier to an agent and those which subsidize its removal or replacement. Among the first group would be (a) an increase in taxation of cigarettes and alcohol to achieve a four- to five-fold increase in price and (b) taxation of foods high in saturated fats to increase their relative costs. The second group would include (c) assistance to farmers to change cattle feed in order to produce beef low in saturated fats, (d) subsidies to lower the relative price of foods rich in unsaturated fats, and (e) financial and other support to help farmers transfer the use of their land from tobacco and alcohol to nonlethal crops.

A simple reading of these proposed measures should convince even the most ingenuous that they will be difficult to legislate and implement. Those opposed to them will be far more influential than the physicians and merchants in the past who, fearing loss of trade, resisted public health activities and regulations for the prevention of infectious diseases. They will include the tobacco industry, the spirits, wine and beer industries, and industry in general because of the costs of prevention of occupational diseases and accidents and the control of air pollution. Unless the change to nonlethal crops is subsidized, there will be serious opposition from farmers. If the loss in advertising revenues caused by the ban on tobacco and alcohol advertising is not compensated by an equivalent use of the mass media for health education about these lethal substances, there will be strong opposition from the opinion-makers in the newspaper, magazine, and advertising industries.

There is little doubt, therefore, that any serious attempt to fulfill the promise of the second epidemiologic revolution will immediately pit the public interest—the health of the people of the United States—against formidable private interests. The outcome of such a confrontation will depend largely on whether health departments move boldly to secure the support of the nation's citizens. That support can be achieved and the resistance can be overcome because the public's stake in these issues is very great. Once the public really understands this point, it will be difficult for anyone, no matter how powerful, to continue to delay the implementation of its demand that effective public health measures be taken.

Screening

During the first epidemiologic revolution, the screening of well persons for early detection and treatment of disease was widely used in tuberculosis and syphilis control. In the noninfectious diseases, the concept has been expanded to include not only the detection of disease but the identification of risk factors as well. Examples of screening for disease include the use of cytology for cancer of the cervix, clinical examination and mammography for breast cancer, and blood pressure determination for hypertension. The determination of serum cholesterol level and the taking of smoking and drinking histories are examples of screening for risk factors.

Screening is valuable only if the tests are relatively cheap, easy to do, and score well on sensitivity and specificity. From the point of view of prevention as distinct from epidemiologic investigation, the tests should be done only if the disease they uncover can be treated effectively. Controlled outcome studies have already demonstrated the value of screening for hypertension and for breast cancer. For the risk factors in ischemic heart disease, the outcome studies are now under way. No controlled studies have been done in cancer of the cervix, but recent evidence indicates a significant correlation of declines in incidence and mortality of cervical cancer with annual rates of cytologic screening.

A full discussion of the value of screening in a wide variety of diseases cannot be undertaken here. It should be noted, however, that screening can also be used effectively for the detection and correction of impairments. Screening for visual defects is particularly useful because of the ease of testing and the availability in most instances of relatively inexpensive corrective lenses.

Treatment following screening presents special problems. When the patient seeks care for an illness, the motivation to accept treatment is relatively high. When there is no manifest illness, as is usual in screening programs, and when treatment must often be maintained over a long period of time, motivation depends on an understanding of possible future outcomes by the patient that is equivalent, or almost equivalent, to that of the physician. Education, therefore, becomes essential. Equally important is the removal of impediments to treatment such as fee-for-service payments, long waiting periods, and lack of personal attention. Easy access to services must be assured—for this reason, long-continued treatment and supervision will probably be most effective at the workplace. Occupational health services will therefore take on new dimensions during the second epidemiologic revolution.

Health Education

It is clear from the discussion so far that we have entered a new period in the history of public health in which health education will again occupy a central rather than a peripheral position. The new programs to prevent ischemic heart disease, cancer, cerebrovascular disease, accidents, cirrhosis of the liver, and chronic obstructive lung disease will all have to rely heavily on health education.

This reliance has two major aspects. The first is the need to educate the public to understand the scientific basis for the new public health programs. Without a well-informed public it will be impossible to counter the opposition of vested private interests who place their own financial welfare above the health of the people. The second aspect is the need to educate individuals to change their behavior in the interest of disease prevention. This can be done most effectively if the countereducation, such as advertising by the tobacco and alcohol companies, is prohibited. Furthermore, the budgets for health education at the federal, state, and local levels need to be at least equivalent to the annual advertising budgets of the tobacco and alcohol companies, which presumably have been somewhere in the $500 million range.

These funds will be used for far more complex tasks than the selling of cigarettes or whiskies. The shifting of dietary habits is not easy to accomplish, although it should be recalled that this has already been accomplished once in this century. "The basic 7" charts that graced every health department clinic and every public health nurse's office should serve as a reminder that health education played an important role in changing the American diet from meat, bread, and potatoes to a more balanced diet in which milk, fruits, and vegetables have a respectable place.

An even more difficult task, perhaps, is educating individuals to take treatment for years when they have no symptoms of disease. In hypertension, for example, treatment has to be continued for the lifetime of the individual, although all that is amiss is a measurement taken by a physician. The magnitude of the task is indicated by the fact that about one sixth of the population age 18 and over has hypertension.

The serious problems of addiction to tobacco, alcohol, and other drugs are known to be difficult to treat. The success that a sizeable proportion of American and English physicians have had in throwing off their tobacco habit, however, indicates that the addiction can be broken. Because physicians may hardly be considered to have stronger wills than their peers in other occupations, one must conclude that superior knowledge and understanding are the basis for their success. Clearly, there is a future for the health education of those already addicted, but of even greater importance will be the use of health education for young people to prevent addiction in the first place.

As we move to meet these responsibilities, it will be essential to conduct health education in a human way, as a transaction between individuals. This caveat should not be necessary, but we live in a nation in which machines seem to have captured and dehumanized men and women. The attempt to solve the problems of decent health care for the American people by good management, operations research, systems analysis, and computerization of everything in sight is a case in point.

Let us not make the same error here by turning everything over to television; if we do so, we shall be sorely disappointed. The mass media should of course be used, including television, radio, newspapers, magazines, and billboards. But in addition we shall need more homely tools, such as pamphlets and leaflets in different languages, movies, slides, filmstrips, posters, exhibits, and classroom materials for teachers. Lectures, talks, study groups, question and answer sessions, and above all personal interviews for education of individual patients should become common practice for public health nurses, hospital and clinic nurses, health educators, nutritionists, dietitions, and even physicians. Indeed, we might take a leaf from the Soviet national health service in which all health workers are required to devote at least four hours a month to health education and in which students in all medical schools, as well as in other schools for health workers, receive classroom and field training in health education.

EPIDEMIOLOGY-BASED HEALTH POLICY: BENEFITS AND COSTS

In 1971–1973, the United States death rate from ischemic heart disease was 327 per 100,000 (9). A number of countries, more or less comparable to the United States in age distribution and industrial development, had considerably lower rates during the same period: Switzerland, 109; Italy, 137; Belgium, 186; Netherlands, 190; and Canada, 229 (10). It is difficult to conceive of these as genetic differences; the weight of evidence points to dietary and other environmental differences as responsible.

Let us now assume that effective public health action is taken in the United States with regard to the major risk factors of serum cholesterol, hypertension, and smoking. It is not too much to assume that the rate can thereby be brought down by about a third, to approximate the relatively high rates of Belgium, Netherlands, and Canada.

There is also good reason to believe that if we seriously undertake to find and treat hypertension on a national scale, the toll from cerebral vascular disease can be lowered by at least a third. Modest successes in removing cigarettes and other carcinogenic agents from the environment could result in a 10% decline in incidence of malignant neoplasms.

The toll from accidents, poisonings, and violence could easily be lowered a third by applying the knowledge that already exists on the epidemiology and control of specific types of trauma. This possibility is not Utopian; from 1973 to 1975, the motor vehicle accident death rate fell 21%, from 26.5 per 100,000 in 1973 to 20.9 in 1975, as a result of the new legislation, enacted because of the gasoline shortage, that established a maximum speed limit of 55 miles per hour on the nation's highways (9).

The control of alcohol consumption would play a major role in the decline of morbidity and mortality from accidents, poisonings, and violence. It would, in addition, sharply reduce the toll from the eighth leading cause of death, cirrhosis of the liver. By appropriate governmental measures aimed primarily at increasing the price of alcohol the United Kingdom lowered its cirrhosis mortality rate from 10 per 100,000 in 1915 to 3 in 1933, a 70% decline in less than 20 years; the rate has remained at this low level ever since. Similar action is badly needed in the United States, for our rate of 15 per 100,000 in 1975 was 25% higher than the rate of 12 in 1915. Such action would undoubtedly save thousands of lives and lower considerably the enormous costs engendered, not only by cirrhosis, but by all the health and social consequences of alcohol consumption.

Chronic obstructive lung disease, now the sixth leading cause of death in the United States, is caused mainly by cigarette smoking. The extent to which a program to prevent cigarette smoking is successful will be the extent to which it will be possible to lower the significant toll from this disease.

Partial and tentative assessment of the costs of preventable illness can now be made using the data prepared by Cooper & Rice on the costs of broad categories of illness in the United States in 1972 (11). These are rough approximations, but they indicate that an effective preventive program could, by a conservative estimate, save each year at least 400,000 lives, 6 million person-years of life, and $5 billion in medical costs (Table 1).

What will be the costs of carrying out this preventive program? These can and should be estimated, but at this point the data are not readily available. We know that secondary prevention programs such as hypertension control will generally be more expensive than those keyed to primary preventive measures. The cost of lowering the maximum speed limit to 55 miles per hour has been minimal indeed, yet this single measure saved 11,000 lives in 1975.

Furthermore, some of the proposed measures, such as heavy taxation of cigarettes and alcohol to increase their price, are actually revenue-producing even though this is not their aim. Such revenue can and should be earmarked for the total preventive program.

With an annual estimated saving of at least 400,000 lives, 6 million person-years of life, and $5 billion in medical costs, it is difficult to conceive that the costs of prevention will even remotely begin to approach the benefits, regardless of how comprehensive and expensive the program may be.

The criticism has been made, however, that the preventive programs will simply save people now to die later at a presumed greater cost to society. From this viewpoint the cost-benefit analysis should be longitudinal rather than cross-sectional in character. Implicit in this approach is doubt concerning the value of adding 10 or 20 years to an individual's life, plus the fear that he or she will end as a burden to society.

This negative attitude toward prevention is based on a static view of both costs and benefits. The benefits of the preventive programs may surprisingly turn out to be far greater than they are now conceived. For example, the prevention of atherosclerosis may have a highly significant effect on brain function in later life. Should this occur, much of the behavioral pathology and mental deficit in the older age groups may disappear, and the lengthening of life may also result in a more fruitful and happier life span. Similar

Table 1 Estimate of potential savings in lives, person-years, and direct costs of illness as a result of selected preventive programs, United States, 1972[a]

Disease	Estimated prevented (%)	No. deaths	No. deaths prevented	Person-years lost	No. person-years saved	Direct costs of illness (in millions)	Direct costs of illness saved (in millions)
Circulatory system	30[b]	1,046,000	314,000	12,152,000	3,646,000	$10,919	$3,276
Malignant neoplasms	10	353,000	35,000	5,701,000	570,000	$ 3,872	387
Accidents, poisonings, and violence	33.3	163,000	54,000	5,471,000	1,824,000	$ 5,121	$1,707
Cirrhosis of the liver	25	33,000	8,000	—	—	—	—
Chronic obstructive lung disease	10	39,000	4,000	—	—	—	—
			415,000		6,040,000		$5,370

[a] For methodology, see reference (11).
[b] 33.3% of ischemic heart disease and cerebral vascular disease, which comprise 90% of total circulatory system disease.

considerations apply to the physical disabilities caused by cerebrovascular disease, which will undoubtedly decline as the result of hypertension and atherosclerosis control programs.

These changes will also affect the cost side of the cost-benefit analysis because a lessening of physical and mental disability will decrease the burdens on society. It is hazardous therefore to undertake a cost-benefit analysis that bases future costs and benefits on actual or presumed current experience. Even if the data on current experience are accurate, the analysis is bound to be as invalid as the use of a life table based on the age-specific death rates of 1980 to predict the true expectation of life of the children born that year.

Funding the Policy

There are two possible approaches to financing an effective national policy based on epidemiology. One requires a change within the health field, the other requires a change in areas external to health.

Large sums are potentially available within the health field to finance prevention. In 1940, total national health expenditures were $3.9 billion, or 4.1% of the Gross National Product. By 1977 they had risen to $162.6 billion, or 8.8% of the GNP (1). Almost all of the latter went for medical care; 5% was spent for research and construction of medical facilities, whereas only 2% was spent on government public health activities.

Unfortunately, the massive expenditures on medical care have been only partially productive: physicians have disappeared from rural areas and the poor sections of the cities, primary medical care has become difficult to obtain even for the well-to-do, and the lack of services for some has been balanced by a plethora of unnecessary services, both surgical and medical, for others. The $154 billion spent for medical care in 1977 was used primarily for care provided by physicians in solo practice, a type of practice that has been obsolete for at least a quarter of a century. The funds are spent almost entirely on a fee-for-service basis, a form of payment in which the negative phenomena described above are inevitable, in which fees tend to grow faster than service, and in which the practitioner tends to be enriched far beyond his genuine and well-recognized value to society.

A good deal of waste occurs in the funds spent for medical care, and there is need to take a sensible way out of the morass. Instead of payment by fee-for-service, practitioners in the health field should be paid like the great majority of Americans, receiving salaries consistent with their training, service, and merit. In the interest of quality of care, they need to work together with other health personnel in community health centers that are linked with hospitals and other services to form a rational health care network serving communities in every part of the country.

Given this kind of rational system, it will be possible to provide effective health service for the nation for much less than 8.8% of the GNP. It is difficult to estimate how much would be saved. Whatever the amount, at least part of the funds should be kept in the health sector, not only to pay for the preventive program, but to improve the health services. It will be essential to build health centers, to further equality of hospital care by converting wards into one- and two-bed rooms, to create in every community an emergency medical service worthy of the name, to develop a serious postgraduate education program not only for physicians but for all types of health personnel, and to establish comprehensive programs in the neglected areas of chronic illness and aging, mental disease, and dental care.

The other alternative is to seek outside the health area for the funds necessary for prevention. It would be unfortunate if public health personnel were to do so by competing with other agencies that serve the needs of the population. Education, libraries, housing, welfare, recreation, parks—all have a major impact on health, and they and the public health agencies, working together, form the real partnership for health.

Individuals and agencies that are concerned with the financing of health and other human services face a major obstacle in the apparent sanctity of the military budget. In fiscal 1973, the last year of the Vietnam War, the military budget was $74 billion. In fiscal 1979, at a time when the nation was not at war, the military budget was $115 billion, or about 55% higher than in 1973. The president's proposed military budget for fiscal 1980 is $126 billion, 10% greater than for 1979 (12). A significant reaction to this increase is the statement by the Reverend Theodore M. Hesburgh, President of the University of Notre Dame, "It makes me feel bad when social priorities give way to military priorities" (12).

A modest approach to changing the priorities is the Transfer Amendment, which proposes to take $12 billion from the military budget and use it for domestic needs (13). Another is to adopt as national policy the reduction of federal funds for fee-for-service medical care and to reassign these funds to government public health activities. Such a "Health Transfer Amendment" could be used to double the 2% of health funds available for prevention. In 1977 this would have created a public health budget of $7.46 billion (1), and could have made possible the first big steps forward toward realizing the potential of the second epidemiologic revolution.

These transfer proposals are eminently reasonable. They would undoubtedly save hundreds of thousands of American lives. But they will not come about without leadership and the education of public opinion. Hermann Biggs, the creator of the eminently practical motto that "Public Health is Purchasable," had a profound understanding of the dynamics of public health victories. All who are interested in prevention and in the development of sound health policy based on epidemiology, need to think and act upon his analysis:

> No duty of society, acting through its governmental agencies, is paramount to this obligation to attack the removable causes of disease. The duty of leading this attack and bringing home to public opinion the fact that the community can buy its own health protection is laid upon all health officers, organizations and individuals interested in public health movements. For the provision of more and better facilities for the protection of the public health must come in the last analysis through the education of public opinion so that the community shall vividly realize both its needs and powers (3).

Literature Cited

1. Gibson, R. M., Fisher, C. R. 1978. National health expenditures, fiscal year 1977. *Soc. Secur. Bull.* 41:3–20
2. Smillie, W. G. 1952. The period of great epidemics in the United States (1800–1875). In *The History of American Epidemiology.* St. Louis: Mosby
3. Winslow, C.-E. A. 1929. *The Life of Hermann M. Biggs.* Philadelphia: Lea & Febiger
4. Fuchs, V. R. 1974. *Who Shall Live? Health, Economics, and Social Choice.* New York: Basic
5. LaLonde, M. 1974. *A New Perspective on the Health of Canadians, A Working Document.* Ottawa: Gov. of Canada
6. Ryan, W. 1971. *Blaming the Victim.* New York: Vintage
7. Smith, S. 1973. *The City That Was.* NY Acad. Med. Repr. Metuchen, NJ: Scarecrow Repr. Corp.
8. Dougherty, P. S. 1974. Advertising: Making bids for youth market. *New York Times.* Dec. 26, 1974
9. Annual summary for the United States, 1975. DHEW, Public Health Serv. 1976. *Monthly vital stat. Rep., Provisional Stat.* 24 (13).
10. United Nations. 1975. *Demographic Yearbook.* New York: United Nations
11. Cooper, B. S., Rice, D. P. 1976. The economic cost of illness revisited. *Soc. Secur. Bull.* 39:21–36
12. *New York Times.* Jan. 23, 1979
13. *New York Times.* Letters, April 3, 1978

Ann. Rev. Public Health 1980. 1:345–93

SCIENTIFIC BASES FOR IDENTIFICATION OF POTENTIAL CARCINOGENS AND ESTIMATION OF RISKS[1]

*Interagency Regulatory Liaison Group,
Work Group on Risk Assessment*[2, 3]

INTRODUCTION

This document describes the best judgments of the scientists in the agencies comprising the Interagency Regulatory Liaison Group (IRLG) on the scientific concepts and methods currently in use to identify and evaluate substances that may pose a risk of cancer to humans. These are fundamental steps in any program regulating carcinogens. The document was prepared by the Risk Assessment Work Group of the IRLG agencies and senior scientists from the National Cancer Institute (NCI) and the National Institute of Environmental Health Sciences.

[1]Originally published in the *Journal of the National Cancer Institute,* Vol. 63, No. 1. The US Government has the right to retain a nonexclusive, royalty-free license in and to any copyright covering this paper.

[2]Address reprint requests to Executive Assistant, Interagency Regulatory Liaison Group, Room 500, 1111 18th Street NW, Washington DC 20207.

[3]Work group members: Eula Bingham (Assistant Secretary of Labor for Occupational Safety and Health); Joseph V. Rodricks (Food and Drug Administration); Elizabeth L. Anderson (Environmental Protection Agency); David W. Gaylor (Food and Drug Administration, National Center for Toxicological Research); Richard A. Heller (Consumer Product Safety Commission); Anson M. Keller (Occupational Safety and Health Administration); Frank Kover (Environmental Protection Agency); Joseph McLaughlin (Consumer Product Safety Commission). Additional participants in the work group: Roy E. Albert (Environmental Protection Agency); Richard R. Bates (National Institute of Environmental Health Sciences); David G. Hoel (National Institute of Environmental Health Sciences); Umberto Saffiotti (National Cancer Institute); Marvin A. Schneiderman (National Cancer Institute).

The document describes (*a*) the basis for qualitative evaluation whether a particular substance presents a carcinogenic hazard and how the results of epidemiologic studies and animal bioassays, along with other types of information, are used in making that evaluation, and (*b*) the methods used for quantitative estimates of the carcinogenic risk posed by the substance, if such risk estimates are appropriate or required.

This document will provide a valuable scientific tool, to be considered with other information, in the evaluation of risk and ascertainment of the adequacy of experimental and epidemiologic methods used in that evaluation. It is an important step in ensuring that the regulatory agencies evaluate carcinogenic risks consistently. The four IRLG agencies caution, however, that this document presently has no regulatory status. Its use will, of course, depend upon the statutory requirements of the individual agencies.

The agencies have subjected this document to scientific peer review through the submission of the document to the *Journal of the National Cancer Institute.* In addition, a public notice and comment procedure has been initiated by publication in the *Federal Register.* Since the Occupational Safety and Health Administration (OSHA) has already received extensive public comment on these and other issues regarding the development of its cancer policy rule-making and will soon promulgate its policy, only the Consumer Product Safety Commission (CPSC), the Environmental Protection Agency (EPA), and the Food and Drug Administration (FDA) will participate in the public notice and comment procedure on this document. At the conclusion of the notice and comment procedure, OSHA will consider whether revisions to its final cancer policy are appropriate. The four agencies emphasize that the goal of this process is to articulate a consistent policy on the scientific principles applicable to the identification and evaluation of substances that may pose a carcinogenic risk to humans.

This document goes on to discuss the qualitative determination that a substance poses a carcinogenic hazard and the quantitative estimation of risk.

THE QUALITATIVE DETERMINATION THAT A SUBSTANCE POSES A CARCINOGENIC HAZARD

The methods used for regulatory purposes in making a qualitative determination that a substance poses a carcinogenic hazard to humans are based on a substantial scientific consensus that has emerged from experience, research, debate, and review. Although some points need further clarification and definition, substantial agreement exists among the federal regulatory agencies on criteria for evaluating the carcinogenicity of a substance.

In addition to determining that a substance may pose a hazard of cancer, regulatory agencies must consider other possible health hazards, and in some instances they are required to balance considerations of risk with other factors (such as possible health benefits or economic costs and benefits) in reaching regulatory decisions.

Definition and Extent of the Problem

NATURE OF CARCINOGENESIS AND CARCINOGENIC RESPONSES
The characteristic toxicologic event in carcinogenesis is a change in the regulatory mechanism of the target cells, resulting in self-replicating cell lesions. The carcinogenic event so modifies the genome and/or other molecular control mechanisms in the target cells that these can give rise to a progeny of permanently altered cells. This progeny of cells constitutes the basis of the neoplastic disease. The expression of the toxic injury therefore does not derive from the same cells originally hit by the toxic agent or from their functional products but rather from the proliferation of a new population of altered cells.

The critical molecular injury caused by specific carcinogens may be quantitatively extremely limited—even to a few cells—and may therefore not be detectable. What will make it manifest, through the subsequent growth of a clinically detectable neoplasm, is the proliferation of the altered cell population. The intensity of the pathologic response in a subject (i.e. the growth rate and spread of a cancer) depends on conditions of the host subsequent to the initial carcinogenic event and can be modified by other factors, such as enhancing agents and dietary factors. The continued progression of clinical manifestations of the carcinogenic process can occur in the absence of continued exposure to the carcinogen. Carcinogenic effects are therefore self-replicating toxic effects different from the common terminal toxic effects in which the manifestations of toxicity are due to altered functional products, degenerative changes, or death of the target cells themselves (1).

A rigorous methodology must be followed in obtaining, reviewing, and documenting the data required for a determination of carcinogenicity from observations on humans and experimental studies. Both epidemiologic observations and experimental studies need to be correlated with information on the chemical and physical nature of the agents under consideration, their reactivity, and their fate in the environment and in the exposed organisms. Evidence of carcinogenicity can be obtained from three sources:

1. epidemiologic evidence from exposed human populations;
2. experimental evidence from long-term bioassays in animals;

3. suggestive evidence derived from studies of chemical structure, reactivity, DNA damage and repair, mutagenicity, neoplastic transformation of cells in culture, induction of preneoplastic changes, or from other short-term tests that correlate with carcinogenicity.

In the evaluation of the results of carcinogenesis studies, the evidence obtained from epidemiologic observations or from experimental bioassays does not necessarily fall sharply into the two categories of positive and negative: In many instances the evidence may be insufficient for a definitive assessment.

ESTIMATION OF THE NUMBER OF CARCINOGENIC SUBSTANCES
Relatively few chemicals have been found to be carcinogenic. In fact, available evidence indicates that most substances do not cause cancer. The NCI's "Survey of Compounds Which Have Been Tested for Carcinogenic Activity" (2–8) and other literature surveys and reviews provide results of long-term animal bioassays on about 7,000 chemicals. Evidence of carcinogenicity on the basis of currently accepted experimental testing methods is available for less that 1,000 chemicals and possibly for as few as 600–800 (9–34). Many of these substances were selected for testing because of their structural similarity to known carcinogens. Thus these data considerably overstate the true proportion of carcinogenic substances in the human environment. A critical review of the literature on carcinogenicity of chemicals has been undertaken by the International Agency for Research on Cancer (IARC) with the support and collaboration of NCI (9–25). Of 368 chemicals evaluated in volumes 1–16 of the IARC monographs, some evidence of carcinogenicity was found for 247 (35).

A small number of chemicals has been adequately studied by epidemiologic methods to determine whether a carcinogenic hazard exists. By one recent estimate, 26 chemical substances or processes have been identified as responsible for cancer induction in humans (9–25, 35). Of those 26 substances, 6 were first identified as carcinogenic by tests in animals, whereas 20 were first identified by epidemiologic evidence.

Of the 368 substances for which carcinogenesis data were reviewed by the IARC, 221 showed some evidence of carcinogenicity from tests in animals, but these substances had not received adequate epidemiologic study to evaluate their effects in humans (35). In addition, 15 occupational categories have been reported to be associated with excess cancer incidences without identification of a specific etiologic agent (36–50).

ENHANCING FACTORS   Experimental and epidemiologic data suggest that some agents may not be carcinogenic alone but substantially contribute to the development of cancer in subjects that have been exposed to carcinogens. Depending on experimental circumstances, these agents have been referred to as cocarcinogens, promoting agents, syncarcinogens, or more generally, modifying or enhancing factors (51, 52).

Research on this category of agents suggests that they may work through a number of mechanisms of action, including (51, 52): (a) alteration of the uptake and/or distribution of carcinogens, (b) modification of the metabolic activation of carcinogens, (c) enhancement of the susceptibility of target tissues, and (d) acceleration of neoplastic progression.

Current evidence suggests that some of these agents act by a mechanism that may be specific for particular organs or conditions of exposure. Because of the possible specificity of their mechanisms of actions, the activity of these agents may not be recognized by conventional bioassays. Since no common general pathway of action has been recognized, it is not expected that tests based on a single-mechanism end point will be applicable for the identification of a broad range of these substances.

Enhancing mechanisms may be a major factor in the development of human cancers; therefore, their identification and control may be important in cancer prevention. Since no general methodology yet exists for testing and evaluation of this entire group of substances, the special circumstances under which each may act must be carefully evaluated. Interpretation of a positive effect in a carcinogenesis bioassay as being due to one of these mechanisms would require rigorous documentation that a full carcinogenic process is not involved.

VARIABILITY OF EFFECTS OF CARCINOGENS   Variability in the action of carcinogens may be due to inherent differences in susceptibility among species and strains of test animals and within populations of humans, and also to variability in the intrinsic differences in carcinogenic reactivity of individual agents. For example, aflatoxin B_1 is strongly carcinogenic in rats but is ineffective in several strains of adult mice (53). β-Naphthylamine is carcinogenic for humans, dogs, and several other species, but this compound has not produced tumors in rats (54). With some other carcinogens, there is a greater concordance of results among species: Dimethylnitrosamine has been found to be carcinogenic in all of the strains of vertebrates tested (55).

Species and strain differences in susceptibility to carcinogens may be due to factors that affect transport and metabolism, which in turn determine the effective dose of the ultimate form of the carcinogen delivered to target cells. These differences may also be due to inherent variations in susceptibility to neoplastic transformation of different organs in different species (56).

Differences in the level of carcinogenic effect of individual agents can only be compared with precision under strictly defined conditions of dosage and biologic end points. Frequently the level of effects, even under strictly defined conditions, will show marked variability depending on the test system used. Nevertheless, in the extreme, some carcinogens are clearly more effective than others by several orders of magnitude (9–25). However, such comparative potency estimates must be made with caution.

Epidemiologic Evidence

Evidence of carcinogenic activity of an agent can be obtained from epidemiologic studies when evaluation of the observations shows that the test agent causes an increased incidence of neoplasms or a decrease in their latency period.

Evidence from studies of human populations identifies carcinogenic chemicals to which those populations were exposed in the past. Many substances that have been identified as carcinogens in humans were discovered by epidemiologic studies of exposed workers; this evidence dates from 18th-century observations of cancer in chimney sweeps to more recent observations on dye workers, asbestos workers, and workers in certain chemical industries (31). It was noted early that clinical signs of cancer are delayed for a long time after initial exposure to carcinogens. This period of latency—often 5–40 years from initial exposure until the disease appears— makes prompt detection of newly introduced carcinogenic substances by epidemiologic studies nearly impossible.

As more substances are introduced into the human environment and as more are tested experimentally, it is expected that a larger proportion will be identifed as carcinogenic; this will be followed by adequate control measures, so that epidemiologic confirmation may become impossible.

TYPES OF EPIDEMIOLOGIC EVIDENCE   Types of epidemiologic evidence of carcinogenicity in humans include neoplastic response directly related to duration and dose of exposure, incidence or mortality differences related to occupational exposure, incidence or mortality differences between geographic regions related to environmental rather than genetic differences, altered incidence in migrant populations, time trends in incidence or mortality related to either the introduction or removal of a specific agent from the environment, case-control studies, and the result of retrospective-prospective and prospective studies of the consequences of human exposure. Clinical case reports may also provide early warning of a potential carcinogen (57).

The two main types of epidemiologic studies used to establish evidence of a carcinogenic hazard are cohort studies and case-control studies (58). Epidemiologic cohort studies involve the comparison of groups differently exposed to a substance. The comparison may include (a) totally unexposed versus exposed groups, (b) groups having distinctly different levels of exposure, or (c) rates in exposed groups versus rates prevailing in the general population. The groups need to be comparable for demographic factors such as age, sex, and race, and controlled for exposure to known carcinogens.

Epidemiologic case-control studies involve comparison of people with a given cancer type versus people without the disease but otherwise comparable with respect to appropriate demographic variables, to ascertain if they differ in exposure to the cancer hazard under investigation.

Epidemiologic findings gain greater force with increasing numbers of well-conducted studies that show similar effects from a given substance under different circumstances.

Absence of a positive statistical correlation does not by itself demonstrate absence of a hazard. Whereas negative epidemiologic data usually do not adequately establish the noncarcinogenicity of suspected materials, such negative data obtained for a given agent from epidemiologic studies of sufficient extent and duration may indicate the upper limits for the rate at which a specific type of exposure could affect the incidence and/or mortality of specific human cancers under the conditions of observation.

The detectability of a carcinogenic effect in a group of humans depends on several factors, including the duration and extent of exposure, size of the exposed population, and background rate of cancer in the target organ. Evaluation of epidemiologic studies requires a knowledge of the smallest possible increase in tumor incidence detectable under the conditions of each study. Such information has rarely been included in published reports. This information is, however, of critical importance in the evaluation of apparently negative studies.

The larger the number of persons in the exposed and control groups and the greater the similarity of these groups for factors other than exposure to the suspect carcinogen, the more likely will an effect be detected. Often, only a small number of humans exposed to a substance can be studied, conditions of exposure are inadequately defined, and records are incomplete. Thus a carcinogenic effect can be easily missed by epidemiologic methods, especially when common types of cancer (such as cancer of the lung, breast, colon, or rectum) are studied, inasmuch as these types often require a large excess of risk before a causal relationship can be identified for the exposure to a particular substance. Substances distributed widely in commerce or in the environment are particularly difficult to study by epidemiologic methods unless high risk ratios are observed, because it is often impossible to identify unexposed groups as controls or to separate groups with high and low exposure. The problem of adequate controls is further compounded by the long latency of cancer, during which multiple opportunities exist for exposure to other potentially carcinogenic substances and modifying factors. The effects of such other exposures on rates of cancer are rarely known, although in some instances they are found to be more than additive (22).

DISEASE ASCERTAINMENT   Because the effect under consideration is cancer morbidity or mortality, it is important to establish the validity, consistency, and reliability of the methods used to ascertain that neoplastic disease is clinically present or that it causes death.

Disease classification is also important, and uniform criteria of tumor nomenclature are needed. Some types of cancer may be classified under a generic name in such a way that changes in their frequency may be missed if only the generic classification is used. Some members of a population may be "lost" to a study if their disease conditions cannot be adequately ascertained.

Specific uniform procedures are not recommended here, but careful attention needs to be given to the extent to which these problems may affect comparison of relevant characteristics between groups.

In the statistical evaluation of cancer incidence or mortality differences, there has been a strong tendency for particular confidence levels (e.g. 95%) and particular probability values (e.g. $P = 0.05$ or $P = 0.01$) to be used as standard points for a finding of statistical significance. It is recognized that probability values fall along a continuum and should be so reported. The uniform use of a standard probability value is not suggested. Regulatory needs are best served by accurate estimates of the possible role of chance in accounting for observed differences.

The most important parameter in the assessment of an epidemiologic study is the magnitude of the effect measured; its interpretation is tempered by considerations of biologic plausibility, bias, confounding factors, and chance.

Evidence from Experimental Animals

Evidence of the carcinogenic activity of an agent can be obtained from bioassays in experimental animals showing that the test substance causes either an increase in the incidence of neoplasms or a decrease in the latency period.

The experimental design and conduct should be reviewed for quality and accuracy, and the results should be evaluated statistically for significance, with the only major experimental variable between control and experimental groups being the presence of the test substance. Positive results observed in more than one group of animals or in different laboratories and the demonstration that the occurrence of neoplasms follows a dose-dependent relationship provide additional confirmation of carcinogenicity. Determination that a causal relationship exists between a test treatment and the responses observed in a bioassay is a complex judgmental activity that includes evaluation of the identity of the test agent and the biologic test system, the conditions of exposure, the methods of observation, and the qualitative and quantitative nature of the pathologic response. The assessment of carcinogenicity therefore relies upon the judgment and experience of professionals. The following discussion refers to aspects of experimental design and conduct that concern evaluation of results. They are not intended as a prescription of protocols.

CRITERIA FOR EVALUATION OF EXPERIMENTAL DESIGN AND CONDUCT   *Experimental design*   Commonly recommended requirements for a thorough assessment of carcinogenic potential in experimental animals generally include (*a*) two species of rodents, (*b*) both sexes of each, (*c*) adequate controls, (*d*) a number of animals sufficient to provide an adequate resolving power to detect a carcinogenic effect, (*e*) treatment and observation extending to most of the lifetime of the animals at a dose range including one level likely to yield maximum expression of carcinogenic potential, (*f*) detailed pathologic examination, and (*g*) statistical evaluation of results (9–25, 27, 31, 32, 57, 59–73).

Positive results obtained in one species only are considered evidence of carcinogenicity. Positive results in more limited tests (e.g. when the observation period is considerably less than the animal's lifetime), but by experimentally adequate procedures, are acceptable as evidence of carcinogenicity. Negative results, on the other hand, are not considered evidence of lack of a carcinogenic effect, for operational purposes, unless minimum requirements have been met.

Choice of the animal model   The animals used most often for carcinogenesis bioassays are mice, rats, and hamsters. These animals are used extensively because (*a*) their natural life-spans are short, (*b*) they are easier to breed and handle in large numbers than larger animals, (*c*) they are inexpensive and easy to care for, (*d*) inbred strains exist that are genetically homogeneous for such traits as "background" cancer rates, susceptibility to carcinogens at specific organ sites, longevity, and response to husbandry systems. Adequately designed and performed studies in other mammalian species may also provide useful information on carcinogenicity. For human risk evaluation, data obtained from bioassays with the use of nonmammalian species can presently provide only suggestive evidence if positive but permit no conclusion if negative.

Experience on the background incidence of tumors in the colony of animals used for testing, obtained over a period of years by extensive observation of untreated animals under the same general maintenance conditions (historical colony controls), is useful in assessing the relevance of experimental findings, such as the appearance of rare tumors.

Rodents with different types of genetic homogeneity have been used for carcinogenesis bioassays. These include (*a*) inbred strains, (*b*) first-generation hybrids of parents of inbred strains, (*c*) randombred animals from a closed colony, (*d*) noninbred animals, and (*e*) animals of unspecified strains or origins. As the genetic and/or environmental variation increases, so does the need for concern about the variation of background tumor incidence.

A particular problem is posed by the use of certain strains of rodents in which particular tumor types reach a high frequency, often well above 50%, in untreated controls. Examples of such strains include mice of strain A for lung adenomas, strain AKR for lymphomas, strain C3H/HeN males for liver cell tumors and C3H females for mammary tumors, and females of several rat strains for mammary fibroadenomas. Although viral factors have been identified in the etiology of mouse AKR leukemia and C3H mammary tumors, no such factors are known to be at work for the other types mentioned above. The effect of carcinogens has been clearly demonstrated in all of the above strains by detection of substantial decreases in the latency period, by definite increases in incidence or multiplicity of these tumor types, and by the induction of tumors of other histologic types in the same or other organs (2–25). Caution must be used, however, in evaluating the significance of a higher incidence of these tumors in a treated group compared with concurrent controls when the incidence in the treated animals falls within a range commonly seen in historical controls from the same colony.

Background incidence rates for tumors of the lung, liver, mammary gland, and hematopoietic tissues are much lower in many other strains of mice, and for tumors of the mammary gland in other strains of rats. In these other strains, no unique biologic trait distinguishes the types of tumors mentioned above from many others, and no reason has been demonstrated for considering that they have any different significance than tumors in other organs as indicators of a carcinogenic response, under otherwise appropriate test conditions.

Number of animals   The number of animals in each group to be effectively considered for the evaluation of carcinogenesis test results is the number in which detection of carcinogenic effects could be expected. This number is obtained by subtracting from the number of animals started on the test the number of those lost to adequate observation (e.g. by intercurrent death followed by cannibalism or autolysis). The number of animals on which complete pathologic examination is conducted is important in the evaluation of tumor pathology.

Positive results can be obtained in tests with the use of a small number of animals if the test is otherwise adequately designed and conducted and if the tumor response is significant. For example, in a group of 15 animals, if 12 show a well-defined neoplastic lesion of a kind rarely seen either in matched or historical controls, the finding is positive. However, a negative finding in a group of 15 animals is not adequate evidence that the test agent is not carcinogenic.

Ideally, the number of animals required to provide adequate negative evidence would be such that an excessive risk would not arise if the test failed to detect carcinogenicity. The likelihood that such a risk would not arise increases both with the number of animals on test and the extent to which human exposure levels are exceeded. The probability of a false negative finding also depends on the background tumor rate in the control animals. For example, if a one-sided level of statistical significance of 5% is used with 55 animals, there is an 80% chance of detecting a tumor rate of 20% in the treated animals for whom the control rate is 5%, whereas 130 animals are required to detect the same difference if the control rate is 30%. The number of animals tested may need to be increased if the number of humans exposed is large or if a small margin of safety exists between the animal dose and the human exposure.

In practice, resource limitations often require a trade-off between the number of animals used and the number of substances tested in order to control the total cancer burden resulting from chemical carcinogens. This is particularly true with substances whose toxicity limits the test dose to a low multiplicity of human exposure levels. In those instances, it may be necessary to accept a lower than ideal degree of "negative evidence."

Route of administration   A key factor in the comparison of an experimental result to the human situation is to assess whether cells capable of malignant transformation are exposed to the reactive carcinogenic agent(s) in both the human and the experimental animal, regardless of whether transformation occurs in identical organs and cell types. Although this comparison is most readily made from experiments with animals in which the route of administration is the same as that in humans, other routes of administration may also be comparable and provide results useful for evaluation of the human hazard. For example, some chemicals are rapidly absorbed by inhalation, circulated through the body, and metabolized by the same pathways that occur following intravenous exposure (74).

Some routes of administration in animals may fail to provide adequate metabolic activation or exposure of target tissues and therefore may lead to false-negative results. This possibility should be assessed in evaluating negative results obtained when the route of administration in animals differs from the route of human exposure.

Generally, the route should be one that leads to absorption and distribution of the test substance. The induction of tumors at a remote site in the animal is evidence of absorption, distribution, and possible metabolic activation of the test substance. If exposures of both humans and animals involve absorption of the substance, any route of administration in animals may be regarded as relevant for a qualitative demonstration of human hazard unless there is evidence that the route of administration in the test species results in the production of carcinogenic substances (from degradation or metabolism) which does not ever occur with human exposure.

When tumors appear only at the site of injection or implantation, careful review is necessary. If there is reason to believe that the tumors occur as a result of "solid state" carcinogenesis (75, 76), the results may be inappropriate for extrapolation to human exposure. If, however, the test material produces tumors at the site of injection or implantation as a result of its chemical reactivity, this response is an indication of carcinogenicity.

There are a number of practical reasons for studying certain substances in animals by a route of administration different from the expected route of human exposure. If a substance under test is highly volatile, accurate administration in food may be difficult because of evaporation; often feeding through a stomach tube is used so that the dose may be measured with greater accuracy. Even for nonvolatile test substances, a stomach tube may be used when it is important to know the exact amount of a substance administered to the test animals. The administration of high doses of a test substance with a disagreeable odor or taste may require the use of routes other than ingestion.

Thus experimental exposures need not necessarily be by the route of human exposure in order to be meaningful, but possible physiologic and metabolic differences related to routes of absorption and distribution should be considered in the assessment of their relevance.

Identity of the substance tested   Substances to which humans are exposed through their occupations, the environment, and the products they use vary widely both in the number and the proportion of contaminating impurities. A full assessment of the carcinogenicity of an impure mixture ideally requires that each component be tested individually at an adequate dosage and that the mixture itself be tested in order to detect cumulative or synergistic effects. Limitation of resources makes this ideal approach impractical as a routine. It is common, therefore, simply to rely on tests either of the product to which humans are exposed, including the impurities present, or of the purified principal chemical substance(s). Because the products may vary according to procedures used in manufacture and processing, tests for one commercial product may not be applicable to another product containing a different set or level of impurities. Change in the manufacturing process of a product may require additional tests to confirm the safety of the new product if the change involves the introduction of different impurities or a substantial increase in the amount of any single component of the product. Even though it is accepted practice to test mixtures, the nature of any impurities known or likely to be present as a result of the manufacturing process is important and may require separate examination or testing. Information on the carcinogenicity of any single chemical in a mixture is an indication of potential hazard of the entire mixture. However, negative results obtained on a component of a mixture may not reflect the potential carcinogenicity of the entire mixture.

Dose levels "Testing should be done at doses and under experimental conditions likely to yield maximum tumor incidence." This recommendation of an FDA advisory committee summarizes the issue of test doses (68).

Bioassays with the use of a few dozen or even a few hundred animals have relatively low sensitivity for detection of carcinogenic effects. Millions of people of varying degrees of sensitivity or exposure may be exposed to the substances under evaluation. Although a test animal cannot be strictly viewed as a "surrogate" of a large number of people without oversimplification, the role of animal tests is to provide maximum detectability of carcinogenic effects within the already narrow confines of test sensitivity. Under otherwise identical conditions, the greater the ratio of test exposure to human exposure, the greater is the safety margin provided by a negative result in a carcinogenesis bioassay.

It is generally recommended that more than one dose level be tested. Most carcinogenic effects show a positive dose-response relationship, but maximum tumor incidence in test animals may not occur at the highest dose when competing toxicity prevails. The highest test dose that can be effectively used in a carcinogenesis bioassay is limited by the conditions of absorption, by the amount that the animal can tolerate during lifetime administration without unwanted toxic side effects, and by the effects on nutrition when the chemical constitutes too large a proportion of the diet.

Results of bioassays done at doses and under conditions permitting maximum expression of carcinogenicity provide a sound basis for the identification of a carcinogenic hazard or its absence.

It is important to estimate the highest dose level that will be tolerated by the test animals during lifetime administration, i.e. the estimated maximum tolerated dose (EMTD). The EMTD is defined as the highest dose that can be administered to the test animals for their lifetime and that is estimated not to produce (a) clinical signs of toxicity or pathologic lesions other than those related to a neoplastic response, but which may interfere with the neoplastic response, (b) alteration of the normal longevity of the animals from toxic effects other than carcinogenesis, and (c) more than a relatively small percent inhibition of normal weight gain (not to exceed 10%) (71).

The EMTD is determined on the basis of prechronic tests and other relevant information. If the test reveals that the EMTD is too high to meet the conditions defined herein, positive results obtained above the EMTD are acceptable as evidence of carcinogenicity unless there is convincing evidence to the contrary. Alternatively, negative results obtained above the EMTD are considered inadequate unless particularly strong and specific scientific reasons justify their acceptance as negative. Positive results obtained at or below the EMTD provide evidence of carcinogenicity.

Age at treatment   Because of the long latency period required for induction and manifestation of tumors, treatment should be started in young animals, and the animals should be observed for a carcinogenic response through most of their expected life-spans. The older the age at first treatment, the shorter is the remaining life-span available for tumor development; consequently, the smaller is the chance of detecting delayed carcinogenic effects.

Although treatment is often started in young adult animals soon after weaning, some protocols call for treatment soon after birth (neonatal) or during fetal development (transplacental). The rationale for exposing test animals transplacentally or neonatally is based on the greater susceptibility of certain organs to carcinogens during early development. Such susceptibility has been demonstrated in several species, including those commonly used for bioassays (77, 78). Animals first treated during the perinatal period must be also treated and observed throughout their life-spans to obtain a valid negative response.

Virtually any agent that is carcinogenic in adult animals can be expected to have some carcinogenic effect when administered to young animals including the neonate and the fetus. Unless a substance is demonstrated to be exclusively carcinogenic when administered to the fetus or neonate, enhanced perinatal susceptibility to carcinogens should be considered not a separate and distinct toxicologic property; rather, it should be a means for increasing the sensitivity of conventional bioassay procedures by extension of the exposure period to these earlier and more susceptible portions of the life-span.

It should be emphasized that these protocol modifications greatly complicate dose selection and experimental design. An agent may be significantly more toxic to the fetus, the neonate, or the pregnant or lactating female animal than to the normal young adult of either sex. This requires independent determination of the toxicity and EMTD. Furthermore, individuals in the litter of a treated pregnant animal cannot be considered independent units for statistical evaluation of effects.

Conduct and duration of bioassays in animals   A long-term bioassay for carcinogenesis in animals is a complex procedure requiring control of many variables for several years. Professional experience and knowledge of the relevant biologic parameters are needed for adequate quality control. Detailed guidance on procedures is provided by reports such as the FDA's "Good Laboratory Practice Regulations" (79) and the NCI's "Guidelines for Carcinogen Bioassays in Small Rodents" (71).

Review of the observations made during the bioassay (on food intake, weight, clinical course, and pathologic conditions of the animals) provides a basis for determining whether these experimental variables are recorded in sufficient detail and are internally consistent to permit independent assessment of their validity.

The purpose of these bioassays is primarily to provide maximal opportunity for detection of a neoplastic response; therefore, the longer the period of observation the better is the chance of detecting delayed effects. A "point of diminishing return" can be reached when intercurrent disease and/or survival considerations make the observation or evaluation of old animals particularly difficult. It is expected that the animals will be observed for most of their life-spans. The best negative evidence for the carcinogenicity of a substance is obtained from tests in which both exposure and observation last through all or nearly all of the expected life-spans of the animals under study.

Negative results decrease in value as the exposure and observation periods are shortened, and they become practically meaningless if these periods are shorter than half the life-spans of the animals. When some animals die early in the course of a test, the value of the test is reduced as a function of the percentage of animals dying without tumors at periods markedly shorter than the life-span of the species. Sometimes, a positive carcinogenic response may be definitely demonstrated in a shorter period of observation if the experiment is adequately controlled; in such cases the test is considered valid even if it is shorter than usual (80).

Accepted procedures include (*a*) the observation of all animals in the study (treated and control groups) until their spontaneous death, (*b*) the sacrifice of animals that show clinical signs of severe illness or impending death (sacrifice of moribund animals prevents losses due to autolysis and provides better observation of tissue pathology), and (c) terminal sacrifice at a scheduled date near the end of the life-span (e.g. after 24 mo on test).

CRITERIA FOR EVALUATION OF PATHOLOGY   *Pathology examination* The evaluation of carcinogenesis bioassay results rests on the extent and accuracy with which organs and tissues of both treated and control animals are examined for morphologic changes. After the termination of a bioassay, the only physical evidence that can be used to permit reevaluation of results, even years afterwards, is represented by the written descriptive and diagnostic records, the graphic or photographic records of gross or microscopic observations, and most importantly, the original slides of tissue sections for microscopic examination. The histologic slides are of critical importance as a lasting direct documentation of the conditions of normal and abnormal tissues and organs, both for scientific and regulatory purposes. Quality and extent of pathologic documentation are therefore major factors in establishing the validity of bioassays in animals (71, 79).

Although a well-conducted pathologic examination cannot generally rescue a poorly designed or badly conducted bioassay, inadequate pathologic examination can significantly reduce or eliminate the value of an otherwise well-conducted experiment. Among the factors to be considered in evaluation of the pathologic examination are:

1. the care and thoroughness of gross tissue examination and the qualifications of the persons conducting this examination to recognize abnormalities,
2. the quality of preservation, sectioning, and staining of tissues,
3. the accuracy of the record-keeping system used for labeling tissues as they are moved from the animal through slide-processing to final diagnosis and reporting,
4. the extent of selection of normal and abnormal tissues for microscopic examination,
5. the qualifications of the pathologist making the microscopic examination.

The numbers of tumors or other lesions diagnosed by the pathologist are not a thorough assessment of incidence unless each factor is adequately considered, controlled, and documented.

The strength of evidence provided by a bioassay also depends on the number of tissues examined. Failure to observe excess tumors in treated animals cannot be considered evidence of the absence of a carcinogenic hazard unless all organs have been examined grossly and all grossly visible suspect lesions have been examined microscopically. In a large organ, the taking of a single random section for histologic examination can result in failure to detect small tumors. Thus multiple cuts through such organs should be made.

It is also important to open and search the entire cavity of all hollow organs for abnormalities. For example, the entire length of the gastrointestinal tract should be opened and inspected. Grossly visible lesions should be selected for histologic examination, and if they are not subsequently observed on tissue slides, preparation of additional sections may be necessary until the gross lesion is verified histologically.

Furthermore, histopathologic examination should be made of major organs in the treated groups and matched controls, and specific organs should be studied in detail in all dose groups and controls in which there is either gross or microscopic evidence of lesions. Major organs are defined in the NCI's "Guidelines for Carcinogen Bioassays in Small Rodents" (71). Positive evidence of carcinogenicity may be valid for a particular organ if it has been adequately examined in both treated and control groups. Negative reports are inadequate for any organ that has not received careful gross examination in all animals and histologic examination of suspect lesions. The more limited the number of organs examined grossly and microscopically, the less the value of the experiment in providing evidence of a negative result.

Evaluation of pathologic results The evaluation of bioassay results and their quality requires a detailed review and expert judgment of all the experimental conditions and observations, including the identity of the test substance; the conditions of administration; the identity, source, and characteristics of the test animals; the accuracy and systematic recording of observations; the extent of pathologic examination; and the competence of the investigators. Meticulous and detailed documentation is of great importance.

Several criteria are applied in the evaluation of bioassay results.

1. Internal consistency of the data is important in reviewing the conduct of the test. Apparent inconsistencies should be investigated by analysis of records.

2. Reproducibility of test results can be demonstrated within a single experiment (in different groups of similarly treated animals or in different dose-level groups) or in separate bioassays conducted with the same experimental design in the same or in different laboratories. Evidence of reproducibility adds greater confidence to the evaluation of results. Statistical considerations provide an estimate of the level of detectability of an effect

and the consequent level of probability that the effect may be missed in a repetition of the test in a given number of animals. Apparent contrary results in any two tests may be simply an effect of chance variation and may be fully compatible with an identical mechanism and level of activity of the test compound.

3. Evidence of a positive dose-response relationship adds further confidence to the evaluation of a positive test, but lack of it may be due to testing in a portion of the dose-response curve with a shallow slope or even with a declining slope due to competing risks. In the presence of positive results in well-designed, well-conducted tests, evidence of reproducibility and positive dose-response relationships is not necessary to reach a conclusion of carcinogenicity.

4. Concordance of results obtained under differing test conditions (e.g. different species, different routes of administration, or markedly different basal diets) provides greater confidence in the evaluation of both positive and negative studies, but it has a different meaning from "reproducibility" within the same tests or under the same conditions. Lack of concordance from tests performed under different conditions does not, in itself, detract from the validity of the positive test. Reasons for a discordance in observation may be identified by evidence obtained during a test or may be sought through further research.

The response to carcinogens in different animal species and even strains is known to vary greatly because of genetic, metabolic, nutritional, and other factors that affect susceptibility in a given test animal. Present knowledge indicates that a substance that is clearly carcinogenic in one test species is likely to be carcinogenic in other species, that it may take extensive tests in several species to demonstrate this correlation, and that the responsive target tissues or organs and the types of tumors induced in different species may vary greatly. Therefore, although concordance of positive results (even if different tumor types are involved) adds support to an evaluation of carcinogenicity, the finding of negative results in some other species generally does not detract from the validity of a positive result as evidence of carcinogenicity for the test substance.

In this respect, positive results supersede negative ones. The assessment of such apparent discrepancies in results requires consideration of all experimental variables, since apparently negative results may derive from limitations in the sensitivity of the test (e.g. early scheduled sacrifice, limited extent of pathologic examination, and statistical probability). If the positive result is itself not fully conclusive or if reasons exist for questioning its validity as evidence of carcinogenicity, the result is generally classified as "inconclusive" or "only suggestive" even in the absence of other negative test results.

5. Evaluation of tumor incidence is made on the basis of the pathologic findings and therefore depends on professional diagnostic judgment. Tumor incidence is evaluated by consideration of all tumors of specific organ sites or anatomically or physiologically related systems. At present there is considerable uncertainty about the interpretation of carcinogenic responses in terms of the total tumor yield in contrast to the response in terms of a statistically significant increase of tumors in specific target organs or tissues. Traditionally, carcinogens have been recognized in studies on humans and animals by a decisive increase in tumors of target organs. However, it is conceivable that a general increase in total tumor yield, in the absence of an excess incidence in one or more target tissues, could occur—for example, by a promoting effect that generally increases the spontaneous incidence of tumors in test animals or by the action of a multipotent carcinogen whose response did not reach statistical significance in any one organ even at the maximum tolerated dose. In some instances, however, control animals may have a high frequency of tumors at certain sites (e.g testicular tumors in F344 male rats). In such instances, a simple cumulative count of tumor-bearing versus tumor-free animals may fail to reveal carcinogenic effects in the treated groups. Prudent judgment is needed on the appropriate categorization of tumors used to evaluate induced effects.

A positive result in a carcinogenesis bioassay can be based on evidence of the induction of an increased incidence or a substantially decreased latency period. The latter is often difficult to establish. Determination of the latency period can be made by various techniques of observation during a bioassay. If both test and control animals are sacrificed at a fixed time, only the early part of a temporal distribution curve may be observable; consequently, the estimate of the average latency period for all tumors or tumor-bearing animals may be artificially altered. If the test and control groups are allowed to live out their life-spans, the comparison of latency periods must take into account the relative survival and the number of animals at risk, particularly in the case of competing risks.

The methods used in estimating the latency period must be defined in the context of each bioassay. It is always difficult to determine the exact onset of a neoplasm. Morphometric criteria may be used for tumors (e.g. skin or subcutaneous tumors) detectable during clinical observation of the animals and a minimum size may be established as a criterion for identification. For neoplasms of the internal organs it is practically impossible to determine an adequate time of onset: Methods such as palpation of the abdomen are highly subjective and generally unreliable. Serial sacrifice studies provide excellent data on time to tumor induction, but they should not be substituted for adequate numbers of animals under lifetime observation. In most instances, what is referred to as latency period is the time between the beginning of the exposure and the observation of a tumor at death. This parameter is obviously influenced by all the factors that determine time of death, e.g. intercurrent diseases, other tumors, or growth rate of individual tumors. Here too, the judgment of experienced pathologists may provide critical evaluation of such aspects as tumor size, location, cell differentiation, and invasion; these factors may contribute to an estimate of temporal sequence.

The observation in treated groups of tumors that are considered rare in untreated and historical controls may raise considerable suspicion even when their incidence is below the required level of statistical significance. Careful review and cautious judgment are necessary in their evaluation; often the rarity of a tumor type is estimated on the basis of a small control population. The occurrence of one or a few neoplasms of a kind, however rare, is not necessarily evidence that a substance is carcinogenic in the absence of other supporting evidence.

6. Evaluation of tumor morphology in the final analysis of bioassay results is highly dependent on the way in which pathology data are categorized. It is incorrect, for example, to subdivide diagnoses into so many individual categories based on different stages of disease or different morphologic features that no single category is large enough to be statistically significant. At the other extreme, it is incorrect to group unrelated end points in a way that maximizes the opportunity to find statistical significance, whether or not such groupings are biologically meaningful.

Carcinogenic and chronic toxic effects of a chemical on an organ, tissue, or cell develop through a series of stages from minimal changes to advanced and possibly fatal end points (81). The stage reached at any particular time is related to the dose of the substance, the conditions of exposure, the time elapsed since beginning of exposure, and host susceptibility factors. Early lesions that are pathognomonic of a disease process resulting from toxic chemicals should be grouped with more advanced lesions, whether or not the animal has survived long enough for the process to develop to the latest stages. The carcinogenic process may go through early stages including atypical hyperplasia, carcinoma in situ, and/or histologically benign tumor before progressing to a clearly malignant stage. Although the stage of development is of critical importance in clinical oncology for assessing the prognosis of a patient at the time of therapy, it is not relevant in deciding whether a chemical is capable of inducing cancer as long as the induction of lesions recognized as neoplastic is conclusively demonstrated.

The induction of preneoplastic lesions in the process of cancer development is an indication that the test substance is capable of inducing cancer in a susceptible host given sufficient exposure and time for cancer to arise. Care must be taken, however, to distinguish atypical hyperplasias that are pathognomonic of neoplastic progression from other nonspecific or reactive hyperplasias.

In the evaluation of bioassays, the concern is with the capability of a test substance to react with a biologic system to give rise to a neoplastic response that may develop through all stages to malignancy. One issue is whether or not the response is the kind that stops at the benign stage and never evolves further to the invasive and metastasizing stage. Few if any tumor types are presently known to belong to this category, which could be called "permanently benign" tumors. For benign tumors, no specific mechanism of induction is known that can be distinguished from the mechanisms of induction of other neoplasms. Moreover, no established body of evidence exists showing that certain substances or groups of substances are capable of inducing exclusively permanently benign tumors without ever inducing any more malignant ones. The mammary fibroadenoma is generally considered to be a benign tumor in both the human (82) and the rat (83), and it has been suggested that its experimental induction provides little evidence that the inducing agent can cause cancer. X-rays or carcinogenic polycyclic aromatic hydrocarbons, however, which principally induce fibroadenomas in some rat strains, induce mostly malignant adenocarcinomas in other strains; the genetic characteristics of the animal rather than the inducing agent determine whether benign or malignant tumors develop (84). Thus the induction of benign tumors, even of a type that rarely progresses to a malignant stage, must be considered a warning that the inducing chemical may be capable of causing cancer in some humans. The induction of benign neoplasms, even if they were demonstrated to be of a permanently benign type, would therefore be considered evidence of carcinogenic activity unless definitive evidence is provided that the test chemical is incapable of inducing malignant neoplasms.

Neoplasms at a benign stage may jeopardize the health and life of the host. Furthermore, it is extremely difficult to rule out the presence of malignant changes simply on the basis of a limited histologic examination of the primary tumor, because focal malignant change or local invasion may have occurred in other areas of the tumor that were not examined microscopically. Similarly, it is very difficult to rule out the metastatic spread of a neoplasm that may be biologically capable of metastasizing without an extremely detailed search for metastases, which can begin as small foci of one or a few cells lodged in the arteriolar walls of peripheral organs (85). The frequency of observation of such metastases depends directly on the amount of peripheral tissue that is examined (86).

Another case to be considered is the combination of neoplasms diagnosed as benign and malignant. This may include instances in which the incidence of histologically malignant tumors is only a relatively small fraction of the total tumor incidence but represents the most advanced stages of the neoplastic response. Although the number of tumors diagnosed as malignant may not reach statistical significance as such in the number of animals at risk, the total neoplastic response (benign and malignant) may be clearly significant.

Some common types of neoplasms found in carcinogenesis bioassays in laboratory rodents are among those often diagnosed as being at a benign stage when observed in test animals. Examples include lung adenomas, skin and bladder papillomas, liver cell adenomas (hepatomas), and hemangiomas in various organs. All of these tumor types are known to progress to frank malignant stages. No pathogenetic mechanisms have been identified that could demonstrate that the induction of such tumors, whether in a benign or malignant stage, in otherwise appropriate, comparable, and well-controlled experimental conditions, provides any different kind of evidence for carcinogenesis than the induction of other tumor types. In the evaluation of tumor incidence, therefore, neoplasms in different stages of progression are counted together.

7. General evaluation of neoplastic pathology for carcinogenesis bioassays includes consideration of the total number of animals with tumors in each group, the total number of individual tumors, and the index of tumor multiplicity in tumor-bearing animals. The tumor response can be further characterized by a detailed observation of the tumor morphology and related preneoplastic changes. The extent of tumor growth and spread and special morphologic characteristics may give useful indications of the time of development of the neoplastic response. The quality of the pathologic response is determined by a comprehensive evaluation of all the pathologic changes observed in both treated and control animals. Special attention is required in the evaluation of toxic effects other than carcinogenicity, because their pathologic manifestations have to be distinguished from those due to the neoplastic response.

The organs and tissues that are the targets of carcinogens may vary greatly in different species and even under different exposure conditions; therefore, no direct analogy of morphologic response can be expected from a carcinogen in animals of different species and in humans. Examples are known both of widely different target sites [e.g. benzidine induces bladder carcinoma in humans and cholangiomas and liver cell carcinomas in hamsters and rats (87)] and of similar responses [e.g. vinyl chloride induces the same type of angiosarcomas of the liver in humans, rats, and mice (88)].

Special conditions of tissue exposure or reaction may result in a tumor response by mechanisms that appear due to physical rather than chemical properties of the test material. The following conditions are evaluated differently in this respect:

1. The induction of sarcomas around a "solid state" implant of the test substance into a connective tissue is not considered an indication of the carcinogenicity of that substance when it is administered in another physical form (75, 76).
2. The induction of a carcinogenic response by asbestos and other fibrous materials by a mechanism linked to certain physical characteristics such as fiber length and diameter is recognized as a basis for categorizing the exposure to such fibrous materials as a carcinogenic hazard (22).
3. The effect of particulate materials in the induction of respiratory neoplasms, when they are administered jointly with certain carcinogens (probably through their capacity to absorb and retain carcinogens, to penetrate the respiratory tract tissues, and to stimulate early cellular responses) is not recognized as evidence of carcinogenicity of these substances but rather as an indication of their role as cofactors in carcinogenesis; particulate materials require careful but separate consideration as a potential hazard (89, 90).
4. The induction of a neoplastic response by a substance because of its radioactivity is recognized as a cancer hazard.

Other factors are sometimes suggested to be sufficient to refute the presumption of positive evidence of a carcinogenic effect. These factors must be critically examined to avoid false-negative judgments based on unsubstantiated hypothetical explanations of the circumstances of tumor induction. The following factors are considered in this respect:

1. Indirect mechanisms of action requiring special exposure levels or conditions. An example has been suggested in the case of substances that may induce bladder neoplasms only in the presence of bladder stones resulting from high levels of intake and urinary excretion of the test substance (91). Support for such a mechanism as an explanation for development of bladder tumors is provided by determination of a specific association of tumors with stones, a dose-response correlation between stones and tumors, and the absence of other chemical or biological indications that the substance might be carcinogenic by other mechanisms. In evaluation of the relevance of such experimental observations to the assessment of human hazard, special consideration is needed for mechanisms by which exposures or intercurrent diseases in the human may act as the cofactor (e.g. in bladder stone induction), thus producing a susceptible state for the possible carcinogenic activity of the test substance.

2. The action of promoting agents only on tissues previously initiated by carcinogens (51, 52). Few examples are well documented, such as the phorbol esters in epidermal carcinogenesis in mice. Criteria of risk evaluation need to be defined and dose-response relationships considered. Any

claim that a substance acts only by this mechanism and thus is of less concern to humans needs to be supported by experiments showing the mechanism of action and demonstrating that the effect does not occur at human exposure levels.

3. Metabolic pathways of carcinogen activation (92), which are suggested as occurring exclusively under certain test conditions in experimental animals but not under other test conditions or in other species. This situation would be important if thorough studies demonstrate that the metabolic pathways for carcinogenic activation of a substance in animals do not occur in humans. Another important situation would be the demonstration that the metabolic pathways of activation of a particular carcinogen identified by studies at high levels of exposure are exclusively formed at such high levels but are absent at lower dose levels.

STATISTICAL ANALYSIS OF RESULTS   Statistical hypothesis testing provides an estimate of the likelihood that an experimental observation may or may not be a result of chance alone. The 95% confidence level is widely accepted as a reasonable assurance that the observed effect is real, but confidence that an increased incidence of tumors is a true indication of the carcinogenicity of a substance increases with increasing statistical significance of the results. Thus the level of statistical significance should be reported rather than the fact that a result is statistically significant or not significant at a single preassigned level of confidence. Failure to detect an increase of tumors in a bioassay may be due to an insufficient number of animals tested and does not unequivocally prove that a substance does not pose a risk of cancer.

Tumors rarely seen in experimental animals may raise considerable suspicion even if the statistical significance is well below the 95% confidence level.

Because of the frequent use in chronic studies of both sexes, more than one species or strain, and more than one dosage level, and because many different tissues are examined, a large number of statistical comparisons are possible between control and treated animals. Thus the results from a chronic study must be interpreted cautiously to control the rate of false positives arising from the large number of possible statistical comparisons (93).

Lifetime animal experiments are often difficult to interpret because of competing causes of death, which may alter the pattern of the observation period of the tumor type under study. A common but inadequate form of presenting tumor data is a report only of the proportion of animals in which particular tumor types were observed during the study. This proportion may contain a mixture of three types of observations: (a) The tumor causes the death of an animal and is subsequently observed upon necropsy, (b) an animal dies due to some cause other than a particular tumor and the tumor is observed upon necropsy, or (c) the tumor is observed when an animal is necropsied at the time of a scheduled sacrifice, generally at the termination of an experiment. Simply combining tumors observed under these three situations makes interpretation difficult, and in fact the data may be misleading if the mortality pattern is altered by the toxicity of the substance.

Serial or terminal sacrifices provide an opportunity to compare the prevalence of tumors in various groups of animals unperturbed by mortality. However, sacrifice data do not provide an opportunity to study the effect of a substance on survival or on causes of death.

The analysis of a bioassay is limited by the quantity and quality of data. Such studies must include the age of each animal at the beginning of the experiment, its age at time of removal from the experiment, reason for removal (death, moribund condition, scheduled sacrifice, or others), and all clinical and pathologic observations, including gross and microscopic examination.

When survival curves of control and treated animals differ due to competing causes of death, adjustment of the number of animals at risk may be necessary. For a tumor type generally leading to the death of an animal, statistical analyses of survival experiments should incorporate life-table or competing risk techniques in order to estimate and test tumor incidence. This approach requires assumptions concerning the independence of the competing causes of death. If all the animals are utilized from a survival study, including sacrificed animals, the net probability of death due to a tumor type can be estimated as though that were the only cause of death of a group of animals. Statistical tests for differences between control and treated groups can be performed on the adjusted tumor incidence rates (94–96).

For a tumor type that is unlikely to kill the animals, methods of analysis based on life-table techniques are not appropriate for adjusting the number of animals at risk. These tumors are observed conditionally as a result of other events occurring first: death of the animal or a scheduled sacrifice. To estimate prevalence rate of these tumors, mortality is assumed to be unrelated to the presence of the tumor. Statistical methods for the analysis of tumors that are not generally life-threatening are discussed by Hoel and Walburg (94) and Peto (95).

Short-term Tests for Carcinogens

Carcinogenesis tests have traditionally been based on the experimental induction of tumors in laboratory animals. Such tests usually involve the observation of treated animals for most of their life-spans.

Recently, short-term methods have been developed to provide more rapid markers for the tentative identification of carcinogenic effects. These methods are directed toward the study of mechanisms underlying neoplastic transformation as well as toward provision of reproducible and rapid methods for testing chemicals and physical agents for potential carcinogenic activity. The use of short-term methods for the evaluation of carcinogens was the subject of a recent review (97) from which the following discussion is largely derived.

METHODS BASED ON GENETIC ALTERATIONS   The analysis of mutagenic effects has been developed mainly to assess the ability of a substance to induce genetic alterations. The resulting information can be used for estimating the genetic hazard of chemical agents for man.

Because of the similarities of basic molecular mechanisms by which chemical mutagens and most chemical carcinogens appear to induce genetic effects (i.e. molecular alterations of DNA), it has been postulated that mutagenic effects can be used to predict carcinogenicity.

The use of a battery of short-term genetic tests is usually recommended in order to minimize false-negative and false-positive results and to select compounds that require further long-term investigations. This battery of tests may include (a) tests for mutations in bacteria and eukaryotic microorganisms, (b) tests for mutations in somatic mammalian cells, (c) tests for effects on chromosomes in higher eukaryotes, including mammals, and (d) evaluation of DNA repair synthesis.

For screening purposes, preference has usually been given to tests that have already been validated with a large sample of compounds belonging to different chemical groups.

Among the mutagenicity tests on microorganisms, the one most widely used and validated is the Ames reversion test in *Salmonella*. Tests in *Escherichia coli, Saccharomyces, Neurospora,* and *Aspergillus* are also being used. Mutagenicity testing is also being conducted in *Drosophila.*

Several other methods currently being evaluated may be used to monitor genetic damage in mammalian cells by carcinogens in vivo and in vitro. These methods include the production of sister chromatid exchanges as well as measurement of the induction of direct damage to DNA and its subsequent repair.

Various short-term mutagenesis tests, some of which are used to provide supportive evidence of carcinogenicity, are discussed in (98).

METHODS BASED ON NEOPLASTIC CELL TRANSFORMATION   Several systems are now available at the mammalian cell level for the identification and study of substances that represent a possible cancer hazard (99).

In recent years a number of systems have been developed to test for neoplastic cell transformation by chemical and physical carcinogenic agents. Some of these systems are being used in several laboratories with good reproducibility; other systems are still being developed. Those that have been most widely studied are (*a*) the golden hamster embryo cell system and (*b*) the mouse embryo fibroblast cell line systems.

In the golden hamster embryo cell system, primary and/or secondary cultures of normal embryo cells are used. Transformation is determined 7–10 days after treatment of cells seeded for colony formation. Quantitation is based on the frequency of morphologically altered colonies.

In the mouse embryo fibroblast systems, established homogeneous cell lines are used. Thus cloned populations of cells can be grown in large quantities and used by many laboratories. Transformants are identifiable 4–6 weeks after exposure to the carcinogen. They may be scored quantitatively by morphologic criteria (focus assay), which correlate highly with tumorigenicity in animals. Among these established lines, the C3H 10T½ Clone 8 cell system has been the most widely studied.

In these tests for neoplastic transformation, the cells derived from transformed colonies or foci, when inoculated into syngeneic or immunosuppressed animals, can grow as malignant tumors. Although the definitive evidence for neoplastic transformation of cells in culture remains their tumorigenicity in animals, a number of phenotypic changes of the cultured target cells are commonly used as indicators.

Other in vitro systems are being developed with the use of specialized cell types such as epithelial cells from liver, epidermis, and other organs. Neoplastic transformation of well-defined epithelial cells by chemicals has been achieved in vitro; conditions for quantitative studies are under development. Such systems may be needed to identify critical target cell populations within target tissues closely correlated with carcinogenesis in vivo.

To be effective, most chemical carcinogens require metabolic activation by cell enzymes to an ultimate reactive metabolite. In mammals metabolic activation of carcinogens takes place in many organs and tissues. Cells in culture can retain enzyme activities, but specific culture systems or preparations may lack or lose the enzyme activity necessary to activate certain chemicals. Therefore, adequate consideration should be given to the effectiveness of metabolic activation functions in each test system used.

EVALUATION OF SHORT-TERM RESULTS The study of carcinogensis at the cell level presently offers an effective means to identify carcinogenic effects and mechanisms. In vitro mammalian cell transformation systems are simple models for the study of the mechanisms of chemical and physical carcinogensis.

As these systems become more widely used as test methods, they will lead not only to better development and definition of screening techniques but also to better understanding of the underlying mechanisms of carcinogensis.

Short-term tests for chemical carcinogens presently do not, in the absence of animal bioassays and epidemiology data, constitute definitive evidence that a substance does (or does not) pose a carcinogenic hazard to humans. However, positive responses in these tests are considered suggestive evidence of a carcinogenic hazard.

Such positive results also supply supporting evidence to positive animal bioassays or epidemiology results. In some instances results from short-term tests may conflict with animal bioassay data. If an animal bioassay shows a positive response, it cannot be dismissed because a negative response was observed in these tests. However, positive responses in such short-term tests are ordinarily sufficient to provide suggestive evidence of carcinogenicity, even if the substance tested has shown only negative responses in some animal bioassays. As the degree of certainty attached to the negative responses in animal bioassays increases because the observation is reproduced in other animal species and strains or under more rigorous test conditions, the suspicion about the chemical as a result of short-term tests may be reduced and eventually eliminated. These conclusions are in accord with those of the National Cancer Advisory Board's Subcommittee on Environmental Carcinogenesis (57):

> At the present, none of the short-term tests can be used to establish whether a compound will or will not be carcinogenic in humans or experimental animals. Positive results obtained in these systems suggest extensive testing of the agent in long-term animal bioassays, particularly if there are other reasons for testing. Negative results in a short-term test, however, do not establish the safety of the agent.

Molecular Structure as Supporting Evidence in Identification of Carcinogens

Information useful in identifying possible carcinogens is provided by their molecular structures. It is well established that certain groupings of atoms (functional groups) in some molecules may impart carcinogenic properties —e.g. some polynuclear aromatic systems, hydrazine groups, N-nitroso groups, and α, β-unsaturated lactones. There is a moderately substantial base of empirical data that permits conclusions about carcinogenic potential on the basis of molecular structure (33, 100).

Similarly, some functional groups have never been shown to impart carcinogenic properties to molecules, although the data base for such negative correlations is much smaller and probably inconsequential. The reason for the absence of a strong empirical data base for noncarcinogens is that structure has frequently been used as a guide to testing chemicals for carcinogenicity, and priorities for testing have often been based on the suspected cancer-inducing properties of chemicals.

In some instances, the predictive power of molecular structure of functional groups known to be correlated with carcinogenic properties has proved unsatisfactory. Therefore, the general consensus of the scientific community appears to be that chemical structure has limited value in identifying carcinogens and is to be used in carcinogenesis hazard assessment only as corroborative supporting evidence.

In the absence of other data, however, there are instances in which structure may provide suggestive evidence that a risk of carcinogenesis exists. When structure is to be used as suggestive evidence, well-documented support should be presented and qualified where necessary by complete notation of substances of similar structure that have been adequately studied for carcinogenic activity.

Qualitative Judgmental Factors in Evaluation of Total Evidence

Evidence that a substance poses a carcinogenic hazard is contributed by each source discussed in the preceding sections of this report: epidemiologic studies, studies on experimental animals, and studies based on short-term and other tests that have been shown to correlate with carcinogenicity; this includes studies of biochemical pathways and chemical structure. For some substances data may be available from all three sources; for others, there may be data from only one or two sources. Each source of relevant data needs to be critically evaluated by consideration of the many aspects discussed in this document.

The judgment that a substance poses a carcinogenic hazard derives from the evaluation of the total evidence provided by all of the sources. Different data sources may not contribute equally to the cumulative evaluation, depending on the specific nature and extent of the data, the scientific quality of the studies, and the adequacy of their documentation.

Conclusions on the carcinogenicity of a substance may be reached on the basis of evidence provided by epidemiologic studies, bioassays in animals, or both. Suggestive evidence is provided by the other types of studies.

In the absence of adequate epidemiologic or animal evidence, a positive response in any of the short-term in-vitro tests that correlate with carcinogenicity is considered suggestive of a carcinogenic hazard. Suggestive evidence may also derive from considerations of chemical structure or biochemical pathways.

Ordinarily, if a substance has produced positive results in a single adequately designed and conducted animal bioassay and no other data are available, the conclusion is that the substance is likely to pose a risk of cancer to humans. These results may be further confirmed by data on chemical structure, in vitro testing, or relevant biochemical studies that suggest a carcinogenic potential. However, negative data from the latter three sources do not override adequate positive data from an animal bioassay. Further confirmation that the substance poses a carcinogenic hazard to humans is obtained from bioassay data showing reproducibility of results, positive dose-response relationships, and concordance of results (see "Evaluation of Pathologic Results").

Because of biologic variability among species, the conclusion that the evidence is positive on the basis of results obtained in one animal species is not altered by negative data obtained in other species or strains of test animals. Moreover, negative epidemiologic data, questionable because of limitations in the power of detection of such studies, do not deny the conclusion of carcinogenicity on the basis of animal bioassays. Negative evidence from properly designed and conducted epidemiologic studies may, however, be used to set an upper limit on human risk to comparable populations under analogous conditions of exposure.

It should be stressed that the qualitative judgment whether a substance poses a carcinogenic hazard is based on the evaluation of cumulative evidence from all pertinent data sources. The reasons for specific conclusions need to be clearly detailed.

The terms "strong" and "weak" have been used in the literature to describe both the nature of the hazard or risk and the extent and quality of the evidence. A certain confusion may have ensued, since one could refer to weak evidence of a strong effect or to strong evidence of a weak effect. The two categories are clearly not equivalent and should not be confused.

THE QUANTITATIVE ESTIMATION OF RISK

The previous section of this document dealt with the issue of the likelihood that a substance poses a carcinogenic hazard to humans. In some instances a regulatory agency may be required, or may find it useful, to estimate quantitatively the cancer risk of such a substance in exposed humans if the compound is assumed to be a human carcinogen.

Quantitative assessment of human cancer risk may be based on epidemiologic or animal data. In either instance, methodologic problems arise because of the need to extrapolate from effects observed under one condition and level of exposure and in one population group or biologic system to arrive at an estimate of the effects expected in the human group or individual. Because extrapolations are involved, uncertainties are necessarily attached to the cancer risk estimates that can be made with current methodologies. Furthermore, uncertainties arise from other sources, particularly from attempts to identify accurately conditions and levels of exposure of the human group or individual.

Despite the uncertainties, risk estimates can be and are being made, not only by some regulatory agencies but by other scientific bodies. Because of the uncertainties, however, and because of the serious public health consequences if the estimated risk were understated, it has become common practice to make cautious and prudent assumptions wherever they are needed to conduct a risk assessment. This approach has a precedent in other areas of public health protection where similar problems arise because of gaps in knowledge (101, 102). Thus current methodologies, which permit only crude estimates of human risk, are designed to avoid understatement of the risk. It must be recognized, however, that in some circumstances this cannot be guaranteed because of other factors that may enhance human response, such as synergistic effects. Thus risk assessments should be used with caution in the regulatory process.

If data on animals are used as the basis for estimating human risk, data obtained from the most sensitive animal species or strain tested are commonly recommended as the starting point for extrapolation. Of the available data, these are clearly the least likely to understate human risk. Use of data from less sensitive species or strains is justifiable only if there are strong reasons to believe that the most sensitive animal model is completely irrelevant to any segment of the exposed human population.

A limited comparison of human and animal data for carcinogens is contained in a report of the National Academy of Sciences (103). Data were compared for benzidine, chlornaphazine, diethylstilbestrol, aflatoxin B_1, vinyl chloride, and cigarette smoke. The authors stated that "as a working hypothesis, in the absence of countervailing evidence for the specific agent in question, it appears reasonable to assume that the lifetime cancer incidence induced by chronic exposure in man can be approximated by the lifetime incidence induced by similar exposure in laboratory animals at the same total dose per body weight." These preliminary observations suggest that current methodologies may not lead to serious errors.

Whether quantitative risk assessment is based on data from animals or humans, there is uncertainty about the shape of the dose-response relationship at the (usually low) levels of actual human exposure. Mathematical extrapolation models are discussed in detail later in this section. The linear nonthreshold dose-response model is most commonly used at the present time. Of the various models, it appears to have the soundest scientific basis and is less likely to understate risk than other plausible models. It has, for many of the same reasons, a long history of use in protection against radiation (101, 102).

The most favorable foundation for quantitative risk assessment is based on well-characterized responses in human populations with well-defined exposures. Unfortunately, the exposure estimates are often unavailable or crude. Negative epidemiologic studies on populations for which usable exposure estimates are available can be valuable in conjunction with animal data; the studies on animals provide evidence for carcinogenic hazard, and the epidemiologic data may provide upper limits of response for cross-comparison with the animal data. Although extrapolation from the observed human population group to other groups carries less uncertainty than extrapolations from animals to humans, the possibility of significant differences in the characteristics and conditions of exposure of the two population groups must be recognized. Any such differences that may affect the estimate of risk should be noted, although information is rarely available that will permit specific integration of these factors into the risk assessment methodology.

To the extent currently possible, the methods described in the following section permit a crude order-of-magnitude estimate of risk for substances that may pose a cancer hazard to humans. As more knowledge develops, risk assessment methodologies should be improved. Some of the kinds of information and knowledge that will likely prove useful in the future are discussed in the sections to follow. At present, most such information is not available and thus cannot ordinarily be used in risk assessment without the imposition of numerous assumptions. Caution is needed in risk assessment as long as these gaps in knowledge exist.

Much has been written about threshold doses for carcinogenic effect, but unfortunately, there is no recognized method for determining their existence. A model recently proposed by Cornfield (104) permits the inclusion of thresholds. However, as Cornfield stipulated originally and again recently (105), a threshold could be derived from this model only if there were instantaneous and complete deactivation of the material before any carcinogenic effect occurs—an improbable event.

Since threshold doses for carcinogenesis have not been established, a prudent approach from a safety standpoint is to assume that any dose may induce or promote carcinogenesis. Some of the mathematical models proposed to describe the dose-response relationship for carcinogenesis are discussed in the following section.

With the present state of knowledge, the quantitative assessment of cancer risks provides only a rough estimate of the magnitude of the cancer risks; this estimate may be useful in setting priorities for control of carcinogens and in obtaining a very rough idea of the magnitude of the public health problem posed by a given carcinogen.

Mathematical Models for High-to-Low Dose Extrapolation Within a Single Biologic System

Mathematical models were developed in the last two decades for estimating the effects of exposure levels well below levels for which test data were available, with the goal of ensuring that the risk will not be underestimated. These models of dose-response relationships make use of data obtained in a given biologic system to extrapolate from high to low doses. Consideration must be given to the many biologic variables that influence the level of response in different species or under different exposure conditions.

THE MODELS   In order to extrapolate outside the experimental range of exposure levels, some mathematical formulation relating response to dose must be available. The two categories of mathematical models commonly used to depict the relationship between response and dose are dichotomous-response models and time-to-response models. In the dichotomous-response situation the response of interest is the presence or absence of some specified condition. Time-to-response models attempt to relate dose level to distribution of the time until the occurrence of a given event, such as tumor observation or death. (Both categories of models are completely specified except for a few unknown parameters, which are typically estimated from a given set of experimental data.)

A variety of different approaches have been proposed to deal with the problem of low-dose extrapolation involving a dichotomous response. Included are the Mantel-Bryan procedure, the one-hit model, linear extrapolation, and various extensions of the multistage model developed by Armitage & Doll (106).

Mantel & Bryan (107, 108) proposed an extrapolation technique based on the log-probit model, which had long been used for bioassays to estimate median lethal doses. They selected this model because it seemed to provide a reasonable fit to a large body of experimental carcinogenesis data and not because of any mechanistic arguments in its support. Under this procedure, extrapolation is conducted from the upper confidence limit on the observed experimental response along a probit log-dose line with a preassigned slope of one to some specified low level of risk. By using the upper confidence limit and fixing the slope at one (a shallower slope than they had typically seen with their experimental data sets), Mantel & Bryan hoped to generate an upper bound on the estimated dose associated with the predetermined risk level, regardless of the true form of the underlying and unknown dose-response curve. However, subsequent theoretical and applied research has demonstrated that the Mantel-Bryan procedure is not as conservative as once thought and may underestimate risk in some situations (109, 110).

The one-hit model is based on the concept that a tumor can be induced after a single susceptible target or receptor has been exposed to a single effective dose unit of a substance (109, 110). Thus, unlike the Mantel-Bryan procedure, there is an assumed biologic mechanism of action for the carcinogen underlying the one-hit model. This action implies that the probability (P) that a tumor will be induced by exposure to a chemical at dose d is given by the equation $P(d) = 1-\exp(-\lambda d)$, where λ is an unknown non-negative constant. When λd is small (i.e. in the low-dose region), it can readily be shown that $P(d) \approx \lambda d$, i.e. for low dose levels the one-hit model is well approximated by a simple linear model in which the probability of tumor observation is directly proportional to dose.

If the unknown (true) dose-response curve is assumed to have a sigmoidal shape—an assumption supported by a wealth of toxicologic data—then the response will curve upward in the low (or, typically, environmental) dose region. Thus a linear model will provide an upper bound to curves of this shape and, it is hoped, a conservative estimate of the dose associated with any specified level of risk (111). A line connecting zero with a point on the dose-response curve for the excess tumor rate above background will always lie above the true dose-response curve for the convex portion of the curve. An additional degree of conservatism is introduced by extrapolating back to zero from an upper confidence limit (UCL) for the net excess tumor rate above the background rate. In the linear model the tumor rate is assumed to be proportional to dose: $P(d) = \lambda d$. The upper confidence limit for the slope λ is UCL $\div$ experimental dose. Thus the maximal risk for a given dose d may be estimated by the equation maximal risk = (UCL/d_e) $\times$ d, where d_e is the experimental dose. Conversely, the equation for a predicted dose for a maximal level of risk is: predicted dose = (risk $\times$ d_e)/ UCL.

A number of investigators have published papers (112–115) based on the Armitage & Doll (116) formulation of the multistage model of carcinogenesis. Under the multistage model it is assumed that the cancer originates as a "malignant" cell, which is initiated by a series of somatic-like mutations occurring in finite steps. It is also assumed that each mutational stage can be depicted as a Poisson process in which the transition rate is approximately linear in dose rate. Then the lifetime probability of tumor induction can be expressed approximately as $P(d) = 1-\exp(-\lambda_0-\lambda_1 d- \ldots -\lambda_k d^k)$, where $\lambda_i \geq 0$ for all values of i, and k corresponds to the number of transitions or mutational stages. (Highly sophisticated computer algorithms have been developed for fitting the multistage model to laboratory data with the use of a restricted maximum likelihood approach which does not require that the value of k be prespecified.)

Both the total incidence of tumors and the time at which tumors occur are important. Tumors leading to early death and life-shortening need to be considered.

Time-to-tumor is the time at which a tumor is detected or observed by palpation or by gross or microscopic examination of an animal at the time of death or sacrifice. Time-to-tumor is not used here to indicate the instant at which a pretumorous condition becomes a tumor. Time-to-observance is better terminology.

Some hope for improving risk estimates has been based on use of the time-to-observance of tumors in addition to use of the proportion of animals possessing tumors. On the basis of Druckrey's work (117), the median time to tumors appeared to increase as the dose decreased. It was hoped that low doses could be found that would result in median times-to-tumor observation well beyond the expected lifetime; this might result in the identification of "practical thresholds." Albert & Altshuler (118) expanded on the use of median time-to-tumor observation by employing distributions of time-to-tumors for individual animals. Chand & Hoel (119) showed that use of a log-normal time-to-tumor distribution leads to a probit-log dose relationship, and use of a Weibull time-to-tumor distribution leads to an extreme value model for the proportion of animals with tumors: $P(d) = 1-\exp[-\exp(\alpha+\beta \log d)]$, where alpha and beta are constants. Schneiderman et al (120) demonstrated that even though the median time-to-tumor may be well beyond the expected lifetime, a significant proportion of animals or humans may still develop tumors within the normal lifespan. Peto (121) examined human data and questioned the concept that lower doses result in longer latency. Whittemore & Altshuler (122), analyzing data on cigarette smoking, concluded that it was not possible to distinguish between the log-normal and the Weibull models.

The available data do not permit a conclusion as to whether lower doses lengthen the latency periods. Animal experiments at high doses may induce more tumors resulting in easier and therefore earlier detection, and this may not be due to an actual decrease of latency period.

Time-to-observance response models have not received the same degree of attention as dichotomous-response models in carcinogenesis risk extrapolation. One of the major factors underlying this relative lack of emphasis may be that studies in which animals were given the substance in their feed have not generated sufficient information to determine the relationship between age and cumulative cancer incidence.

PROCEDURES   In the preceding section it was noted that the Mantel-Bryan procedure is essentially empirical and lacks biologic relevance with respect to current knowledge about carcinogenesis. Since risk extrapolations developed by the Mantel-Bryan technique tend to zero much more rapidly in the low-dose region than do extrapolations based on somatic mutation models, the Mantel-Bryan procedure would certainly not be appropriate if the carcinogen under study were thought to act directly on cellular DNA (109).

Initially, extrapolation based on a multistage model appears to offer significant advantages over linear extrapolation procedures. Under the multistage approach, no assumptions are made a priori about the exact form for the mathematical extrapolation. Instead, the experimental data are used to estimate the shape of the dose-response curve. However, Crump et al (109, 114) and Guess et al (110) have shown that the upper confidence limit on estimated risk becomes essentially linear for generalized polynomial extrapolation in the low-dose region. This approximate linearity holds even when the maximum likelihood estimate of excess risk does not contain a linear component (estimated). Therefore, there is some question whether the mathematical refinements of generalized polynomial extrapolation are justified for application to animal bioassays, which may be only crude approximations to the human situation (109).

As an interim procedure, it has generally been recommended (106) that whenever quantitative risk analysis is deemed necessary, linear extrapolation should always be included among any methods used unless there is reason to believe that the experimental (observed) response does not fall in the convex portion of the dose-response curve. If the response is in the concave portion of the curve, the one-hit model is suitable. At low observed responses the linear and one-hit models yield nearly identical results. An added degree of protection can be achieved by starting the extrapolation from the upper confidence limit of the response.

The mathematical procedures per se are intended to provide upper limit estimates of risk from a statistical standpoint. However, the risk estimates as applied to humans should not be regarded as upper limit estimates because of large biologic uncertainties (see "Extrapolation from Observed Effects to Estimates of Risk for the Observed Population").

Characterization of Population Exposure

The estimation of total population exposure to a given substance (and/or to its decomposition and metabolic products) requires consideration of the following aspects: (a) sources of human exposure (occurrence, production, uses, and environmental distribution), (b) analytical methods for detecting and measuring exposures in the environment and in the population, (c) routes and conditions of exposure, (d) duration, frequency, and intensity of exposure, and (e) size and characteristics of the exposed populations.

During examination of exposure data, important qualitative and quantitative factors beyond definable numerical values of dose level and population size will emerge; although such information may not be usable directly in a mathematical calculation of risk estimate, it will frequently provide additional perspective and insight during risk evaluation. Because of the great diversity in sources and estimating procedures available in various situations, it does not seem practicable at this point to set minimum detailed specifications for the reliable estimation of exposures or to identify recommended or approved methods and procedures for producing exposure estimates. The following general considerations indicate the kind of data useful for assessment of population exposures. The better defined these data are, the higher will be the confidence that a realistic estimate of risk for the exposed populations has been made (123).

SOURCES OF HUMAN EXPOSURE   Two types of exposure sources are considered: primary sources and human contact sources.

Primary sources of exposure to a chemical are those that determine its release into the human environment, and they include natural occurrence, extraction from natural products, mining, chemical synthesis, manufacture or production, and specific uses.

Human contact sources are those that bring about the contact of the substance with the human body, and they include items or preparations containing the chemical (such as foodstuffs or consumer products), vehicles, or a medium in which the chemical is present (such as ambient air or drinking water).

Some substances may originate from a single primary source and be present in a wide range of human contact sources; conversely, a specific human contact source may be traced to several different primary sources. It is important that for each substance the entire range of sources and environmental distribution be examined.

Frequently, there is more than one source of human exposure, and an individual may be exposed to a substance of concern from an array of sources depending upon the circumstances. Analysis of environmental distribution and exposure pathways allows identification of the most significant sources, so that both the size of the population exposed and the intensity of exposure can be established. In some instances, it is possible to estimate combined exposure to the same substance from different sources, primarily where the populations affected by these different sources are the same. Frequently, however, differences in the populations exposed from various sources are so large that any attempt to combine the estimates may produce an unrealistic or unclear description of the actual human exposure conditions. Then it is preferable to consider each source separately and subsequently use whatever knowledge is available on multiple sources of exposures to interpret these observations.

Estimates of the total level of production of a substance can be useful indicators of the extent of exposure, particularly over time. Dates of first synthesis and commercial production of a substance are useful in the evaluation of delayed toxic effects and allow an estimate of the time before which no human exposure could have occurred. The accuracy of data on national production and foreign trade of individual substances (which are often difficult to obtain) needs to be ascertained.

Uses of a substance are important descriptors of its environmental distribution and the extent of human exposure. Whenever possible, all uses of carcinogenic substances should be identified.

An important distinction is that between uses for which human exposure is intended (intentional exposures) and that for which it is not intended (unintentional exposures). Individual exposure or consumption of a substance may be voluntary or involuntary. The sociologic bases and implications of these definitions are beyond the scope of this report.

ANALYTICAL METHODS FOR DETECTION AND MEASUREMENT OF EXPOSURES The specificity and limit of detection of analytical procedures for the identification of many carcinogenic substances, both in the environment and in exposed organisms, have been remarkably improved in recent years. Progress in analytical chemistry is expected to undergo further refinement and improvement in the near future.

The limit of detection of analytical methods varies considerably for different substances and different conditions of analysis, and this is a critical factor in assessing a source of exposure. It is important to consider that the agent may not be measurable but may still be present below the minimum detectable level. The minimum detectable level of a substance may vary depending on different vehicles, media, and conditions of exposure.

Quantitative determinations of the level of a substance in various exposure sources should consider time and space distribution and variations, and ranges of values may be useful to estimate the conditions of exposure.

The chemical and physical properties of the substance should be identified. Such characteristics as particle size distribution for aerosols and dust should be determined insofar as possible.

Analytical determination of the levels of a substance in exposed organisms, particularly in the exposed population, is of great value but not always obtainable. Available data on the levels of substance (or its metabolites) in the target tissues or body fluids should be considered.

The dose of an ultimate carcinogen at the site of action in the tissues or cells, which is measured at all times after its introduction ("target tissue dose") is ideally the dose that should be estimated and correlated with expected effects. This target tissue dose usually cannot be closely estimated because of many variables and uncertainties (102). The relationship between target tissue dose and exposure dose may vary considerably under different conditions. To the extent practicable, documentation of the analytical methods, the sampling conditions, the limits of detectability, and the range of observed values is desirable.

ROUTES AND CONDITIONS OF EXPOSURE   All possible routes of exposure associated with each source should be identified. If any routes of exposure are considered irrelevant for estimation of effective doses, the circumstances should be specified. Careful consideration of sources of exposure—e.g. product use patterns, environmental or occupational situations, and background—may suggest or reveal routes of exposure not immediately apparent. For example, a chemical may also be absorbed through the skin or by ingestion when inhalation is apparently the primary route.

For estimation of animal-to-human correlations in the evaluation of test data on animals, it is necessary to obtain the human dose level in units consistent with those used to describe the effective dose in the animal bioassay being used for comparison. In some instances, any necessary conversion from the actual measurement at the source to the needed units describing exposure dose can be straightforward (e.g. by simple application of observed or estimated food ingestion rates to a chemical's concentration in a food). In other instances, complex calculations or modeling procedures may be necessary, as in the estimation of effective exposure distributions from ambient air on the basis of monitoring data or emission inventories for point sources. This conversion or translation step, often necessary in the estimation of human exposure, should always be explicitly identified and reported. When available data show substantial differences between the route and conditions of exposure in test animals and in humans, it is necessary to rely on estimates of comparability and to attempt to establish an acceptable equivalent dose. In the absence of satisfactory equivalent dose data, only defensible conservative assumptions should be used in such a way that the possible risk is not underestimated.

DURATION, FREQUENCY, AND INTENSITY OF EXPOSURE   An important factor in the quantitative evaluation of population exposure is the length of time during which exposures occur. Although the time of exposure may vary considerably within a population, there are cases in which it can be reasonably well-defined. These include cases of specified duration of exposure (e.g. to certain drugs or certain occupational carcinogens) or continuous lifetime exposure to widely disseminated environmental carcinogens (e.g. polycyclic aromatic hydrocarbons).

Effective exposure rates corresponding to typical patterns of individual exposure, whether short-term or long-term temporal trends, must be reported wherever significantly different patterns exist. The two components of the estimated level or amount of exposure—the effective rate per unit time or per incident of exposure and the frequency-duration pattern— should be explicitly identified for each exposure pattern considered.

SIZE AND CHARACTERISTICS OF EXPOSED POPULATIONS   The total number of people exposed to any level of a carcinogenic substance represents a major indicator of the extent of risk related to that substance. Because combinations of exposures to different carcinogens may contribute to the cancer risk in the same population or individual, and because no threshold level for exposure to a carcinogen can presently be reliably determined for a population, a contributory risk level from any exposure level, however small, must be assumed.

Age of exposure should be considered, i.e. whether exposure is essentially lifelong (at more or less constant rates) or is concentrated in certain age ranges. The relationship between total lifetime exposure in each exposure pattern and the amount of this exposure that may be concentrated in any specific age ranges should be identified. Wherever feasible, the degree of stratification of exposed populations should be identified to permit distinctions between effective exposure amounts by age (e.g. childhood, working age, and elderly age groups) and by sex. As noted above, populations having high-risk age groups should be identified. Attention should be given to exceptional exposure groups of special concern, such as infants, children, and pregnant women, as well as to groups with special genetic conditions or concurrent disease. In addition, in descriptions of certain population subgroups, the smoking habits, dietary and alcohol consumption patterns, and other cultural and environmental characteristics should be considered if possible.

Extrapolation from Observed Effects to Estimates of Risks for Exposed Population

The quantitative estimation of risk from a carcinogenic substance for the entire exposed or potentially exposed population may be conducted with the use of observations on the effects of the substance in (a) a defined human population group and (b) experimental animal tests.

In both situations the extrapolation will take into account the factors that characterize and distinguish the groups observed and the factors to which the extrapolation applies.

CORRELATIONS FROM OBSERVED HUMAN POPULATION GROUPS TO OTHERS   The problem to be considered here is the estimation of present or potential risks for all people exposed to a given substance by means of data obtained from observations in a defined population group. The observed group may be small and its exposure conditions may be well defined, as for certain studies of drugs or for occupational exposures. In other situations the observed group may be poorly defined, even if larger. In analyzing the correlation between observed and estimated population effects, it is desirable where feasible to review the critical differences between the two conditions, such as age and sex distribution of the population; genetic, racial, and ethnic differences; environmental differences and migration patterns; dietary and cultural habits; smoking patterns; alcohol consumption; patterns of intercurrent disease; and particular susceptibility states including pregnancy and fetal and neonatal exposures. Many of these complex variables are considered under "Epidemiologic Evidence" and "Characterization of Population Exposure" above.

ANIMAL-TO-HUMAN CORRELATIONS   Although a close qualitative similarity has been established in the nature of the response of laboratory animals and humans to carcinogenic substances, a quantitative correlation is more uncertain because of the marked variation of susceptibility in different animal species and among individuals in the human population. It is not possible to reduce the variables to a single safety factor for general use (106).

Several species-conversion factors should be considered in estimating risk levels for humans from data obtained in another species. Species-conversion factors are affected by many variables, such as body surface, body weight, metabolic pathways, nutritional conditions, genetic variability, and bacterial flora as well as tissue distribution and the retention and fate of the chemical. In evaluating exposures to the general population, one should consider all ages, transplacental exposures, concurrent disease conditions, and special susceptibility states.

Other conversion factors should also be considered when observations are obtained for test species under exposure conditions markedly different from those in the population (e.g. different routes or modes of exposures, vehicles, modifying factors, variations in age, sex, perinatal exposures, disease states, and single vs multiple exposures). The limits of uncertainty should be stated whenever possible (102, 106).

Different carcinogens tested under comparable experimental conditions show a wide range of response; if extreme cases are included, the range of variation is more than one millionfold. Changes in experimental conditions, particularly ones that alter the effective dose, can markedly affect the observed level of effect of a carcinogen within the same genetic strain of animal. Exposure of experimental animals to certain other chemicals in addition to a carcinogen under test may change the observed effect in either direction and at the extremes up to one hundredfold or even one thousand-fold (124). Differences between species can be even greater. On the other side of the correlation, the human response to carcinogens as well as to many other chemicals and drugs may also show great quantitative variations among individuals. Studies on the metabolic activation and chemical interaction of carcinogens in human tissues in vitro have shown interindividual quantitative variations of about one hundredfold in relatively small population samples (125–127). Individuals resistant or sensitive to one carcinogen may not be equally resistant or sensitive to another carcinogen or to combined effects of several exposures. Such wide interindividual variations are also well known from many pharmacokinetic studies.

A number of variables are relevant to the correlation of animal and human conditions. Some problems inherent in the use of animals must be kept in mind when animal studies are used for estimation of the quantitative carcinogenic potential of a substance for humans. A concise statement of some of these factors is contained in "Drinking Water and Health," prepared by the Safe Drinking Water Committee, Advisory Center on Toxicology, National Research Council, National Academy of Sciences (56). Factors discussed in this document include the rate of chemical absorption, distribution within the body, metabolic differences among exposed animals, effect of intestinal bacteria, rates of excretion and reabsorption, differences in molecular receptor sites for the carcinogen, environmental and genetic differences, and number of exposed animals and susceptible cells.

Metabolism and pharmacokinetics account for major differences in sensitivity to chemical carcinogens between species. In principle, this information could be used in estimating the relative sensitivity of humans compared to experimental animals. In practice, detailed metabolic pathways in humans are not known for many carcinogens; moreover, the marked variation in metabolism and sensitivity among individuals of different ages, states of health, and other biologic conditions require more information on the heterogeneity of human metabolic and pharmacokinetic responses than is usually available. It is hoped that future research will clarify these important correlations in much greater depth. Such information, if available, should be used to correct for an underestimate of human risk, but it should be used to correct for an overestimate of human risk only when there is substantial information on diversity of human response.

The contribution of animal test data to the estimation of the risk level for humans should be based on experiments with the most sensitive species available. Confidence that this procedure will not underestimate the human risk increases with the number of experiments and the number of species and strains studied.

Lack of Predictable Thresholds for an Exposed Population

The self-replicating nature of cancer, the multiplicity of causative factors to which individuals can be exposed, the additive and possibly synergistic combination of effects, and the wide range of individual susceptibilities work together in making it currently unreliable to predict a threshold below which human population exposure to a carcinogen has no effect on cancer risk.

Observation of the marked individual differences in the response of human subjects to carcinogens shows that some individuals do not develop cancer in their lifetime, whereas others develop it readily after the same exposure to a carcinogen. Although these observations are compatible with the existence of different "thresholds" for individual subjects in certain conditions, they are not a basis for predicting a no-effect level of a carcinogen in other individuals or under different conditions. There is no presently acceptable way to determine reliably a threshold for a carcinogen for an entire population.

Individual human subjects in the population are exposed throughout life to a number of carcinogens, which may be considered to provide a background of carcinogenic risk; exposure to any amount of a single carcinogen, however small, is regarded as capable of adding to the total carcinogenic risk (109). Cancer susceptibility varies greatly among individual members of human populations due to genetic, racial, and ethnic factors; to environmental and dietary exposure; and to other modifiers.

Variability among individuals makes it very difficult to have confidence that an observed no-effect level of exposure in animals or even in a specific human population (for which individual variation may be small in comparison to the total population) will be applicable to the total human population at risk. A large number of factors (e.g. age, sex, race, nutritional status, immunologic status, general state of health, previous exposure to the substance in question or to other substances) could affect individual susceptibility. Even if thresholds for carcinogens could be demonstrated for certain individuals or for a defined population, no reliable method is known for establishing a threshold that could apply to the total human population (67).

SUMMARY OF RISK ESTIMATION   For a given substance, the usefulness of dose-response data obtained from a specific human population group or from animal tests for estimation of risk in the general population is limited by the consideration that general population exposures to one substance are usually only a component of the total carcinogenic burden derived from multiple sources, with their possible interactions.

Recognition of these limitations, however, does not imply that no attempt should be made to develop reasonable risk estimates for different conditions of human exposure. The several components of quantitative risk assessment include the following:

1. definition and quantification of exposures,
2. characterization of the exposed populations in quantitative terms,
3. chemical and physical properties of the substance and its chemical reactivity in relation to exposure,
4. prudent quantitative mathematical extrapolation of the responses from observed to estimated exposure ranges within the observed biologic system,
5. qualification of the estimated risk in light of identifiable biologic and toxicologic differences that may be present in the exposed human population.

Literature Cited

1. Saffiotti, U. 1977. Scientific bases of environmental carcinogenesis and cancer prevention: Developing an interdisciplinary science and facing its ethical implications. *J. Toxicol. Environ. Health* 2:1435–1447

2. Hartwell, J. L. 1951. *Survey of Compounds Which Have Been Tested for Carcinogenic Activity. Natl. Cancer Inst., Public Health Serv. Publ. No.* 149. Washington DC: GPO

3. Shubik, P., Hartwell, J. L. 1957. *Survey of Compounds Which Have Been Tested for Carcinogenic Activity.* Natl. Cancer Inst., Public Health Serv. Publ. No. 149: Suppl 1. Washington DC: GPO

4. Shubik, P., Hartwell, J. L., Peters, J. A., eds. 1969. *Survey of Compounds Which Have Been Tested for Carcinogenic Activity.* Natl. Cancer Inst., Public Health Serv. Publ. No. 149: Suppl. 2. Washington DC: GPO

5. National Cancer Institute. 1973. *Survey of Compounds Which Have Been Tested for Carcinogenic Activity, 1961–1967.* Public Health Serv. Publ. No. 149. Washington DC: GPO

6. National Cancer Institute. 1971. *Survey of Compounds Which Have Been Tested for Carcinogenic Activity, 1968–1969.* Public Health Serv. Publ. No. 149. Washington DC: GPO

7. National Cancer Institute. 1974. *Survey of Compounds Which Have Been Tested for Carcinogenic Activity, 1970–1971* vol. Publc Health Serv. Publ. No. 149. Washington, DC: US GPO

8. National Cancer Institute. 1975. *Survey of Compounds Which Have Been Tested for Carcinogenic Activity, 1972–1973* vol. Public Health Serv. Publ. No. 149. Washington DC: US GPO

9. International Agency for Research on Cancer: 1972. *Inorganic substances, chlorinated hydrocarbons, aromatic amines, N-nitroso compounds, natural products, miscellaneous.* IARC Monogr. Eval. Carcinog. Risk Chem. Man. 1:1–184

10. International Agency for Research on Cancer. 1973. *Some Inorganic and Organometallic Compounds.* IARC Monogr. Eval. Carcinog. Risk Chem. Man. 2:1–181

11. International Agency for Research on Cancer. 1973. *Certain Polycyclic Aromatic Hydrocarbons and Heterocyclic Compounds.* IARC Monogr. Eval. Carcinog. Risk Chem. Man. 3:1–272

12. International Agency for Research on Cancer. 1974. *Some Aromatic Amines, Hydrazine and Related Substances, N-Nitroso Compounds and Miscellaneous Alkylating Agents.* IARC Monogr.

Eval. Carcinog. Risk Chem. Man. 4:1–286

13. International Agency for Research on Cancer. 1974. *Some Organochlorine Pesticides.* IARC Monogr. Eval. Carcinog. Risk Chem. Man. 5:1–241

14. International Agency for Research on Cancer. 1974. *Sex Hormones.* IARC Monogr. Eval. Carcinog. Risk Chem. Man. 6:1–243

15. International Agency for Research on Cancer. 1974. *Some Anti-thyroid and Related Substances, Nitrofurans and Industrial Chemicals.* IARC Monogr. Eval. Carcinog. Risk Chem. Man. 7:1–326

16. International Agency for Research on Cancer. 1975. *Some Aromatic Azo Compounds.* IARC Monogr. Eval. Carcinog. Risk Chem. Man. 8:1–357

17. International Agency for Research on Cancer. 1975. *Some Aziridines, N-, S-, and O-Mustards and Selenium.* IARC Monogr. Eval. Carcinog. Risk Chem. Man. 9:1–268

18. International Agency for Research on Cancer. 1976. *Some Naturally Occurring Substances.* IARC Monogr. Eval. Carcinog. Risk Chem. Man. 10:1–353

19. International Agency for Research on Cancer. 1976. *Cadmium, Nickel, Some Epoxides, Miscellaneous Industrial Chemicals, and General Considerations on Volatile Anesthetics.* IARC Monogr. Eval. Carcinog. Risk Chem. Man. 11:1–306

20. International Agency for Research on Cancer. 1976. *Some Carbamates, Thiocarbamates and Carbazides.* IARC Monogr. Eval. Carcinog. Risk Chem. Man. 12:1–282

21. International Agency for Research on Cancer. 1977. *Some Miscellaneous Pharmaceutical Substances.* IARC Monogr. Eval. Carcinog. Risk Chem. Man. 13:1–255

22. International Agency for Research on Cancer. 1977. *Asbestos.* IARC Monogr. Eval. Charcinog. Risk Chem. Man. 14:1–106

23. International Agency for Research on Cancer. 1977. *Some Fumigants, the Herbicides 2,4-D and 2,4,5-T, Chlorinated Dibenzodioxins and Miscellaneous Industrial Chemicals.* IARC Monogr. Eval. Carcinog. Risk Chem. Man. 15:1–345

24. International Agency for Research on Cancer. 1978. *Some Aromatic Amines and Related Nitro Compounds—Hair Dyes, Colouring Agents and Miscellaneous Industrial Chemicals.* IARC Monogr. Eval. Carcinog. Risk Chem. Man. 16:1–400

25. International Agency for Research on Cancer. 1978. *Some N-Nitroso Compounds.* IARC Monogr. Eval. Carcinog. Risk Chem. Man. 17:1–365

26. National Institute for Occupational Safety and Health. 1975. *Suspected Carcinogens.* A subfile of the NIOSH Toxic Substances List. DHEW Publ. No. (NIOSH) 75–188. Rockville, MD: US DHEW

27. Arcos, J. C., Argus, M. F., Wolf, G. 1968. *Chemical Induction of Cancer: Structural Bases and Biological Mechanisms,* vol I. New York/London: Academic

28. Arcos, J. C. Argus, M. F. 1974. *Chemical Induction of Cancer: Structural Bases and Biological Mechanisms,* vol IIA. New York/London: Academic

29. Arcos, J. C., Argus, M. F. 1974. *Chemical Induction of Cancer: Structural Bases and Biological Mechanisms,* vol IIB. New York/London: Academic Press

30. Berenblum, I. 1969. Carcinogenesis as a Biological Problem. Vol 34, *Frontiers of Biology.* Amsterdam: North-Holland

31. Hueper, W. C., Conway, W. D. 1964. *Chemical Carcinogenesis and Cancers.* Springfield, Ill: Thomas

32. Clayson, D. B. 1962. *Chemical Carcinogenesis.* Boston: Little, Brown & Co.

33. Searle, C. E., ed. 1976. Chemical Carcinogens. American Chemical Society Monograph 173. Washington, DC: Am. Chem. Soc.

34. Teichmann, B., Schramm, T. 1973. Substanzen mit kanzerogener Wirkung. Berlin-Buch: Zentralinstitut für Krebsforschung der Akademie der Wissenschaften der DDR.

35. Tomatis, L., Agthe, C., Bartsch, H., Huff, J., Montesano, R., Saracci, R., Walker, E. and Wilbourn, J. 1978. Evaluation of the carcinogenicity of chemicals: a review of the monograph program of the International Agency for Research in Cancer (1971 to 1977). *Cancer Res.* 38:877–85

36. National Cancer Institute, National Institute of Environmental Health Sciences, National Institute for Occupational Safety and Health 1978. Estimates of the Fraction of Cancer in the United States Related to Occupational Factors. US Dept. Labor, Occupational Safety and Health Admin., Docket No. H-090. Washington, DC

37. Rockette, H. E. 1977. Cause specific mortality of coal miners. *J. Occup. Med.* 19:795–801

38. Li, F. P., Fraumeni, J. F., Jr., Mantel, N. and Miller, R. W. 1969. Cancer mortality among chemists. *J. Nat. Cancer Inst.* 43:1159–1164

39. Koskela, Riita-Sisko, Hernberg, S., Karava, R., Jarvinen, E. and Nurinen, M. 1969. A mortality study of foundry workers. *Scand. J. Work Environ. Health* 2 (suppl. 1):73–89

40. Gibson, E. S., Martin, R. H., Lockington, J. N. 1977. Lung cancer mortality in a steel foundry. *J. Occup. Med.* 19:807–812

41. Moss, E., Lee, W. R. 1974. Occurrence of oral and pharyngeal cancers in textile workers. *Br. J. Ind. Med.* 31:224–232

42. Lloyd, J. W., Decoufle, P., Salvin, L. G. 1977. Unusual mortality experience of printing pressmen. *J. Occup. Med.* 19:543–550

43. Wagoner, J. K., Miller, R. W., Lundin, F. E., Jr., Fraumeni, J. F., Jr., and Haij, M. E. 1963. Unusual cancer mortality among a group of underground miners. *N. Engl. J. Med.* 269:284–289

44. Redmond, C. K., Strobino, B. Y., Cypress, R. H. 1976. Cancer experience among coke by-product workers. *Ann. NY Acad. Sci.* 271:102–115

45. Lemon, R. A., Lee, J. S., Wagoner, J. K. and Blejer, H. P. 1976. Cancer mortality among cadmium production workers. In *Occupational Carcinogenesis.* (Saffiotti, U. and Wagoner, J. (Eds.). *Ann. NY Acad. Sci.* 271:274–279.

46. Monson, R. R., Nakano, K. K. 1976. Mortality among rubber workers. I. White male union employees in Akron, Ohio. *Am. J. Epidemiol.* 103:284–96

47. Acheson, E. D. 1976. Nasal cancer in the furniture and boot and shoe manufacturing industries. *Prev. Med.* 5:295–315

48. Brinton, L. A. 1976. A death certificate analysis of nasal cancer among furniture workers in North Carolina. *Cancer Res.* 37:3473–3474

49. Aksoy, M., Erdem, S., Dincol, G. 1974. Leukemia in shoe-workers exposed chronically to benzene. *Blood* 44:837–841

50. Cole, P., Goldman, M. B. 1975. Occupation. In *Persons at High Risk of Cancer* ed. J. F. Fraumeni, Jr. pp. 167–184. New York: Academic

51. Slaga, T. J., Sivak, A., Boutwell, R. K., eds. 1978. Mechanisms of Tumor Promotion and Cocarcinogenesis. Carcino-genesis, a Comprehensive Survey, vol. 2. New York: Raven Press

52. Colburn, N. H. Tumor promotion and preneoplastic progression. In *Modifiers of Carcinogenesis, a Comprehensive Survey* (Slaga T. J., ed), vol 7. New York: Raven Press. In press

53. International Agency for Research on Cancer. 1976. *Aflatoxins.* IARC Monogr. Eval. Carcinog. Risk Chem. Man. 10:51–72

54. International Agency for Research On Cancer. 1974. *2-Naphthylamine.* IARC Monogr. Eval. Carcinog. Risk Chem. Man. 4:97–111

55. Magee, P. N., Montesano, R., Preussman, R. 1976. N-Nitroso compounds and related carcinogens. In *Chemical Carcinogens,* C. E. Searle. ed. American Chemical Society Monograph 173. Washington DC: Am. Chem. Soc. pp. 491–625

56. Safe Drinking Water Committee, Advisory Center on Toxicology, National Research Council, National Academy of Sciences. 1977: Drinking Water and Health. 1977. Washington, DC: Natl. Acad. Sci.

57. National Cancer Advisory Board. 1977. General criteria for assessing the evidence for carcinogenicity of chemical substances: Report of the Subcommittee on Environmental Carcinogenesis, National Cancer Advisory Board. *J. Natl. Cancer Inst.* 58:461–465, 1544

58. Fraumeni, J. F. Jr., ed. 1975. Persons at High Risk of Cancer: An Approach to Cancer Etiology and Control. Proceedings of a conference sponsored by the National Cancer Institute and the American Cancer Society, Key Biscayne, Fla., Dec. 10–12, 1974. New York: Academic Press

59. Shubik, P., Sicé, J. 1956. Chemical carcinogenesis as a chronic toxicity test. A review. *Cancer Res.* 16:728–742

60. International Union Against Cancer. 1957. Report of symposium on potential cancer hazards from chemical additives and contaminants to foodstuffs. *Acta Un. Int. Contra. Cancr.* 13:170–193

61. Subcommittee on Carcinogenesis, Food Protection Committee, Food and Nutrition Board, National Academy of Sciences National Research Council: Problems in the evaluation of carcinogenic hazard from use of food additives. *Cancer Res.* 21:429–456, 1961

62. Joint FAO/WHO Expert Committee on Food Additives. 1961. Fifth report of the Joint FAO/WHO Expert Commit-

tee on Food Additives. Evaluation of Carcinogenic Hazards of Food Additives. *WHO Tech. Rep. Ser.* 220:1–32
63. WHO Expert Committee on the Prevention of Cancer. 1964. Report of the WHO Expert Committee on the Prevention of Cancer. *WHO Tech. Rep. Ser.* 276:1–53
64. Berenblum, I., ed: 1969. Carcinogenicity Testing. Union Internationale Contre le Cancer Tech. Rep. Ser., vol. 2. Geneva, Switzerland: UICC
65. WHO Scientific Group. 1969. Report of the WHO Scientific Group on Principles for the Testing and Evaluation of Drugs for Carcinogenicity. *WHO Tech. Rep. Ser.* 426:1–26
66. Advisory Panel on Carcinogenicity of Pesticides. 1969. Carcinogenicity of pesticides. *In* Report of the Secretary's Commission on Pesticides and Their Relationship to Environmental Health, U.S. Dept. Health, Educ., Welfare. Washington DC: U.S. Govt. Print. Off., 1969, pp. 459–506
67. Ad Hoc Committee on the Evaluation of Low Levels of Environmental Carcinogens: Evaluation of environmental carcinogens—report to the Surgeon General. 1971. *In Chemicals and the Future of Man.* Hearings before the Subcommittee on Executive Reorganization and Government Research of the Committee on Government Operations of the U.S. Senate, 92d Congress, 1st session. Washington DC: U.S. Govt. Print. Off., pp. 171–183
68. Food and Drug Administration Advisory Committee on Protocols for Safety Evaluation: Panel on carcinogenesis report on cancer testing in the safety evaluation of food additives and pesticides. 1971. *Toxicol. Appl. Pharmacol.* 20: 419–438
69. Health and Welfare, Canada: The Testing of Chemicals for Carcinogenicity, Mutagenicity, and Teratogenicity. 1973. Ottawa, Canada: Ministry Health Welfare
70. WHO Scientific Group. 1974. Report of the WHO scientific group for the assessment of the carcinogenicity and mutagenicity of chemicals. *WHO Tech. Rep. Ser.* 546:1–19
71. Sontag, J. M., Page, N. P., Saffiotti, U. 1976. Guidelines for carcinogen bioassays in small rodents. Natl. Cancer Inst. Carcinogenesis Tech. Rep. Ser. No. 1. Natl. Inst. Health, DHEW Publ. No. (NIH) 76–801. Washington DC: GPO
72. Albert, R. E., Train, R. E., Anderson, E. 1977. Rationale developed by the Environmental Protection Agency for the assessment of carcinogenic risks. *J. Natl. Cancer Inst.* 58:1537–1541
73. Hiatt, H. H., Watson, J. D., Winsten, J. A. eds. 1977. Origins of Human Cancer. Cold Spring Harbor Conferences on Cell Proliferation, vol. 4. Cold Spring Harbor, N.Y.: Cold Spring Harbor Laboratory
74. Klaassen, C. D. Absorption, distribution and excretion of toxicants. In *Toxicology, the Basic Science of Poisons* (Casarett L. J., Doll J., eds). New York: Macmillan, 1975, pp. 26–44
75. Bischoff, F., Bryson, G. 1964. Carcinogenesis through solid state surfaces. *Prog. Exp. Tumor Res.* 5:85–97
76. Brand, K. G. Foreign body induced sarcomas. 1975. In *Cancer, a Comprehensive Treatise* (Becker F. F., ed), vol. 1. New York and London: Plenum Press, pp. 485–511
77. Rice, J. M. 1976. Carcinogenesis: A late effect of irreversible toxic damage during development. *Environ. Health Perspect.,* 18:133–139
78. Rice, J. M., ed. 1970. Perinatal Carcinogenesis. Natl. Cancer Inst. Monogr., 51:1–282
79. Food and Drug Administration. 1978. Nonclinical Laboratory Studies. Good Laboratory Practice Regulations. Fed. Register 43: No. 247, 59986–60025
80. Saffiotti, U., Page, N. P. 1977. Releasing carcinogenesis test results: Timing and extent of reporting. *Med. Pediatr. Oncol.* 3:159–167
81. Farber, E., Sporn, M. B., cochairmen: Symposium: Early lesions and the development of epithelial cancer. 1976. *Cancer Res.* 36:2475–2706
82. Stewart, F. W. Tumors of the breast. 1950. In *Atlas of Tumor Pathology,* sect. Ix, fasc. 34. Washington, DC: Armed Forces Inst. Pathol., pp. 7–10
83. Young, S., Hallowes, R. C. 1973. Tumours of the mammary gland. 1973. In *Pathology of Tumors in Laboratory Animals* (Turusov VS, ed), vol. 1, part 1. IARC Sci. Publ. 5:31–74
84. Shellabarger, C. J. 1972. Mammary neoplastic response of Lewis and Sprague-Dawley female rats to 7,12-dimethylbenz(a)anthracene or X-ray. *Cancer Res.,* 32:883–885
85. Baserga, R., Saffiotti, U. 1955. Experimental studies on histogenesis of blood-borne metastases. *Arch. Pathol.* (Chicago) 59:26–34
86. Kyriazis, A. P., Koka, M., Vesselinovitch, S. D. 1974. Metastatic rate of liver tumors induced by diethylni-

trosamine in mice. *Cancer Res.* 34: 2881–86

87. International Agency for Research on Cancer. 1972. Benzidine. IARC Monogr. Eval. Carcinog. Risk. Chem. Man 1:80–86

88. International Agency for Research on Cancer. 1974. Vinyl chloride. IARC Monogr. Eval. Carcinog. Risk Chem. Man. 7:291–318

89. Hanna, M. G. Jr., Nettesheim, P., Gilbert, J. R., eds. 1970. Inhalation Carcinogenesis. Atomic Energy Commission Symp. Ser. No. 18 (CONF-691001). Oak Ridge, Tenn.: U.S. Atomic Energy Comm. Div. Tech. Information Extension

90. Karbe, E., Park, J. F., eds. 1974. Experimental Lung Cancer. Carcinogenesis and Bioassays. Berlin, Heidelberg, New York: Springer-Verlag

91. Clayson, D. B. 1974. Bladder carcinogenesis in rats and mice: Possibility of artifacts. *J. Natl. Cancer Inst.* 52:1685–1689

92. Miller, E. C., Miller, J. A. The metabolism of chemical carcinogens to reactive electrophiles and their possible mechanisms of action in carcinogenesis. *In* Chemical Carcinogens (Searle, C. E., ed). American Chemical Society Monograph 173. Washington DC: Am. Chem. Soc. 1976, pp. 737–762

93. Fears, T. R., Tarone, R. E., Chu, K. C. 1977. False positive and false negative rates for carcinogenicity screens. *Cancer Res.* 37:1941–1945

94. Hoel, D. G., Walburg, H. E. Jr. 1977. Statistical analysis of survival experiments. *J. Natl. Cancer Inst.* 49:361–372

95. Peto, R. 1974. Guidelines on the analyses of tumour rates and death rates in experimental animals. *Br. J. Cancer* 29:101–105

96. Thomas, D. G., Greslow, N., Gart, J. J. 1977. Trend and homogeneity analyses of proportions and life table data. *Comput. Biomed. Res.* 10:373–381

97. Methods for Carcinogenesis Tests at the Cellular Level and Their Evaluation for the Assessment of Occupational Cancer Hazards. 1977. *Proc. Meet. Scientific Comm., Milan, Italy, 1977.* Milan: Fondazione Carlo Erba

98. Working Group on Mutagenicity Testing, Subcommittee on Environmental Mutagenesis, US Department of Health, Education, and Welfare Committee to Coordinate Toxicology and Related Programs. 1977. Approaches to determining the mutagenic properties of chemicals: Risk to future genera-

tions. *J. Environ. Pathol. Toxicol.* 1:301–352

99. Saffiotti, U., Autrup, H., eds. 1978. In Vitro Carcinogenesis. Guide to the Literature, Recent Advances and Laboratory Procedures. Natl. Cancer Inst. Carcinogenesis Tech. Rep. Ser. No. 44. Natl. Inst. Health, DHEW Publ. No. (NIH) 78-844. Washington, DC: US GPO

100. Asher, I. M., Zervos, C., eds. 1978. Structural Correlates of Carcinogenesis and Mutagenesis: A Guide to Testing Priorities? Proceedings of the Second Food and Drug Administration Office of Science Summer Symposium, Annapolis, Md., Aug. 31–Sept. 2, 1977. Rockville, Md.: Food Drug Admin.

101. International Commission on Radiological Protection: Radiation Protection—Recommendations of the International Commission on Radiological protection. 1966. ICRP Publ. 9. Oxford: Pergamon Press

102. Task Group: Air pollution and cancer: Risk assessment methodology and epidemiological evidence. 1978. *Environ. Health Perspect.* 22:1–12

103. Environmental Studies Board, National Research Council, National Academy of Sciences: Carcinogenesis in man and laboratory animals. In *Pest Control: An Assessment of Present and Alternative Technologies.* Vol. 1. Contemporary Pest Control Practices and Prospects: The Report of the Executive Committee. Washington, DC: Natl. Acad. Sci., 1975, pp. 66–82

104. Cornfield, J. 1977. Carcinogenic risk assessment. *Science* 198:683–99

105. Cornfield, J. 1978. Models for carcinogenic risk assessment. *Science* 202: 1107–1109

106. Hoel, D. G., Gaylor, D. W., Kirschstein, R. L., et al. 1975. Estimation of risks of irreversible, delayed toxicity. *J. Toxicol. Environ. Health* 1:133–151

107. Mantel, N., Bryan, W. R. 1961. "Safety" testing of carcinogenic agents. *J. Natl. Cancer Inst.* 27:455–70

108. Mantel, N., Bohidar, N. R., Brown, C. C., Ciminera, J. L., and Tukey, J. W. 1975. An improved Mantel-Bryan procedure for "safety" testing of carcinogens. *Cancer Res.* 35:865–872

109. Crump, K. S., Hoel, D. G., Langley, C. H., and Peto, R. 1976. Fundamental carcinogenic processes and their implications for low dose risk assessment. *Cancer Res.* 36:2973–2979

110. Guess, H. A., Crump, K. S., Peto, R. 1977. Uncertainty estimates for low-

dose-rate extrapolations of animal carcinogenicity data. *Cancer Res.* 37:3475–3483

111. Gross, M. A., Fitzhugh, O. G., Mantel, N. 1970. Evaluation of safety for food additives: An illustration involving the influence of methyl salicylate on rat reproduction. *Biometrics.* 26:181–194

112. Cox, D. R. 1972. Regression models and life-tables. *J. R. Stat. Soc.* [B] 34:187–202

113. Guess, H. A., Crump, K. S. 1976. Low-dose-rate extrapolation of data from animal carcinogenicity experiments—analysis of a new statistical technique. *Math Biosci.* 32:15–36

114. Crump, K. S., Guess, H. A., Deal, K. L. 1977. Confidence intervals and test of hypotheses concerning dose response relations inferred from animal carcinogenicity data. *Biometrics.* 33:437–451

115. Hartley, H. O., Sielken, R. L. 1977. Estimation of "safe doses" in carcinogenic experiments. *Biometrics.* 33:1–30

116. Armitage, P., Doll., R: Stochastic models for carcinogenesis. 1961. In Proceedings of the Fourth Berkeley Symposium on Mathematical Statistics and Probability, Berkeley, Calif., June 20–July 30, 1960 (Neyman J., ed), vol. 4. Berkeley, Calif.: Univ. California Press, pp. 19–38

117. Druckrey, H. 1968. Quantitative aspects of chemical carcinogenesis. In *Potential Carcinogenic Hazards From Drugs (Evaluation of Risks)*, ed., R. Truhart. Unio Internationale Contre le Cancer Monograph Ser., vol. 7. Berlin: Springer-Verlag, pp. 60–78

118. Albert, R. E., Altshuler, B. 1973. Considerations relating to the formulation of limits for unavoidable population exposures to environmental carcinogens. *In* Radionuclide Carcinogenesis (Ballou, J. E. and C. L. Sanders et al, eds), Springfield, Va.: AEC Symposium Series, CONF-72050, NTIS 1973 pp. 233–253.

119. Chand, N., Hoel, D. G. 1973. A comparison of models for determining safe levels of environmental agents. In *Reliability and Biometry: Statistical Analysis of Lifelength,* eds. F. Proschan, R. J. Serfling, pp. 681–700. Philadelphia: Soc. Indust. Appl. Math.

120. Schneiderman, M. A., Decoufle, P., Brown, C. C. Thresholds for environmental cancer—Biological and statistical considerations. *NY Acad Sci.* In press

121. Peto, R. 1977. Epidemiology, multistage models, and short-term mutagenicity tests. In *Origins of Human Cancer.* Cold Spring Harbor Conferences on Cell Proliferation (Hiatt, H. H., Watson, J. D., Winsten, J. A., eds), vol. 4, book C. Cold Spring Harbor, N.Y.: Cold Spring Harbor Laboratory, 1977, pp. 1403–1428

122. Whittemore, A., Altshuler, B. 1976. Lung cancer incidence in cigarette smokers: Further analysis of Doll and Hill's data for British physicians. *Biometrics* 32:805–816

123. Second Task Force for Research Planning in Environmental Health Science: Environmental measurements of chemicals for assessment of human exposure, chap. 7. 1977. *In* Human Health and the Environment. Some Research Needs. Natl. Inst. Health, DHEW Publ. No. (NIH) 77–1277. Washington, DC: Dept. Health, Educ., Welfare, pp. 217–242

124. Bingham, E., Falk, H. 1969. Environmental carcinogens: The modifying effect of carcinogens on the threshold response. *Arch. Environ. Health.* 19: 770–783

125. Harris, C. C., Autrup, H., Stoner, G., Yang, S. K., Leutz, J. C., Gelboin, H. V., Selkirk, J. K., Connor, R. J., Barrett, L. A., Jones, R. T., McDowell, E. and Trump, B. F. et al. 1977. Metabolism of benzo[*a*]pyrene and 7,12-dimethylbenz[*a*]anthracene in cultured human bronchus and pancreatic duct. *Cancer Res.* 37:3349–3355

126. Harris, C. C., Autrup, H., Connor, R., Barrett, L. A., McDowell, E. M. and Trump, B. F. et al. 1976. Interindividual variation in binding of benzo [*a*]pyrene to DNA in cultured human bronchi. *Science.* 194:1067–1069

127. Harris, C. C., Autrup, H., Stoner, G. 1978. Metabolism of benzo(a)pyrene in cultured human tissues and cells. In *Polycyclic Hydrocarbons and Cancer* (T'so, P.O., Gelboin, H.V., eds), vol. 2. New York and London: Academic Press, pp. 331–342

AUTHOR INDEX

SUBJECT INDEX

A

Accidents, 15
  mortality from, 10, 12–13,
    326, 328
  occupational, 266–67
  prevention of, 131–32, 135,
    332–33, 335, 339, 341
  vehicular, 267–68
  statistical studies of,
    194–204
Activities of daily life (ADL)
  measures, 238, 249
Adolescents
  and cigarette smoking, 30
  death by accident of, 12
  nursing services to, 89–90
Age
  and cigarette smoking, 30
  and dental health, 24
  and disability, 26–27
  and heart disease, 18–19
  and hypertension, 16–17
  mortality trends by, 6–8
    for cancer, 11–12
  of nursing home residents,
    233
  US demographic trends in,
    4–5
  utilization expenditures by,
    3–4
  See also Adolescents;
    Children; Elderly;
    Infants
Alcohol abuse
  programs for, 311
  regulation of, 123, 131–33,
    331–36
  risk factors of, 29, 327, 384
Algorithms
  as decision making
    instruments, 48–49, 53
Ambulatory care
  age statistics on, 3
  auditing of, 40, 43, 47, 52,
    58
  frequency of visits for, 15,
    176–78
  nurses' role in, 92
  See also Physicians
American Academy of
  Pediatrics
  competence formulations,
    49–50
American Board of Internal
  Medicine
  competence formulations,
    49–50
American College of Surgeons
  hospital standards, 52

American Medical Association
  Physicians Recognition
    Award, 55
American Public Health
  Association
  policy of, 306, 308–9
  in public health movement,
    297–98, 301–2
  Subcommittee on
    Administrative Practice,
    304
Animal bioassay, 348, 353,
    373–74
  correlations with human
    populations, 374–75,
    383, 385–87
  pathology examination in,
    360–61
  analysis of, 368–69
  evaluation of, 361–68
  research designs in, 353–60
    administration route in,
      355–58, 362, 366–68
    age and time factors in,
      358–60, 362–66,
      368–69
    number of animals in,
      354–57
    susceptibility variations in,
      349, 354, 362–63,
      365–66, 368, 375,
      386–87
    statistical analysis of, 380
Arizona
  in-migration to, 5
Association of State and
  Territorial Health Officials
  (ASTHO), 299–301, 304,
  308–9

B

Benefit-cost analysis, 258–60
  in public health programs,
    339–42
  quantification problems in,
    260–65, 269–71
  See also Economic evaluation
Blood pressure
  See Hypertension

C

California
  health regulation in, 149–50
  health services in, 303
  in-migration to, 5
Canada
  surgical study, 286–91

Cancer
  asbestosis, 31, 361
  of bladder, 21
  of breast, 12, 20–21, 326–27
    336
  cervical, 20–21, 327
    hysterectomy for
      prophylaxis of, 278–79
  chronic, 19–20
  of colon, 21
  of corpus, 20–21
  genesis of, 364
    latency period, 350–51,
      358, 363–64
    metastasis of, 365
    multistage model of,
      378–80
    susceptibility to, 349,
      382–83, 386–87
  incidence and mortality
    trends of, 10–12, 20–21,
    326–27, 350
  leukemias, 12, 20–21
  of lungs, 12, 20–21, 29, 329
  mesothelioma, 31
  neoplasms
    benign, 365–66
    cocarcinogens and, 349,
      367
    impact of, 13, 15
    pathology of, 360–69
  occupational exposure to, 31,
    361
  of ovaries, 20–21
  of pancreas, 20
  prevention programs for,
    341
  of prostate, 20–21
  of rectum, 20–21
  respiratory, 12, 327
  of stomach, 20–21
  treatment preference
    comparisons, 293
  US policy on, 345–46
Carcinogens
  aflatoxin B_1, 349, 375
  benzidine, 366, 375
  dimethylnitrosamine, 349
  industrial, 31, 327, 361
  mutagens as, 370
  β-naphthylamine, 349
  polycyclic aromatic
    hydrocarbons, 365, 372,
    384
  qualitative analysis of,
    346–48
    detectability of, 349, 351,
      382–83
    dose response levels in,
      349–50, 357–59,
      361–62, 364, 367–68

ORDER FORM   ANNUAL REVIEWS INC.

Please list on the order blank on the reverse side the volumes you wish to order and whether you wish a standing order (the latest volume sent to you automatically upon publication each year). Volumes not yet published will be shipped in month and year indicated. Prices subject to change without notice. Out of print volumes subject to special order.

NEW TITLES FOR 1980

ANNUAL REVIEW OF PUBLIC HEALTH   ISSN 0163-7525
    Vol. 1 (avail. May 1980): $17.00 (USA), $17.50 (elsewhere) per copy

ANNUAL REVIEWS REPRINTS: IMMUNOLOGY, 1977–1979   ISBN 0-8243-2502-8
A collection of articles reprinted from recent *Annual Review* series
    Avail. Mar. 1980   Soft cover: $12.00 (USA), $12.50 (elsewhere) per copy

SPECIAL PUBLICATIONS

ANNUAL REVIEWS REPRINTS: CELL MEMBRANES, 1975–1977   ISBN 0-8243-2501-X
A collection of articles reprinted from recent *Annual Review* series
    Published 1978   Soft cover: $12.00 (USA), $12.50 (elsewhere) per copy

THE EXCITEMENT AND FASCINATION OF SCIENCE, VOLUME 1   ISBN 0-8243-1602-9
A collection of autobiographical and philosophical articles by leading scientists
    Published 1965   Clothbound: $6.50 (USA), $7.00 (elsewhere) per copy

THE EXCITEMENT AND FASCINATION OF SCIENCE, VOLUME 2: Reflections by Eminent Scientists
    Published 1978   Hard cover: $12.00 (USA), $12.50 (elsewhere) per copy   ISBN 0-8243-2601-6
                          Soft cover: $10.00 (USA), $10.50 (elsewhere) per copy   ISBN 0-8243-2602-4

THE HISTORY OF ENTOMOLOGY   ISBN 0-8243-2101-7
A special supplement to the *Annual Review of Entomology* series
    Published 1973   Clothbound: $10.00 (USA), $10.50 (elsewhere) per copy

ANNUAL REVIEW SERIES

Annual Review of ANTHROPOLOGY   ISSN 0084-6570
    Vols. 1–8 (1972–79): $17.00 (USA), $17.50 (elsewhere) per copy
    Vol. 9 (avail. Oct. 1980): $20.00 (USA), $21.00 (elsewhere) per copy

Annual Review of ASTRONOMY AND ASTROPHYSICS   ISSN 0066-4146
    Vols. 1–17 (1963–79): $17.00 (USA), $17.50 (elsewhere) per copy
    Vol. 18 (avail. Sept. 1980): $20.00 (USA), $21.00 (elsewhere) per copy

Annual Review of BIOCHEMISTRY   ISSN 0066-4154
    Vols. 28–48 (1959–79): $18.00 (USA), $18.50 (elsewhere) per copy
    Vol. 49 (avail. July 1980): $21.00 (USA), $22.00 (elsewhere) per copy

Annual Review of BIOPHYSICS AND BIOENGINEERING*   ISSN 0084-6589
    Vols. 1–8 (1972–79): $17.00 (USA), $17.50 (elsewhere) per copy
    Vol. 9 (avail. June 1980): $17.00 (USA), $17.50 (elsewhere) per copy

Annual Review of EARTH AND PLANETARY SCIENCES*   ISSN 0084-6597
    Vols. 1–7 (1973–79): $17.00 (USA), $17.50 (elsewhere) per copy
    Vol. 8 (avail. May 1980): $17.00 (USA), $17.50 (elsewhere) per copy

Annual Review of ECOLOGY AND SYSTEMATICS   ISSN 0066-4162
    Vols. 1–10 (1970–79): $17.00 (USA), $17.50 (elsewhere) per copy
    Vol. 11 (avail. Nov. 1980): $20.00 (USA), $21.00 (elsewhere) per copy

Annual Review of ENERGY   ISSN 0362-1626
    Vols. 1–4 (1976–79): $17.00 (USA), $17.50 (elsewhere) per copy
    Vol. 5 (avail. Oct. 1980): $20.00 (USA), $21.00 (elsewhere) per copy

Annual Review of ENTOMOLOGY*   ISSN 0066-4170
    Vols. 7–24 (1962–79): $17.00 (USA), $17.50 (elsewhere) per copy
    Vol. 25 (avail. Jan. 1980): $17.00 (USA), $17.50 (elsewhere) per copy

Annual Review of FLUID MECHANICS*   ISSN 0066-4189
    Vols. 1–11 (1969–79): $17.00 (USA), $17.50 (elsewhere) per copy
    Vol. 12 (avail. Jan. 1980): $17.00 (USA), $17.50 (elsewhere) per copy

Annual Review of GENETICS   ISSN 0066-4197
    Vols. 1–13 (1967–79): $17.00 (USA), $17.50 (elsewhere) per copy
    Vol. 14 (avail. Dec. 1980): $20.00 (USA), $21.00 (elsewhere) per copy

Annual Review of MATERIALS SCIENCE   ISSN 0084-6600
    Vol. 1–9 (1971–79): $17.00 (USA), $17.50 (elsewhere) per copy
    Vol. 10 (avail. Aug. 1980): $20.00 (USA), $21.00 (elsewhere) per copy

(continued on reverse)
*Price will be increased to $20.00 (USA), $21.00 (elsewhere) per copy effective with the 1981 volume.

Annual Review of MEDICINE: Selected Topics in the Clinical Sciences* ISSN 0066-4219
  Vols. 1–3, 5–15, 17–30 (1950–52, 1954–64, 1966–79): $17.00 (USA), $17.50 (elsewhere) per copy
  Vol. 31 (avail. Apr. 1980): $17.00 (USA), $17.50 (elsewhere) per copy

Annual Review of MICROBIOLOGY ISSN 0066-4227
  Vols. 15–33 (1961–79): $17.00 (USA), $17.50 (elsewhere) per copy
  Vol. 34 (avail. Oct. 1980): $20.00 (USA), $21.00 (elsewhere) per copy

Annual Review of NEUROSCIENCE* ISSN 0147-006X
  Vols. 1–2 (1978–79): $17.00 (USA), $17.50 (elsewhere) per copy
  Vol. 3 (avail. Mar. 1980): $17.00 (USA), $17.50 (elsewhere) per copy

Annual Review of NUCLEAR AND PARTICLE SCIENCE ISSN 0066-4243
  Vols. 10–29 (1960–79): $19.50 (USA), $20.00 (elsewhere) per copy
  Vol. 30 (avail. Dec. 1980): $22.50 (USA), $23.50 (elsewhere) per copy

Annual Review of PHARMACOLOGY AND TOXICOLOGY* ISSN 0362-1642
  Vols. 1–3, 5–19 (1961–63, 1965–79): $17.00 (USA), $17.50 (elsewhere) per copy
  Vol. 20 (avail. Apr. 1980): $17.00 (USA), $17.50 (elsewhere) per copy

Annual Review of PHYSICAL CHEMISTRY ISSN 0066-426X
  Vols. 10–21, 23–30 (1959–70, 1972–79): $17.00 (USA), $17.50 (elsewhere) per copy
  Vol. 31 (avail. Nov. 1980): $20.00 (USA), $21.00 (elsewhere) per copy

Annual Review of PHYSIOLOGY* ISSN 0066-4278
  Vols. 18–41 (1956–79): $17.00 (USA), $17.50 (elsewhere) per copy
  Vol. 42 (avail. Mar. 1980): $17.00 (USA), $17.50 (elsewhere) per copy

Annual Review of PHYTOPATHOLOGY ISSN 0066-4286
  Vols. 1–17 (1963–79): $17.00 (USA), $17.50 (elsewhere) per copy
  Vol. 18 (avail. Sept. 1980): $20.00 (USA), $21.00 (elsewhere) per copy

Annual Review of PLANT PHYSIOLOGY* ISSN 0066-4294
  Vols. 10–30 (1959–79): $17.00 (USA), $17.50 (elsewhere) per copy
  Vol. 31 (avail. June 1980): $17.00 (USA), $17.50 (elsewhere) per copy

Annual Review of PSYCHOLOGY* ISSN 0066-4308
  Vols. 4, 5, 8, 10–30 (1953, 1954, 1957, 1959–79): $17.00 (USA), $17.50 (elsewhere) per copy
  Vol. 31 (avail. Feb. 1980): $17.00 (USA), $17.50 (elsewhere) per copy

Annual Review of SOCIOLOGY ISSN 0360-0572
  Vols. 1–5 (1975–79): $17.00 (USA), $17.50 (elsewhere) per copy
  Vol. 6 (avail. Aug. 1980): $20.00 (USA), $21.00 (elsewhere) per copy

*Price will be increased to $20.00 (USA), $21.00 (elsewhere) per copy effective with the 1981 volume.

To ANNUAL REVIEWS INC., 4139 El Camino Way, Palo Alto, CA 94306 USA
(Tel. 415-493-4400)

Please enter my order for the following publications:
(Standing orders: indicate which volume you wish order to begin with)

_____, Vol(s). ____ Standing order ____

_____, Vol(s). ____ Standing order ____

_____, Vol(s). ____ Standing order ____

_____, Vol(s). ____ Standing order ____

Amount of remittance enclosed $_____   California residents please add applicable sales tax.
Please bill me ☐   Prices subject to change without notice.

SHIP TO (include institutional purchase order if billing address is different)

Name _____

Address _____

_____

_____ Zip Code _____

Signed _____ Date _____

☐ Please add my name to your mailing list to receive a free copy of the current Prospectus each year.
☐ Send free brochure listing contents of recent back volumes for *Annual Review(s)* of